Optical Fiber Biosensors

Optical Fiber Biosensors

Device Platforms, Biorecognition, Applications

Daniele Tosi[1,2], Marzhan Sypabekova[1,3], Aliya Bekmurzayeva[1,2], Carlo Molardi[1], Kanat Dukenbayev[1]

[1]*Nazarbayev University, School of Engineering and Digital Sciences, Nur-Sultan, Kazakhstan*

[2]*National Laboratory Astana, Laboratory of Biosensors and Bioinstruments, Nur-Sultan, Kazakhstan*

[3]*Nazarbayev University, School of Medicine, Nur-Sultan, Kazakhstan*

ELSEVIER

ACADEMIC PRESS

An imprint of Elsevier

Academic Press is an imprint of Elsevier
125 London Wall, London EC2Y 5AS, United Kingdom
525 B Street, Suite 1650, San Diego, CA 92101, United States
50 Hampshire Street, 5th Floor, Cambridge, MA 02139, United States
The Boulevard, Langford Lane, Kidlington, Oxford OX5 1GB, United Kingdom

British Library Cataloguing-in-Publication Data
A catalogue record for this book is available from the British Library

Library of Congress Cataloging-in-Publication Data
A catalog record for this book is available from the Library of Congress

ISBN: 978-0-12-819467-6

For Information on all Academic Press publications
visit our website at https://www.elsevier.com/books-and-journals

Publisher: Mara Conner
Acquisitions Editor: Carrie Bolger
Editorial Project Manager: Fernanda A. Oliveira
Production Project Manager: Anitha Sivaraj
Cover Designer: Christian J. Bilbow

Typeset by MPS Limited, Chennai, India

Contents

Section III

Preface

After Nobel Prize winner Prof. Charles Kao discovered fiber optics in 1966, few could think of an application beyond the field of communications, specifically in sensors. However, only 1 year later, what was defined as the first photonic sensor was published. Ten years later, in 1976, one of the most relevant applications from the industrial point of view in relation to fiber optic sensors emerged, the gyroscope. For a couple of decades, numerous and very talented researchers were trying to find new niches. Among other fiber optic sensors, popular applications that jump from the lab to industry are those related to current meters, sensors distributed in intelligent structures, etc. With the emergence of nanotechnology and the availability of more advanced optoelectronic instrumentation, along with the need to detect analytes with decreasing concentrations to diagnose diseases in increasingly early stages, an increase of very important works related to fiber optic biosensors trying to respond to all these challenges are being published. This book is specially designed to cover these aspects that are emerging with the idea of contributing to the development of this new multidisciplinary field that could give rise to the next niche of fiber optic sensors: fiber-optic biosensors.

This book has been structured into three independent blocks: technology, biofunctionalization, and applications, with the aim of attracting researchers and early career scientists to this field of optics and photonics, mainly from engineering and physics, but also from science and biomedicine. The first eight chapters perfectly cover the technological aspects of fiber optic sensors to later explain in the next two chapters those fundamental aspects related to bioreceptors and biofunctionalization to take into account in the development of fiber-optic biosensors. The later chapters try to encourage the reader to take the next step, which is as always to be able to advance in these research works to achieve their real transfer to the market and bring enormous advantages to this biomedical sector in terms of sensitivity, specificity, speed, etc., that fiber optic biosensors are ready to provide.

Acknowledgments

The authors would like to express their gratitude to the Elsevier editorial staff, who continuously assisted during the process of conception, preparation, and production of the book. It has been a pleasure to work with a team that showed great dedication, craftsmanship, and that really supported us during the whole time, making it possible to deliver. We would like to thank in particular Fiona Geraghty (who was the first to contact us, back to an EMBC conference), and Fernanda Oliveira, who assisted us throughout the whole process, as well as Anitha Sivaraj, Praveen Anand, Carrie Bolger, and the many more staff who connected with us.

We would also like to acknowledge the many researchers and colleagues that have worked with us in these years, and contributed to our work with a strong effort. Several students, researchers, faculties contributed to the success of our research, through hard work and brilliant minds. We share an acknowledgments to their contribution, and we are excited to see how they are building great technologies.

The field of fiber optic biosensors has shown a growth from a small niche to a mature research over the course of the last years. While several cornerstones have been displaced, the field has grown with the incessant contributions of many research centers and universities around the world, forming a solid and cohesive scientific community. We would like to thank the many contributors who have worked hard not only to improve the technology but also to form a community around it that continues to be strong and respectful.

And finally, we would like to thank our families and friends, who have been supporting our work from the very beginning, making it possible to achieve our goals.

1

Introduction to optical fiber biosensors

1.1 From biosensors to optical fiber biosensors

Biosensors are at the ground of today's diagnostic and biological sensing, and one of the building blocks of analytical devices. The impact of biosensors has been broad, with medical diagnostic being the main driver: the possibility of using miniaturized sensors for detection of biological analytes has great impact in modern tools: several applications that detect blood saturation, pulmonary capacity, glucose, cancer biomarkers among others make use of biosensors.

The genesis of biosensors dates back to 1953, where Clark et al. designed the first biosensor (Clark, Wolf, Granger, & Taylor, 1953) aimed at the detection of oxygen concentration in liquids; this sensor was the first example of the measurement of a biological analyte, with a rapid detection in situ. This designed, labeled Clark's electrode is the first example of a biological sensor based on a variable electrode, with a Teflon membrane that allows the oxygen gas to reach the cathode, where it is reduced. Subsequently, Clark and Lyons applied the Clark's electrode concept to the continuous measurement of oxygen in blood, which became a fundamental support tool for cardiovascular surgery (Clark & Lyons, 1962). Clark's electrode is a precursor of the electrochemical sensors class (Grieshaber, MacKenzie, Vörös, & Reimhult, 2008), which analyze the current, voltage, potential, or conductance through a reference and a working electrode during chemical reduction processes, and became an important detection method for enzymatic processes.

In parallel, the development of electronic devices such as transistors and chips has pushed the development of biosensors through several generations. Field-effect transistors (FETs) are an excellent and versatile device for biosensors: they are miniaturized, fast, and with low power consumption so that they can be inserted in vivo to operate real-time detection of physical parameters but also to express a detection of other fundamental measurands; for example, MOSFET-type transistors are at the base of chemical radiation dosimeters.

Optical Fiber Biosensors.
DOI: https://doi.org/10.1016/B978-0-12-819467-6.00001-9

By acting on the properties of a FET, it is possible to modify its classical gate-drain-source structure: the ion-suspended FET (ISFET) is a structure in which the transistor gate is suspended in liquid and the gate field is modulated by the ions corresponding to the chemical reactions under analysis; ISFET devices rapidly became an important analytical tool for electrochemical sensing. Today, the field of transistors implementing biological detection has taken the label of "BioFET" (Schöning & Poghossian, 2002): the principle of operation has remained similar to ISFET, using biological analytes to modulate the electrical field at the gate, altering the drain current. Several electronic devices have been used to detect transistors, either by simply reading the output currents or using sweeping functions such as cyclic voltammetry.

The advances in electronics has brought transistors to interface with other functions used to filter, modify, or magnetically attract/repel analytes before their detection. Lab-on-chips have been developed according to this principles: on a single miniature chip, they perform several task that includes microfluidics (used to govern the properties of the analytes under investigation, for example, flowing cells to a detection point), labeling analytes, and introducing other processes (Patel, Nanda, Sahoo, & Mohapatra, 2016). Lab-on-chips in general work for the multifunctional devices, that accumulate a set of biological, electrochemical, or optical tasks on a single chip and then perform a detection.

The flow from electrochemical sensors and their methods, the most notable ones including electrochemical impedance spectroscopy and conductometric analyzers, to transistors and then to lab-on-chips has been noteworthy as sensors expanded in terms of performance, range of detection, and hardware. The advent of portable platforms such as smartphones (Zhang & Liu, 2016) and even wearable sensors (Stoppa & Chiolerio, 2014) has opened up great avenues for low-cost analyzers, exploiting also the connection possibilities given by wireless network protocols operating on low-bandwidth sensors such as bluetooth or low-range wi-fi. Smart garments, measuring skin conductivity and percutaneous parameters, are the topic of several current research efforts, witnessed by the development of many smart textiles such as sensorized t-shirts, smart watches, or implantable devices for semiintermittent sensing.

While electronic biosensors and chips have mostly focused on the low-cost and ease of manufacturability of devices, in parallel optical sensors have established as the biosensing technology behind the most performing analyzers, thanks to the combination between the excellent performance figures (in terms of detection capability, resolving specific analytes at the lowest concentration) and the possibility to embed all the optical hardware into benchtop analyzers, and in some cases portable instruments. In some ways, optical biosensors move the field of electrical detection to the optical domain, at a much smaller wavelength (or at a much larger frequency). While electrical biosensors use the biological elements to modulate electrical circuit elements, such as the impedance between two electrodes or the gate current flowing into a transistor, optical biosensors use light propagation as the key principle, and the biological elements affect the properties of light. Since light propagates in optical circuits as a wave, it has a wider range of properties that can be affected by the analytes under investigation, for example, the power, the reflection or transmission spectrum, the polarization state, or the phase of the waves.

Fluorescence-based methods are the most popular phenomenon exploited for the design of optical biosensors; these sensors show high specificity in the detection of cells and biomolecules, intracellular sensing, and also to study molecular interactions. Fluorescence occurs when a photon is absorbed by an atom and emitted at a lower energy level; biosensors exploit the fluorescence processes occurring when the photon is absorbed and retransmitted by a biomolecule (Bertone, Burford, & Hamilton, 2018). Fluorescent signals have short-time duration, and several techniques for detection have been employed in optical biosensors: the most common are the detection of lifetime of fluorescence spectra, Forster resonance energy transfer, and fluorescence imaging that applies the fluorescence detection over a matrix of photodetectors.

Optical fluorescence biosensors, as well as several lab-on-chip and electrochemical technologies, are based on an activation process, that involves usually an exchange of energy between the analytes itself and other components of the sensor: for example, an optical source is needed for the fluorescence signal to be activated in the biomolecules. In order to perform sensing without the need of an activation, recent optical methods have focused on *label-free* biosensing; this terminology implies that the biomolecules or analytes do not have to be labeled or activated before sensing, but rather the sensor is capable of binding itself to the analyte and detect it in a direct way.

Surface plasmon resonance (SPR) is the most popular method for label-free optical biosensing (Homola, 2008): from the early works of Cullen, Brown, and Lowe (1987) that proved the SPR formation in gold layers interacting with biological analytes to form the first generation of optical immunosensors, to the current days where SPR has been integrated on commercial devices with the capability of processing large scale or immunoassays faster than other methods, SPR has constituted the backbone of label-free optical sensors. In short, SPR is based on the interaction between polarized light incident on a metallic thin film, having thickness much shorter than the wavelength, and electrons that are excited in the metallic film. When the light is incident in SPR condition, it is coupled into the metallic layer (where it rapidly vanishes) rather than reflected backwards: this principle allows measuring the refractive index (RI) of the analytes, but through a proper functionalization it can render a quantitative measurements of the analytes binding to the metallic film surface. Since the metallic layer can both host the SPR sensor and serve as a platform to immobilize bioreceptors, SPR technologies became popular as they allow high-performance sensing with a label-free method that can be fabricated in one process, for example, through high-energy ion sputtering. The SPR technology has been presented in a bulky setup, with interchangeable chips that can rapidly perform biological measurement with excellent precisions, but also in portable handheld instruments, miniaturizing the components (light source and spectrometers); recently, SPR sensors have been reported even on a full-smartphone architecture (Walter, Alwis, Roth, & Bremer, 2020).

The need for miniaturized probes that can work in situ has been the main driver for optical fiber biosensors (OFB), which is the content of this book. Optical fibers have been developed an engineered mainly for telecommunications and imaging, and they are the most popular waveguide for light propagation. In the mid-late 1960s, Charles Kao (who was awarded the Nobel Prize in Physics in 2009) and his group demonstrated the possibility of using the impurity of silica glass, in a cylindrical shape, to guide light over a long distance at relatively low losses. Adding up on the progress on light sources and detectors, as well as on every component of optical circuits, has allowed to create large-scale network that delivers high-speed connectivity, up to several tens of Terabit per second that we well know today (Agrawal, 2012). In parallel, optical fibers have been substantially developed also for imaging systems, broadly used in medical diagnostic for endoscopy and cardiovascular devices as well as for noncontact imaging.

The same optical fiber technologies that gained popularity for telecommunication and imaging have received a growing interest for sensing; in fact, optical fiber sensors have excellent performance and critical advantages over optical and electrical counterparts, but the most important factor in biosensing is that they allow the fabrication of a small compact probe that can work in real time, with rapid in situ detection. So, we can move from a scenario where we analyze with a biosensor a sample retrieved through a collection or a biopsy, to the real-time investigation of proteins, biomolecules, cells, or antibodies (Socorro-Leránoz, Santano, Del Villar, & Matias, 2019). Thanks to the fact that the fiber acts as a cable with tiny size, we can even fabricate sensors that operate intermittently in vivo (Wilson & Gifford, 2005), with the perspective of having a long-term sensing in place.

OFB have a close contact with their free-space or bulky optical counterparts; several sensing methods transpose the optical counterparts into a fiber-optic device. SPR probes, for example, have been largely developed also for optical fibers, maintaining the same working principle but adapting it to the specific fiber geometrical and propagation properties. Another example of similarities is given with optical interferometers: classical methods of interferometry are used in high-precision measurements, and they can be converted into devices that have a similar approach but run through an optical fiber. However, there are other types of fiber-optic sensing devices that instead employ methods specifically suited for waveguides: methods based on fiber Bragg gratings or photonic crystal fibers require an optical fiber for implementing the sensing mechanism.

Looking at the commercial aspects for biosensors, Global Market Insights estimates the 2018 market of biosensor to a total of $18.6B, with a compound annual growth rate of 8% to reach $31.5B in 2025. Fig. 1.1 shows the market shares for each industrial area of biosensors. Almost two-thirds of the market (64%) is addressed toward medical diagnostic and instrumentation, which is by far the most important share; biosensors for medical diagnostic involve both analyzers and in situ probes, and they address the detection of cardiovascular, urologic, diabetes, and cancer biomarkers as main application. Currently, 53% of the biosensors aim at clinical diagnostic, while 11% are medical instruments; in total, about 52% of medical biosensors are benchtop instruments, while the most prominent market (9.3% annual growth) is wearable technologies. The other third of the biosensors market is mainly divided between industrial process control, agriculture, defense, and environmental sensors.

1.2 Optical fiber biosensors

OFB make use of optical fibers both as a sensing element, and to propagate the light from an optical source to a detector; the implementation of OFB resembles the classical optical fiber systems used in telecommunications, adapted for sensing rather than for long-distance transmission; other systems instead are more closely inspired to imaging systems, particularly when using fibers with larger size.

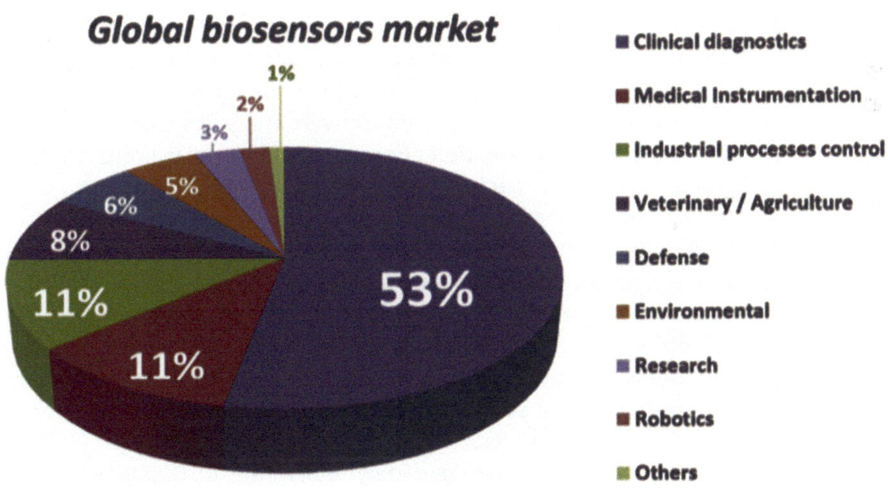

Figure 1.1 Global biosensors market share, arranged by market segments. Source: *Figure reproduced from Socorro-Leránoz, A.B., Santano, D., Del Villar, I., & Matias, I.R. (2019). Trends in the design of wavelength-based optical fibre biosensors (2008–2018).* Biosensors and Bioelectronics: X, 1, *100015 with permission.*

The key advantages in terms of biosensing performance and applications of OFB with respect to electrochemical and optical methods can be summarized as follows:

- *Compact form factor:* Sensors are developed along or on the tip of optical fibers, which have a small size; standard telecom fibers have typically size of 250 μm, about three times the diameter of a human hair, but it is possible to shrink the size further. In fact, most biosensors detect with thin fibers or with structures that reduce the fiber diameter. All the optics of the sensor are enclosed in a small device that can easily fit medical needles or catheters, and in some cases sustain itself a percutaneous insertion.
- *Electromagnetic compatibility*: Optical fiber sensors are immune to external electromagnetic fields. Their readout is unaffected by perturbations such as magnetic fields like the ones used in magnetic resonance imaging (MRI), or by ionizing radiation such as those used in chemotherapies. This is an important factor in clinical applications, since electrical sensors are not MRI-compatible and transistors are also affected by radiation; OFB instead are compliant to any harsh environment.
- *Biocompatibility*: Fibers are made of silica glass, which is a biocompatible material according to ISO10993 standard. Fibers can be therefore used inserted in medical needles for detection without harming the body. Some very recent research has even gone to propose bio-resorbable fibers, that can be absorbed by the body after completing a sensing task (Theodosiou et al., 2019).
- *Safety*: Unlike electrical circuits, fibers are used in a totally passive way, hence they cannot start fires or shock; this is important in implantable sensors.
- *Performance*: Optical fiber sensors have reached a great maturity, and perform extremely well in terms of limit of detection and selectivity. This is often due to the intrinsic advantage of using sensing methods with high sensitivity coupled with telecom-derived analyzers that have great precision. As a result, OFB sensors detecting at subnanomolar limits are frequent, with several devices approaching the femtomolar-level detection.
- *Multiplexing*: In order to detect multiple parameters, or in different locations, when using electrical sensors we would need to use one different sensor for each detection and interrogate them separately. Fiber optics, however, enables the access to sensor multiplexing: it is possible either to interrogate multiple sensors inscribed on the same fiber, or to use a single analyzer to switch between multiple fiber sensors, or even to combine the two methods to form very large sensing networks. Optical fibers offer a great variety of multiplexing techniques.
- *Capability to work in liquids and in air*: Inherently, OFB detect in media that have RI inferior to the fiber itself. This means that fibers can detect in most liquid analytes, including water or liquid samples such as saliva, urine, sweat, or in solid analytes (e.g., detection of several cancer biomarkers inspecting the tissues), as

well as in air. In fact, most sensors have a sensitivity much higher in liquids than in air, while several electrochemical sensors require modifications in order to continuously detect in liquids.

- *Long range*: Optical fibers have an extremely small attenuation, which allows to transmit light over long distances; OFB therefore can work at a very broad distance, for sensing in very remote locations or in harsh environments.

While certainly OFB offer top performance, and a great versatility for biological sensing, the main drawback is implicit in the high cost of optical technologies. Optical fiber interrogators have cost that ranges from the few thousands of dollars up to hundreds of thousands for system having telecom grade; recent research has focused on reducing the cost of the units to a fraction of the current price, but there is still a wide gap compared to cheap electronic sensors. The fiber itself is a disposable and cheap material, having cost of usually few dollars per meter down to few cents for the most popular fibers, but costs rise when we look at the whole system that includes fiber connectors, as well as other components to assemble circuits. For such reasons, OFB are being investigated both with an eye on reducing costs and improving volume manufacturing, but also with the intent of bringing a diagnostic to applications where traditional technology would fail to perform, or would be inconclusive.

OFB originate from environmental sensors, and their working principles are based on refractometers. Fig. 1.2 shows the typical working principle of OFB. Improperly, we can define the biosensor as a selective refractometer, which is a device capable of measuring the RI of the medium in its surrounding (Chiavaioli, Gouveia, Jorge, & Baldini, 2017): for example, we can use a refractometer to inspect the RI of a water solution with great precision. The light propagating in the fiber, in correspondence of the RI sensing location, is forced to interact with the outer medium; at the interface, we observed the changes of light intensity or spectrum that we can detect on the analyzer. An RI sensor is certainly label-free, because it responds to the change of the environment in the proximity of the fiber, but it is not selective: in fact, it would respond to any change of the surrounding environment, without distinguishing any of the analytes that we aim at detecting.

Therefore, in order to perform a selective detection, and convert the principle of a refractometer into a selective biosensor, we apply a *functionalization* to the sensing element. This process involves the deposition of bioreceptors on the surface of the fiber, which bind specifically to the analyte under detection, and ideally do not bind to other analytes (such as controls). The functionalization process usually works on thin metallic films, having thickness of few tens of nanometers, much smaller than the wavelength; for this reason, sensors using SPR principles are particularly common as they can use the metallic layer also to host the sensing principle, but several other OFB configurations use the metallic film simply to host the bioreceptors,

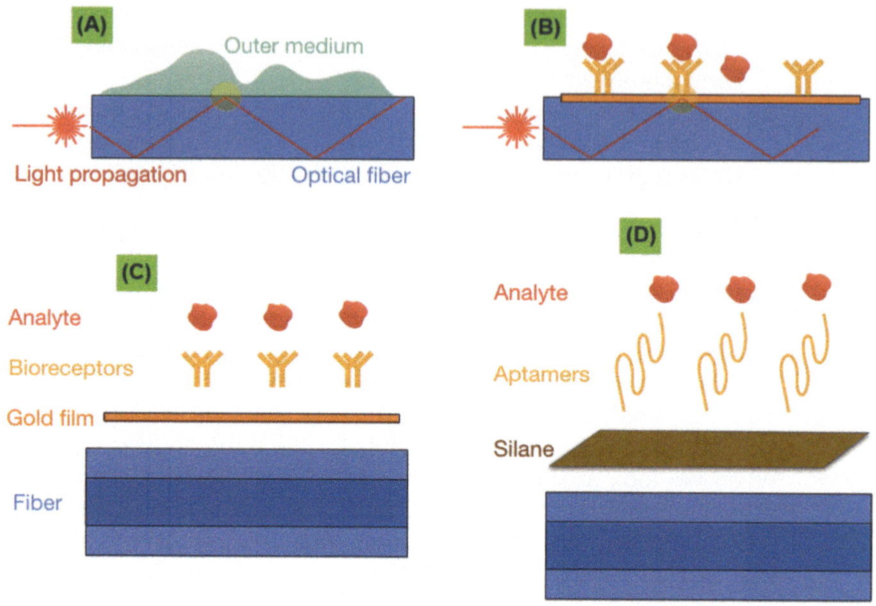

Figure 1.2 Sketch of the working principle of a generic optical fiber biosensor. (A) An OFBG works as the light propagating in the fiber interacts with the surrounding medium, detecting refractive index variations. (B) A biosensor exploits this principle for a selective detection: bioreceptors are immobilized on the fiber surface, and bind on the analyte under investigation; this way, the change of the surrounding environment impacts on the properties of light propagation. (C) Layered view of each building block of a thin film metallic functionalization, with a gold (or silver) film deposited on the fiber surface and immobilizing a bioreceptor. (D) Alternative implementation using a silanization process, for the design of an aptasensors having aptamers as bioreceptors immobilized on the silanized fiber.

encoding the sensing principle in a different part of the sensing unit. In order to efficiently immobilize bioreceptors, two key methods are the deposition of 30–100 nm thick metallic films (Caucheteur, Guo, & Albert, 2015), or a silanization process (Bekmurzayeva et al., 2018), in which the fiber surface is covered with organofunctional alkoxysilane molecules.

Fig. 1.3 shows the main functionalization methods in use in current optical biosensors. The antibody–antigen interaction is a chemical reaction between an antibody and multivalent antibodies that bind through a stable covalent bond, and is used in several sensors (e.g., for detection immunoglobulin G). Another biological sensing methods involve self-assembled monolayers (SAM), which are assemblies of molecules formed on the surface of the fiber by adsorption. Aptasensors make use of aptamers, which are oligonucleotide or peptide molecules that bind to a specific analyte through chemical bond. Aptasensors are becoming increasingly important in the field of OFB (Lobry et al., 2020), as they can exploit the aptamer selection methods already in use in biology.

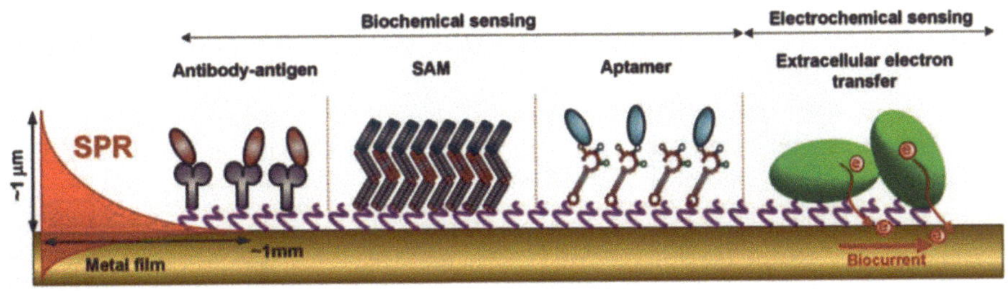

Figure 1.3 Illustration of the main surface functionalization methods in use in optical fiber biosensors. Source: *Image reproduced from Guo, T., González-Vila, Á., Loyez, M., Caucheteur, C. (2017). Plasmonic optical fiber-grating immunosensing: A review.* Sensors, *17(12), 2732.*

1.3 An overview of achievements in optical fiber biosensors

In comparison with the main electrochemical, lab-on-chip, and optical biosensors that adapt well-established technologies of the last century to perform biological detection, OFB are a much more recent topic since most of the technological components on which analyzers and optical networks are based have been developed in the last two decades. Hence, the research in OFB is still in an early-stage era, but with prominent prospects about what is up to come. The last 15 years have seen the whole evolution of this research field, in terms of technologies, implementation, and applications.

Fig. 1.4 gives an outline of some of the main applications of OFB, each visualizing the current technology readiness level (TRL). A flyby of the main applications shows that OFB are applied in the detection of cardiovascular and cancer biomarkers, in urology, in percutaneous sensing, for protein sensing, immunoglobulins, cancer cells detection, and bacterial detection. All of these applications show a TRL ranging from 2 to 5, considering the European Union scale, where TRL2 consists in the validation of the potential application up to TRL5 where the system is validated in a simulated or real environment (e.g., in vitro or in vivo measurements). In general, optical principles behind OFB can be easily validated, as we can simply evaluate the optical performance criteria for biosensors simply as refractometers, by measuring the RI levels of analytes. The next steps are to validate the biological response by measuring the limit of detection, specificity, and in general quantifying how the sensor responds to different concentrations of analytes and controls. The main progress through the TRL is attributed to packaging of the sensor, which allows positioning it at the point of detection, performing in situ diagnostic; researchers have embodied OFB into endoscopic, urologic, or other catheters, as well as designing methods that allow percutaneous insertion of the fiber directly to the sensing point.

An important application for OFB is glucose monitoring, which has significant impact on diabetes early-stage diagnostic (Lobry et al., 2019); here, an

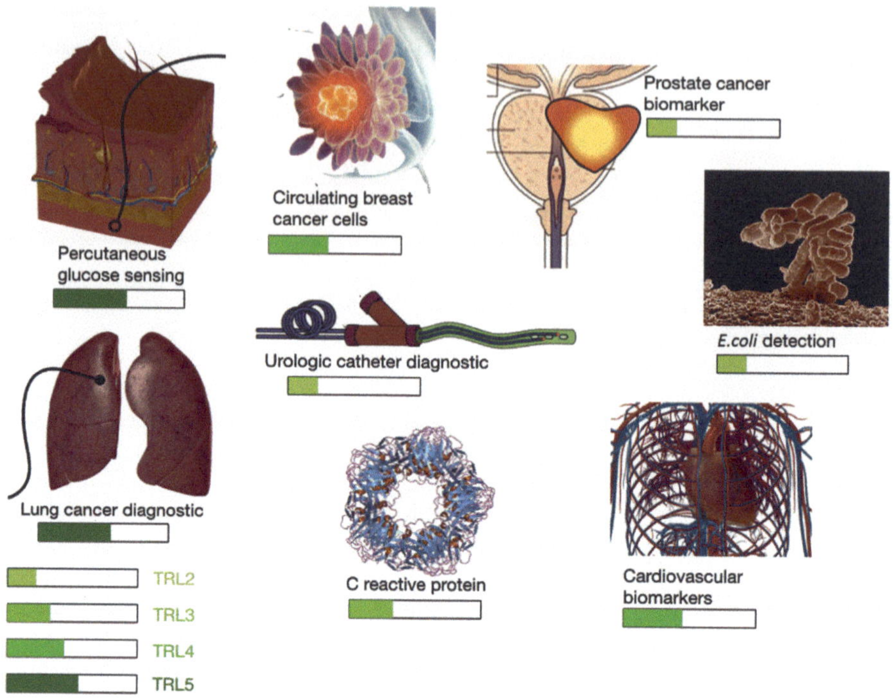

Figure 1.4 An overview of some of the main applications of optical fiber biosensors, each showing the current technology readiness level (TRL).

important progress has been driven by the sencil project (Liao et al., 2008), which demonstrated the development of percutaneous fibers achieved by coating a fiber tip with a hydrogel for intermittent or semipermanent placement through the skin. Similarly, Loyez et al. (2019) have demonstrated the embodiment of a plasmonic grating OFB sensor in an endoscopic catheter, positioned in the lung for cytokeratins-17 biomarker detection. These technologies have shown great prospects both in terms of biological sensing and in the evolution of the packaging, from a lab-based technology to a real-case scenario.

Several other research efforts have been addressed in the identification of biomarkers. Cancer biomarkers have been heavily investigated: in fact, the possibility to perform an early-stage diagnostic offered by optical fiber technology proves to have superior sensitivity at lower concentrations, hence showing a reliable identification of each biomarker. The case of prostate cancer, using a free prostate specific antigen, has been investigated using a monoclonal antibody linked with a SAM as a bioreceptor for the specific detection. The case study of breast cancer has also been heavily researched, both for the direct detection of breast cancer recirculating cells (Loyez et al., 2020), and for the identification of breast cancer biomarkers such as human epidermal growth factor receptor 2 (Sun, Ran, & Wang, 2017). Similarly, the detection of cardiovascular biomarkers using optical fibers is gaining significant traction; recent works have reported an immunosensor for sensitive cardiac troponin I (Liu et al., 2018), while the thrombin marker has been subject of recent studies in aptasensors (Sypabekova et al., 2019). The case study of urological biomarkers is also significant in biosensing technologies, as protein detection in urine content (Guo et al., 2016) plays a significant role in diagnostic, and the packaging of these typologies of sensors in intermittent urologic catheters has been proven in fiber-optic sensors (Poeggel et al., 2015).

Immunosensors cover an important range of applications of OFB (Guo et al., 2017), spanning from the detection of C-reactive protein (Zubiate, Zamarreño, Sánchez, Matias, & Arregui, 2017) to cytokins detection (Zhang, Arman, Anwer, Hutchinson, & Goldys, 2019); this type of sensors highlights the properties of optical fiber surface coatings, as the sensors achieve remarkable selectivity through the use of effective bioreceptors. A similar consideration can be drawn for sensors capable of resolving bacteria, such as the analysis of *Escherichia coli* (Zhou et al., 2018). These areas belong to a lower TRL level, as sensors have proven effective and selective sensing in vitro, but their effectiveness in field measurements has not been achieved to this date.

Fig. 1.5 provides a historical perspective to the evolution of OFB. Prior to 2005, most of the fiber sensing technologies applied to biochemical and biological measurements made use of the fiber as a passive element, simply carrying fluorescence signals or adapting an imaging setup with the use of endoscopic

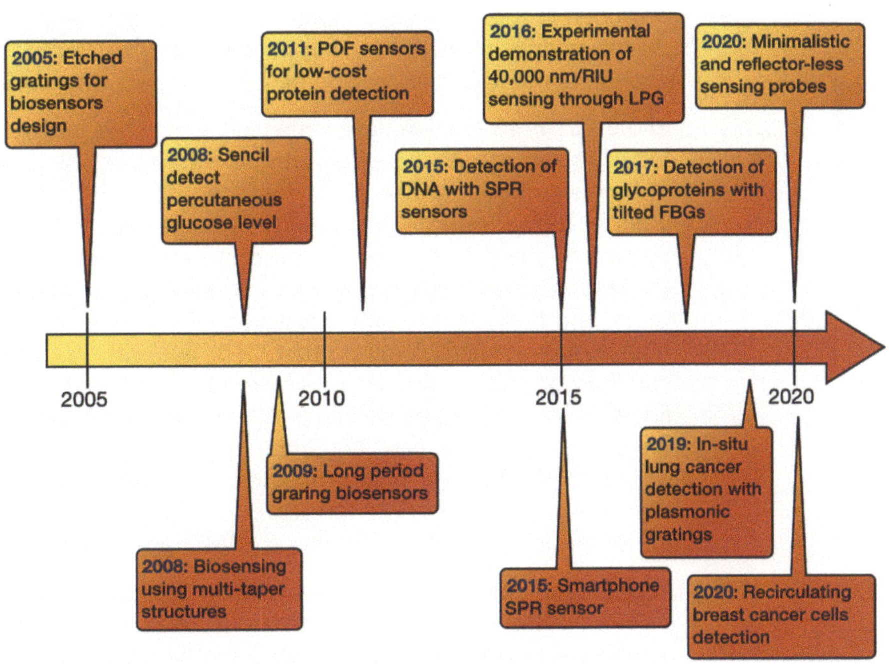

Figure 1.5
A chronology of the main achievements in optical fiber biosensor technology and applications, within 2005–10 timeframe.

fibers. The present days of OFB, which saw the intensification of research efforts in the last 5 years, can be set around 2005–08. In this moment, the developments of fiber Bragg grating technologies have provided scientists and engineers with the very first "fiber-only" type of sensor, which runs only on optical fibers and can be suited for biosensing (Othonos & Kalli, 1999). The development of inscription methods for optical gratings has allowed providing an easy implementation of biosensors; around this time, the first results on chemically etched gratings have been reported. In parallel, the 2008–10 period has brought significant results in terms of sensor packaging, with the previously mentioned sencil project among others to open important avenues for in vivo biosensing using optical fibers. The 2008–10 period has also seen the important achievements of manufacturing methods based on fiber splicing; from the arc-fusion splicers that simply handle telecom-grade fibers, the availability of adanced fusion splicers as well as CO_2 laser-based splicers has brought several instruments capable of fabricating optical devices, both inline on the fiber and around the tip of the fiber. In this period, we see the beginning of tapered fiber biosensors, and multitaper fiber biosensors, as well as for most of the interferometers for RI sensing in the fiber.

Around 2009, several research group has proposed works that perform biosensing using long-period gratings (Pilla et al., 2009); this technology has the capability of working at an excellent performance and sensitivity ratings, much larger than other competing methods, and therefore it has enabled sensing with subpicomolar resolution in the following period. The establishment of an easy and splicer-based manufacturing methods for long-period gratings has certainly provided a great impulse to the following development of high-performance OFB units.

In the 2010–15 era, we have witnessed a constant progress of each of the OFB technologies; rather than a few highlight events, each technology (gratings, SPR, interferometers) benefitted from the developments recorded in terms of manufacturing, optical elements, and packaging. A large emphasis has been posed into the development of low-cost sensors, aimed at reducing the cost of the interrogation unit; rather than using expensive light emitting diodes or lasers, and bulky interrogators, research efforts have been directed to achieving high performance, similar to other OFB, but with units that cost a fraction of commercial units. A first result was achieved through the use of plastic optical fibers, in lieu of glass fibers that are commonly used; these large fibers can couple the light in easier way, and implement simple yet sensitive methods for the detection. In 2011, a platform based on plastic fiber sensors for biosensing using SPR technology was presented, using a low-cost spectrometer and a jminimalistic architecture (Cennamo, Massarotti, Conte, & Zeni, 2011).

Subsequently in 2015, Bremer and Roth (Bremer & Roth, 2015) have reported a SPR sensor optimized for a smartphone; the system uses the flashlight already present on the phone and that spans the whole visible wavelength range, and converts the phone camera into a smartphone by the use of a diffraction grating. This system proved the possibility of combining the benefits of long-range sensing offered by the optical fibers with the portability and cost of a smartphone, and reported the first prototype of a fully working system that integrates the whole sensing mechanism on the phone itself, without the need for an external light source, detector, or amplifier. In 2015, furthermore, Chen et al. (Chen et al., 2015) reported a sensor prototype based on long-period gratings for the DNA analysis; this system allowed proving the detection of oligonucleotides immobilized on the fiber surface, which provided an effective and reliable methods for bonding to DNA and performing a spectrally sensitive detection method.

Moving to the last half-decade, we can identify important achievements on performance, manufacturing methods, and on applications of OFB. At first, we have witnessed the expansion of performance of long-period gratings, using the dispersion tuning regime method, an arrangement that modifies the spectrum of the sensor improving the sensitivity. A theoretical analysis (Del Villar, 2015) showed the possibility to obtain a sensitivity figure over 100,000 nm/RIU (RIU = refractive index units); 1 year later, in 2016, a work from Smietana et al. (Śmietana, Koba, Mikulic, & Bock, 2016) has shown a performance rating of 40,000 nm/RIU obtained experimentally, by chemically etching a long-period grating. While these extremely high sensitivity values have been recorded in a narrow RI range as they are resonant conditions, in general this progress has allowed to push long-period gratings to sensitivity values close to SPR levels, while however employing interrogators with a much better precision.

Another important achievement was reported in 2017, concerning the possibility to use of optical fiber sensors for detection of glycoproteins (Zhang et al., 2017). Glycoproteins can function in OFB both as target analyte, because they have a function in immunoglobulin analysis and immunosensors, but also as a bioreceptor as it binds to several viruses.

In 2019 significant progress was reported for sensor packaging, as the first in situ fully functionalized biosensor was reported by Loyez et al. (2019). The system reported in this work embodies a plasmonic grating sensors into an endoscopic device with semiflexible form factor, that was inserted into lungs for cancer biomarkers detection; the proposed case study was addressed to cytokeratin-17 lung cancer biomarkers, detected directly in the lung tissue. This work progressed biosensing technology upward in terms of TRL, performing both an ex vivo evaluation on human tissue, and an in vivo test on animals, reporting promising results on a small sample set. In a progress of this work, the same team from Universite' de Mons, Belgium, developed a system for the detection of recirculating breast cancer cells (Loyez et al., 2020), employing biosensing in a fluidic setup.

As a final milestone, in 2020 several works have addressed the problem of reducing the complexity of biosensors; rather than fabricating structures with a high sensitivity, but characterized by different devices and inscriptions within the fiber cores, minimalistic biosensors have been proposed; among others, authors from Nazarbayev University, Kazakhstan, reported a reflector-less biosensor (Sypabekova, Aitkulov, Blanc, & Tosi, 2020), which is a reflective probe entirely based on Rayleigh scattering and without the need of any in-fiber device or cavity, and a fiber ball resonator (Shaimerdenova, Ayupova, Sypabekova, & Tosi, 2020) that is fabricated from a standard fiber in few seconds and with a single step. These sensors have spectral characteristics that show a quasi-random pattern, as opposite as the previous sensors that have a well-defined spectral profile, but prove the possibility of manufacturing sensors in high volumes and still obtain a detectable signal.

1.4 Conclusion

A key advantage of OFB over other technologies such as microelectromechanical sensors, FETs, or conductometric sensors, is the capability to work at a rapid detection rate and in a miniature form factor. Over recent years, this capability has been exploited for the fabrication of biological sensors, as well as sensors that combine the biochemical detection with physical parameters (e.g., tactile sensors or breathing rate analysis), that are packaged in a way that ensure in vivo operation, or the application in contact with the patient undergoing diagnostic (Loyez et al., 2019). In this section, we discuss solutions that have been proposed for endoscopic catheters, urologic devices, and percutaneous needles, which represent the most important case scenarios for OFB devices.

References

Agrawal, G. P. (2012). *Fiber-optic communication systems* (2012). John Wiley & Sons.

Bekmurzayeva, A., Dukenbayev, K., Shaimerdenova, M., Bekniyazov, I., Ayupova, T., Sypabekova, M., . . . Tosi, D. (2018). Etched fiber Bragg grating biosensor functionalized with aptamers for detection of thrombin. *Sensors*, *18*(12), 4298.

Bertone, E., Burford, M. A., & Hamilton, D. P. (2018). Fluorescence probes for real-time remote cyanobacteria monitoring: A review of challenges and opportunities. *Water Research*, *141*, 152–162.

Bremer, K., & Roth, B. (2015). Fibre optic surface plasmon resonance sensor system designed for smartphones. *Optics Express*, *23*(13), 17179–17184.

Caucheteur, C., Guo, T., & Albert, J. (2015). Review of plasmonic fiber optic biochemical sensors: Improving the limit of detection. *Analytical and Bioanalytical Chemistry*, *407*(14), 3883–3897.

Cennamo, N., Massarotti, D., Conte, L., & Zeni, L. (2011). Low cost sensors based on SPR in a plastic optical fiber for biosensor implementation. *Sensors*, *11*(12), 11752–11760.

Chen, X., Liu, C., Hughes, M. D., Nagel, D. A., Hine, A. V., & Zhang, L. (2015). EDC-mediated oligonucleotide immobilization on a long period grating optical biosensor. *Journal of Biosensors and Bioelectronics*, *6*(2).

Chiavaioli, F., Gouveia, C. A., Jorge, P. A., & Baldini, F. (2017). Towards a uniform metrological assessment of grating-based optical fiber sensors: From refractometers to biosensors. *Biosensors*, *7*(2), 23.

Clark, J. R. L. C., Wolf, R., Granger, D., & Taylor, Z. (1953). Continuous recording of blood oxygen tensions by polarography. *Journal of applied physiology*, *6*(3), 189–193.

Clark, L. C., Jr, & Lyons, C. (1962). Electrode systems for continuous monitoring in cardiovascular surgery. *Annals of the New York Academy of Sciences*, *102*(1), 29–45.

Cullen, D. C., Brown, R. G., & Lowe, C. R. (1987). Detection of immuno-complex formation via surface plasmon resonance on gold-coated diffraction gratings. *Biosensors*, *3*(4), 211–225.

Del Villar, I. (2015). Ultrahigh-sensitivity sensors based on thin-film coated long period gratings with reduced diameter, in transition mode and near the dispersion turning point. *Optics Express*, *23*(7), 8389–8398.

Grieshaber, D., MacKenzie, R., Vörös, J., & Reimhult, E. (2008). Electrochemical biosensors-sensor principles and architectures. *Sensors*, *8*(3), 1400–1458.

Guo, T., González-Vila, Á., Loyez, M., & Caucheteur, C. (2017). Plasmonic optical fiber-grating immunosensing: A review. *Sensors*, *17*(12), 2732.

Guo, T., Liu, F., Liang, X., Qiu, X., Huang, Y., Xie, C., ... Albert, J. (2016). Highly sensitive detection of urinary protein variations using tilted fiber grating sensors with plasmonic nanocoatings. *Biosensors and Bioelectronics*, *78*, 221–228.

Homola, J. (2008). Surface plasmon resonance sensors for detection of chemical and biological species. *Chemical Reviews*, *108*(2), 462–493.

Liao, K. C., Hogen-Esch, T., Richmond, F. J., Marcu, L., Clifton, W., & Loeb, G. E. (2008). Percutaneous fiber-optic sensor for chronic glucose monitoring in vivo. *Biosensors and Bioelectronics*, *23*(10), 1458–1465.

Liu, T., Liang, L. L., Xiao, P., Sun, L. P., Huang, Y. Y., Ran, Y., ... Guan, B. O. (2018). A label-free cardiac biomarker immunosensor based on phase-shifted microfiber Bragg grating. *Biosensors and Bioelectronics*, *100*, 155–160.

Lobry, M., Lahem, D., Loyez, M., Debliquy, M., Chah, K., David, M., & Caucheteur, C. (2019). Non-enzymatic D-glucose plasmonic optical fiber grating biosensor. *Biosensors and Bioelectronics*, *142*, 111506.

Lobry, M., Loyez, M., Hassan, E. M., Chah, K., DeRosa, M. C., Goormaghtigh, E., ... Caucheteur, C. (2020). Multimodal plasmonic optical fiber grating aptasensor. *Optics Express*, *28*(5), 7539–7551.

Loyez, M., Hassan, E. M., Lobry, M., Liu, F., Caucheteur, C., Wattiez, R., ... Albert, J. (2020). Rapid detection of circulating breast cancer cells using a multiresonant optical fiber aptasensor with plasmonic amplification. *ACS sensors*, *5*(2), 454–463.

Loyez, M., Larrieu, J. C., Chevineau, S., Remmelink, M., Leduc, D., Bondue, B., ... Caucheteur, C. (2019). In situ cancer diagnosis through online plasmonics. *Biosensors and Bioelectronics*, *131*, 104–112.

Othonos, A. S., & Kalli, K. (1999). *Fiber Bragg gratings fundamentals and applications in telecommunications and sensing* (p. 1999) Artech House.

Patel, S., Nanda, R., Sahoo, S., & Mohapatra, E. (2016). Biosensors in health care: The milestones achieved in their development towards lab-on-chip-analysis. *Biochemistry Research International, 2016*.

Pilla, P., Manzillo, P. F., Malachovska, V., Buosciolo, A., Campopiano, S., Cutolo, A., ... Cusano, A. (2009). Long period grating working in transition mode as promising technological platform for label-free biosensing. *Optics Express*, *17*(22), 20039–20050.

Poeggel, S., Duraibabu, D., Tosi, D., Leen, G., Lewis, E., McGrath, D., ... Mirone, V. (2015). Differential in vivo urodynamic measurement in a single thin catheter based on two optical fiber pressure sensors. *Journal of Biomedical Optics*, *20*(3), 037005.

Schöning, M. J., & Poghossian, A. (2002). Recent advances in biologically sensitive field-effect transistors (BioFETs). *Analyst.*, *127*(9), 1137–1151.

Shaimerdenova, M., Ayupova, T., Sypabekova, M., & Tosi, D. (2020). Fiber optic refractive index sensors based on a ball resonator and optical backscatter interrogation. *Sensors*, *20* (21), 6199.

Śmietana, M., Koba, M., Mikulic, P., & Bock, W. J. (2016). Towards refractive index sensitivity of long-period gratings at level of tens of µm per refractive index unit: Fiber cladding etching and nano-coating deposition. *Optics Express, 24*(11), 11897–11904.

Socorro-Leránoz, A. B., Santano, D., Del Villar, I., & Matias, I. R. (2019). Trends in the design of wavelength-based optical fibre biosensors (2008–2018). *Biosensors and Bioelectronics: X, 1*, 100015.

Stoppa, M., & Chiolerio, A. (2014). Wearable electronics and smart textiles: A critical review. *Sensors, 14*(7), 11957–11992.

Sun, D., Ran, Y., & Wang, G. (2017). Label-free detection of cancer biomarkers using an in-line taper fiber-optic interferometer and a fiber Bragg grating. *Sensors, 17*(11), 2559.

Sypabekova, M., Aitkulov, A., Blanc, W., & Tosi, D. (2020). Reflector-less nanoparticles doped optical fiber biosensor for the detection of proteins: Case thrombin. *Biosensors and Bioelectronics*, 112365.

Sypabekova, M., Korganbayev, S., González-Vila, Á., Caucheteur, C., Shaimerdenova, M., Ayupova, T., … Tosi, D. (2019). Functionalized etched tilted fiber Bragg grating aptasensor for label-free protein detection. *Biosensors and Bioelectronics, 146*, 111765.

Theodosiou, A., Pugliese, D., Ceci-Ginistrelli, E., Boetti, N. G., Janner, D., Milanese, D., & Kalli, K. (2019). Femtosecond laser written plane-by-plane Bragg grating sensors in bioresorbable phosphate optical fibres. *Journal of Lightwave Technology, 37*(10), 2363–2369.

Walter, J. G., Alwis, L. S., Roth, B., & Bremer, K. (2020). All-optical planar polymer waveguide-based biosensor chip designed for smartphone-assisted detection of vitamin D. *Sensors, 20*(23), 6771.

Wilson, G. S., & Gifford, R. (2005). Biosensors for real-time in vivo measurements. *Biosensors and Bioelectronics, 20*(12), 2388–2403.

Zhang, D., & Liu, Q. (2016). Biosensors and bioelectronics on smartphone for portable biochemical detection. *Biosensors and Bioelectronics, 75*, 273–284.

Zhang, K., Arman, A., Anwer, A. G., Hutchinson, M. R., & Goldys, E. M. (2019). An optical fiber based immunosensor for localized detection of IL-1β in rat spinal cord. *Sensors and Actuators B: Chemical, 282*, 122–129.

Zhang, Y., Wang, F., Qian, S., Liu, Z., Wang, Q., Gu, Y., … Peng, W. (2017). A novel fiber optic surface plasmon resonance biosensors with special boronic acid derivative to detect glycoprotein. *Sensors, 17*(10), 2259.

Zhou, C., Zou, H., Li, M., Sun, C., Ren, D., & Li, Y. (2018). Fiber optic surface plasmon resonance sensor for detection of *E. coli* O157: H7 based on antimicrobial peptides and AgNPs-rGO. *Biosensors and Bioelectronics, 117*, 347–353.

Zubiate, P., Zamarreño, C. R., Sánchez, P., Matias, I. R., & Arregui, F. J. (2017). High sensitive and selective C-reactive protein detection by means of lossy mode resonance based optical fiber devices. *Biosensors and Bioelectronics, 93*, 176–181.

I

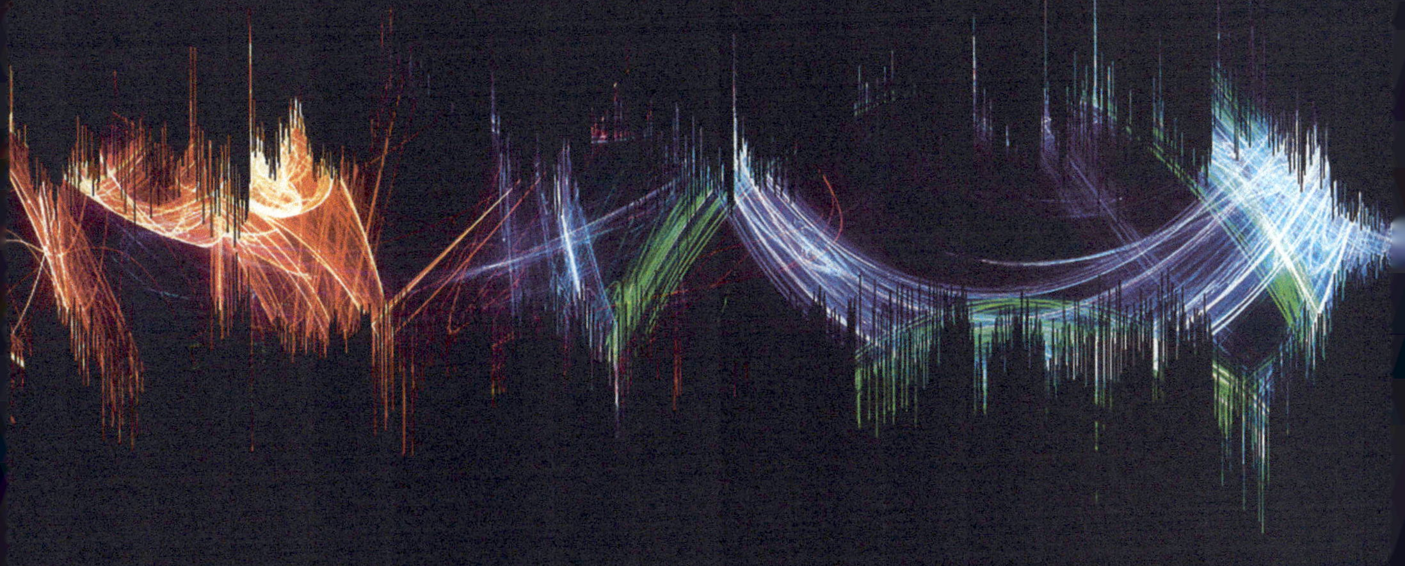

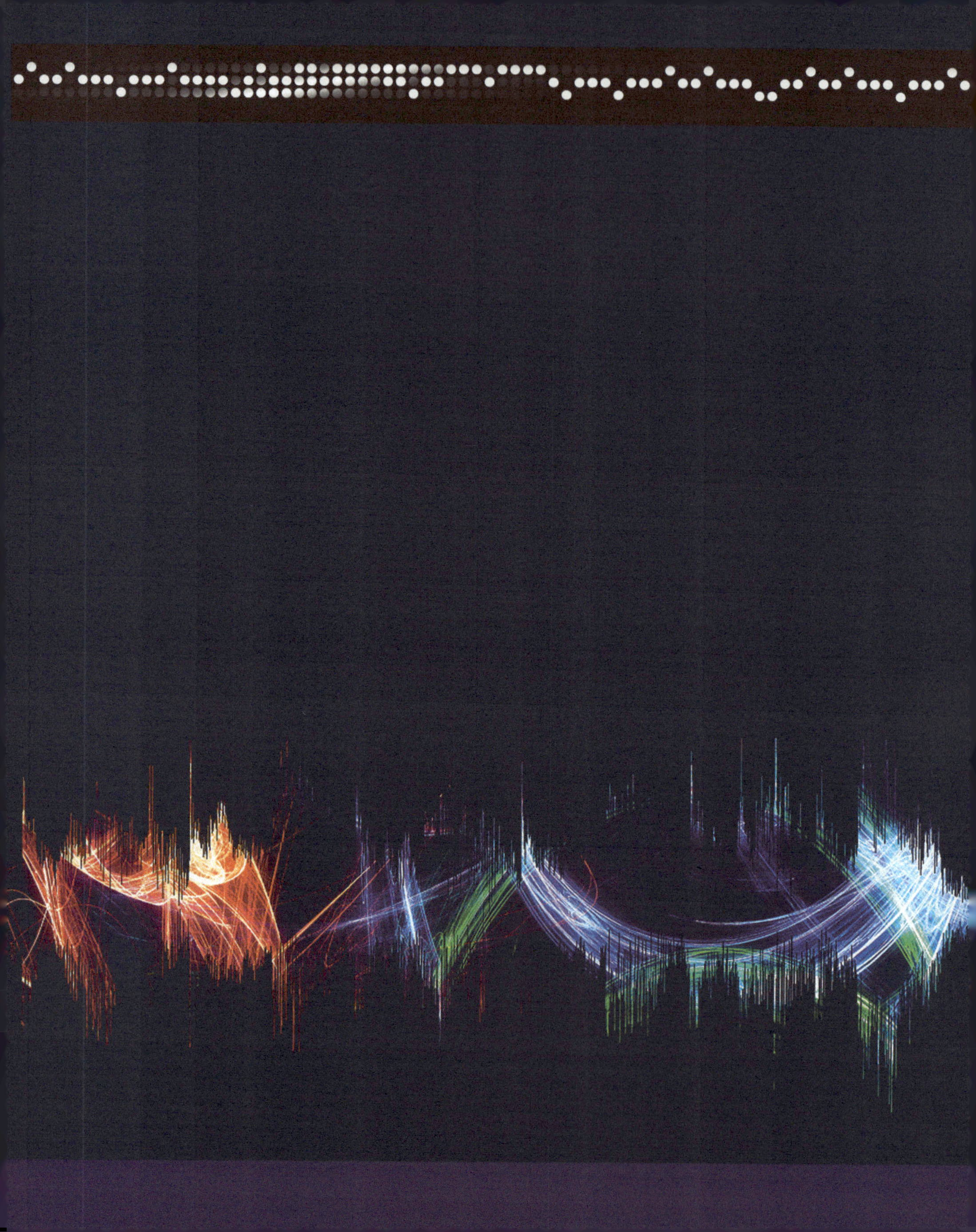

2

Principles of fiber optic sensors

2.1 Fundamentals of optics

To approach the field of optical fiber biosensors, we need first to introduce some of the underlying properties of light propagation, both into free space and into the fiber waveguides. In this section, we focus our attention on providing the key properties of light waves that allow readers building a foundation for the biosensors described in the next chapters; for a more thorough theoretical background, we recommend referring to Saleh and Teich (2019) for free-space and guided light propagation, and Ulaby, Michielssen, and Ravaioli (2010) for the fundamental properties of electromagnetics.

2.1.1 Fundamentals of wave optics

The electromagnetic radiation refers to waves that carry energy that propagates through space; radiofrequency waves, microwaves, light, X-rays, and gamma rays are all examples of electromagnetic radiations—all operating at different frequencies. Light is an electromagnetic radiation that occupies a specific portion of the electromagnetic spectrum as shown in Fig. 2.1—image reproduced from Danciu et al. (2019) with permissions.

Radiofrequencies and microwaves occupy a spectral portion up to 300 GHz; X and Gamma rays occupy the spectral portion having frequency over 3000 THz. The spectrum of light occupies the inner portion, between this range, and is divided into three parts: ultraviolet (UV), visible (VIS), and infrared (IR). The visible part of the optical spectrum corresponds to the range of frequencies that can be detected by human eyes. Rather than the frequency, in optics, the spectrum of the waves is commonly reported using the *wavelength* parameter: for a wave having frequency f, the wavelength λ is defined as

$$\lambda = \frac{c}{f} \tag{2.1}$$

where $c = 3 \times 10^8$ m/s is the light speed in vacuum. The wavelength is not a mere parameter to identify the frequency of the wave, but rather a physical

Optical Fiber Biosensors.
DOI: https://doi.org/10.1016/B978-0-12-819467-6.00016-0

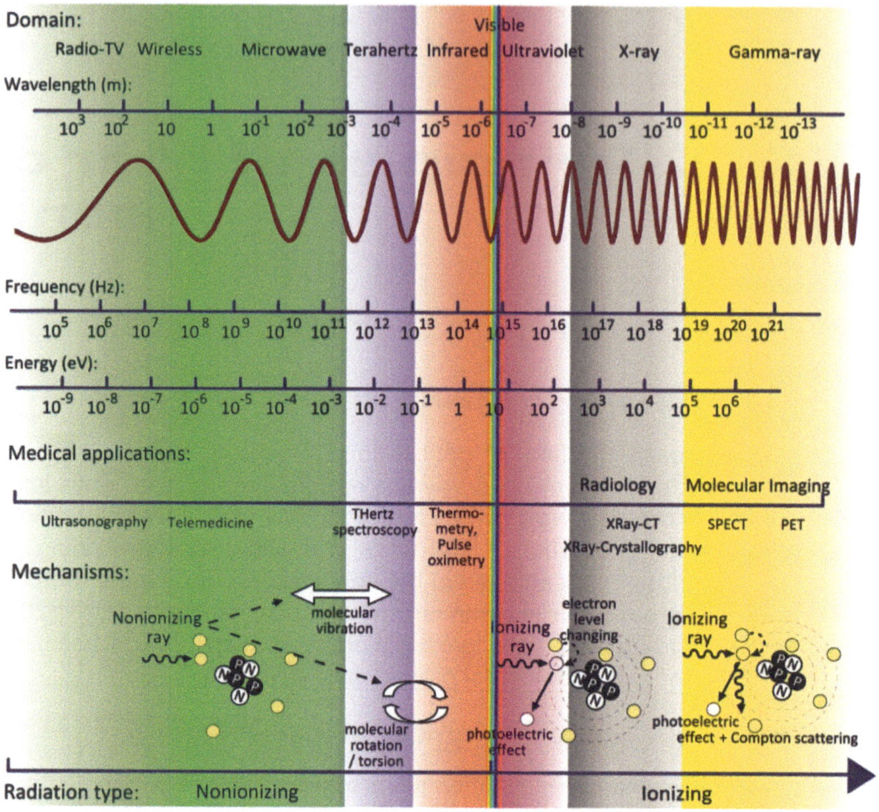

Figure 2.1 Spectrum of electromagnetic radiation, covering radiofrequencies, microwaves, Terahertz waves, infrared, visible, UV, X-ray, and Gamma-ray type of radiations, and some of their medical applications. Source: *Image from Danciu M., Alexa-Stratulat T., Stefanescu C., Dodi G., Tamba B. I., Mihai C. T., . . . Ianole V. (2019). Terahertz spectroscopy and imaging: A cutting-edge method for diagnosing digestive cancers.* Materials, 12*(9), 1519, reproduced with permission.*

parameter that defines the properties of the wave; the size of the optical fibers as well as the elements that compose the sensing device (e.g., the coating of the biosensor) have different behaviors depending on whether they are much smaller, much larger, or having a comparable size with respect to the wavelength of the light interacting with it. As such, UV light ranges between 1 and 380 nm; VIS range is from 380 (red) to 700 nm (blue); and IR range is from 700 nm to 1 mm wavelength.

Optical fiber biosensors usually exploit only a portion of the light spectral range, in which it is appropriate to develop the optical devices and the circuitry. The visible range is convenient because of the wide availability of light sources and detectors, particularly at red and green wavelengths, and is mostly used in low-cost systems and in surface plasmon resonance because of the high sensitivity of devices. Many systems are based on the IR range, usually around the wavelength of 1550 nm or around 1060 nm, in which components of telecommunications and lasers are optimized.

Light waves involve the propagation of electric fields, labeled as ***E***, where the bold font refers to a vector, and magnetic fields labeled as ***H***. Both electric and magnetic fields are vector fields; we can, therefore, write the fields in Cartesian coordinates as

$$\begin{aligned} \boldsymbol{E} &= E_x\hat{\boldsymbol{x}} + E_y\hat{\boldsymbol{y}} + E_z\hat{\boldsymbol{z}} \\ \boldsymbol{H} &= H_x\hat{\boldsymbol{x}} + H_y\hat{\boldsymbol{y}} + H_z\hat{\boldsymbol{z}} \end{aligned} \tag{2.2}$$

where the components E_x, E_y, and E_z represent the electric field intensity in the directions x, y, and z, and the terms $\hat{\boldsymbol{x}}, \hat{\boldsymbol{y}}, \hat{\boldsymbol{z}}$ are the unity vectors that represent the direction of the field (a similar notation for the magnetic fields).

The physical principles that relate the electric and magnetic fields between them, and with the electrical (or optical, in this case) sources are grouped in the Maxwell equations, that link ***E*** and ***H*** (Ulaby et al., 2010):

$$\begin{aligned} \nabla\cdot\mathbf{D} &= \rho_v \\ \nabla\times\mathbf{E} &= -\frac{\partial\mathbf{B}}{\partial t} \\ \nabla\cdot\mathbf{B} &= 0 \\ \nabla\times\mathbf{H} &= \mathbf{J} + \frac{\partial\mathbf{D}}{\partial t} \end{aligned} \tag{2.3}$$

Here, the operator $\nabla\cdot$ refers to the divergence of the field, while the operator $\nabla\times$ is the curl. The field **D**, directly related to **E**, is the electric flux density; the field **B**, related to **H**, is the magnetic flux density. Electric and magnetic sources are represented by the terms ρ_v, the electric charge density per unit volume, and **J**, the charge density per unit area. The Maxwell equations in Eq. (2.3) are comprehensive of all terms: resolving the Maxwell equations allows to determine the fields **E** and **H** that propagate in the structure, taking into account the specific boundary conditions. For example, solving the Maxwell equations for an optical fiber means resolving the system in (2.3) imposing the boundary condition given by the fiber under analysis. In this chapter, we will not aim at solving the full body of Maxwell equations, but rather keep the discussion to the wave fundamentals; for a full solution of the electromagnetics structures, we can recommend the reference Ulaby et al. (2010).

Since light waves have a specific frequency f, which undermines a specific time periodicity, we are interested in resolving the propagation of pulsating light waves in the simplest form, that is, in homogeneous lossless media and with no boundaries (*unbounded* waves). In this case, the solution is given by **plane waves**: a plane wave has a planar wavefront, that is, orthogonal to the direction of propagation. Many wave problems can be approximated to plane waves, and in fact several concepts that apply also to optical fiber sensors can be well explained using this approximation. In a plane wave, the electric field and the magnetic field are orthogonal between each other (*impedance relationship*), and the components along the propagation direction are equal to zero: if a wave propagates along the direction z, then we have $E_z = 0$, $H_z = 0$. If E_0 is the field at the location $z = 0$, then the field at the location z can be expressed as

$$E(z) = E_0 e^{-jkz} \tag{2.4}$$

The term $\exp(-jkz)$, where j is the imaginary unit, corresponds to a phase shift of the wave: while the intensity of the field is not changed, that is, $|E(z)| = |E_0|$, the phase of the field changes as the field propagates along its direction. The term k is a parameter of the wave, called wavenumber; it refers to the spatial periodicity of the wave and is measured in m^{-1} units.

2.1.2 Constitutive parameters of materials

The solution of the wave propagation equations depends on the media in which waves propagate. We now introduce the basic constitutive parameters of the media that are of fundamental importance to study the propagation of waves into the optical fibers and into the biosensors structures. The *constitutive relationships* of waves relate the fields **E** and **D**, as well as **H** and **B**:

$$\boldsymbol{D} = \varepsilon \boldsymbol{E} = \varepsilon_0 \varepsilon_r \boldsymbol{E} \tag{2.5}$$

$$\boldsymbol{B} = \mu \boldsymbol{H} = \mu_0 \mu_r \boldsymbol{H}$$

The term ε is the electric permittivity of a material. It is equal to the product of the electric permittivity in vacuum ($\varepsilon_0 = 8.854 \times 10^{-12}$ F/m) and the relative permittivity of the medium (ε_r) which characterize each type of medium or analyte. Similarly, μ is the magnetic permittivity and is the product of the magnetic permeability in vacuum ($\mu_0 = 1.257 \times 10^{-6}$ H/m) and the relative magnetic permeability of the medium (μ_r). Nonmagnetic media always hold $\mu_r \cong 1$, and therefore in the treating of optical fibers and biosensors, we can always consider $\mu = \mu_0$ unless otherwise stated.

We define η the intrinsic impedance of a medium:

$$\eta = \sqrt{\frac{\mu}{\varepsilon}} = \frac{\eta_0}{\sqrt{\varepsilon_r}} \tag{2.6}$$

where $\eta_0 = (\mu_0/\varepsilon_0)^{1/2} = 377\ \Omega$ is the intrinsic impedance of free space. The intrinsic impedance defines the relationship between **H** and **E**: for a wave propagating in the generic direction $\hat{\boldsymbol{k}}$, we have:

$$\boldsymbol{E} = -\eta \hat{\boldsymbol{k}} \times \boldsymbol{H} \tag{2.7}$$

$$\boldsymbol{H} = \frac{1}{\eta} \hat{\boldsymbol{k}} \times \boldsymbol{E}$$

which shows the orthogonality of **E** and **H** in plane waves, while both are orthogonal to the direction of propagation.

The phase velocity v of a wave defines the speed at which the wave travels in a medium and is defined as the speed at which the wavefront travels along the propagation direction. The velocity v is related to the dielectric permittivity as

$$v = \frac{1}{\sqrt{\mu\varepsilon}} = \frac{c}{\sqrt{\varepsilon_r}} \quad (2.8)$$

where c is the speed in vacuum, previously defined. In optics, rather than using the relative dielectric permittivity, we prefer to use the *refractive index* (RI) definition:

$$n = \frac{c}{v} = \sqrt{\varepsilon_r} \quad (2.9)$$

The RI n is, therefore, the ratio between the light speed in vacuum and the light speed in media, and characterizes the material in which light propagates. In biosensors, where we detect the change of the analyte in the surrounding of a fiber, the RI of the fiber and the RI of its surrounding analyte define the working principle of the device, and we interrogate small changes of the analyte RI. Hence, it is important to evaluate the RI of the analytes and media of interest (such as glass or plastics that constitute the optical fibers), which define the optical properties of the media in which light propagates.

Table 2.1 shows the RI of several media of interest in optics, optical fibers and biosensors, and diagnostic. For a full database of RI values, readers can refer to Refractometer (2020), a database of the RI of several media (particularly, aqueous media, alcohol, and gases that are usually adopted in optics for calibrations). It is important to notice that, while we treat the RI as a constant in the wave propagation analysis, the RI is indeed dependent by the wave properties too. Most notably, n is not constant with the wavelength, but rather we have $n = n(\lambda)$: this effect is called *chromatic dispersion* of the material and is, for example, at the base of the optical prism. Hence, in Table 2.1, we report the RI at specific calibration wavelengths, but their value can differ at other optical wavelengths.

The RI, as it controls the speed of propagation of waves, affects the wavenumber that indicates the spatial periodicity of the wave. The wavenumber k depends on both RI and wavelength:

$$k = \frac{2\pi n}{\lambda} \quad (2.10)$$

2.1.3 Polarization

A plane wave traveling in the direction z can be written as (Ulaby et al., 2010):

$$\mathbf{E}(z,t) = \hat{\boldsymbol{x}} E_x \cos(\omega t + kz) + \hat{\boldsymbol{y}} E_y \cos(\omega t + kz + \delta) \quad (2.11)$$

Table 2.1 Refractive index of several media of interest, at optical wavelengths. The table includes air, water, optical fiber materials (glass, PMMA, sapphire), glucose, sucrose, and ethanol that are used to calibrate the RI in biosensors, and analytes (blood cells, liver, urine) for some biosensing applications.

Medium	RI value	Wavelength (nm)
Vacuum	1	
Air	1.000293 (≅1)	589.29
Water	1.3330	589.29
Silica (quartz)	1.458	589.29
Diamond	2.417	589.29
Glucose (10% in water)	1.3477	589.29
Glucose (20% in water)	1.3635	589.29
Sucrose (10% in water)	1.3478	589.29
Sucrose (20% in water)	1.3639	589.29
Sucrose (30% in water)	1.3812	589.29
Ethanol (10% in water)	1.3395	589.29
Ethanol (20% in water)	1.3469	589.29
Poly(methyl methacrylate) (PMMA)	1.4893–1.4899	380–700
Sapphire	1.762–1.778	VIS–IR
Liver cells	1.369	964
Urine	1.3400–1.3408	1550
Red blood cells	1.402	633

where $\omega = 2\pi f$ is the angular frequency. E_x and E_y describe the magnitude of the wave along x and y directions, and the term δ is the *phase shift*, representing the phase difference between the directions x and y.

The *polarization* of a wave describes the locus traced by the vector **E** at a given point in space as a function of time, or equivalently the locus traced at a given time as a function of space. In general, for a wave having arbitrary values of E_x, E_y, and δ, the polarization describes an elliptical curve, and for this reason, we refer to it as *elliptical polarization*; however, we have some noteworthy polarization states that occur when the elliptical polarization degenerates.

Overall, we can identify three states of polarizations:

1. *Linear polarization*. This occurs when the waves are in phase ($\delta = 0$) or out of phase ($\delta = \pm\pi$). In this case, the ellipses collapses into a line on the xy plane. Noteworthy cases are for $E_y = 0$ (x or horizontal polarization), and for $E_x = 0$ (y or vertical polarization).

2. *Circular polarization.* Circular polarization occurs when $E_x = E_y$, and when $\delta = \pi/2$ (left-hand circular polarization), or $\delta = -\pi/2$ (right-hand circular polarization). In this case, the ellipses degenerates into a circumference.
3. *Elliptical polarization.* For any other case, the polarization is elliptical; the ellipses can be aligned along the *x*/*y* axes (this occurs when $\delta = \pm\pi/2$ but $E_x \neq E_y$) or its main axes can be inclined with respect to the *x*/*y* directions.

Fig. 2.2 shows some example of polarization states, reporting both the trace of the wave (magnitude of E_x and E_y for a generic wave along the direction *z*), and the planar trace that shows E_y as a function of E_x for all values of the location *z*. All the waves in this chart have the same magnitude but different polarization states. The first wave is linearly polarized along the horizontal direction, and we can see that the locus is a horizontal line, while the trace is a sine wave flattened on the horizontal plane. The second wave is a left-hand circular polarization: the locus is a circle, while the trace is a corkscrew that proceeds in the anticlockwise direction. A right-hand circular wave has the same locus, but a trace that instead revolves around the clockwise direction. The third polarization state is linear, at a 45° angle inclination; this occurs as $E_x = E_y$ and $\delta = 0$. The trace of the wave is a sine wave, rotated by an angle with respect to the first wave. The last two waves have elliptical polarization: the locus describes, in both cases, ellipses with different ellipticity and inclination angle, while the trace is a similar to an asymmetrical corkscrew.

The polarization has pivotal role in fiber optic, including the biosensing technologies as entire classes of sensors are based on polarization effects. All waves

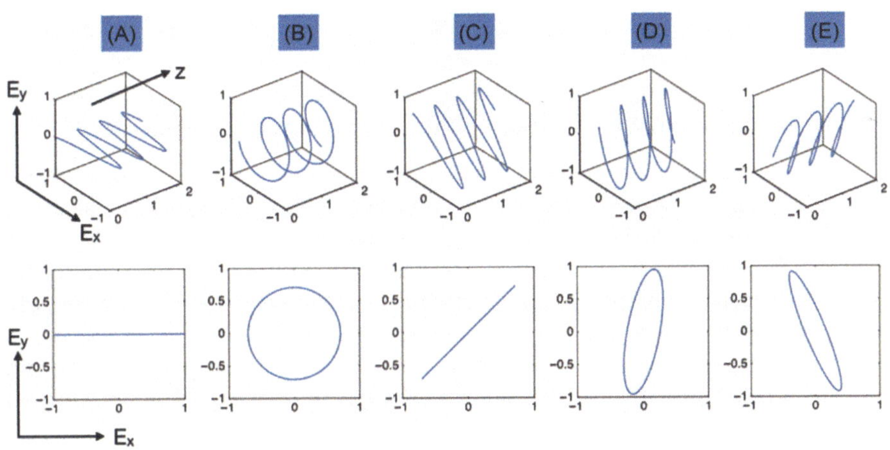

Figure 2.2 Example of different polarization charts of some waves. Upper charts: field intensities E_x and E_y along the direction of propagation *z*; lower charts: locus of the polarization trace, reporting E_x and E_y at a location *z* for a period of the wave. The chart described by the locus describes the state of polarization of the wave. All waves reported in the chart have unitary magnitude, that is, $|E_x|^2 + |E_y|^2 = 1$. (A) *x* (horizontal) polarization; (B) left-hand circular polarization; (C) 45° linear polarization; (D) and (E) elliptical polarizations.

carry the same amount of average power regardless of their polarization state; and in general, optical detectors such as spectrometers and photodiodes do not have a polarization-dependent behavior. However, the light transmitted and reflected at the interface between two media, as well as the plasmonic effects that we will review in the next sections, have a strong dependency on the polarization. In other words, while two waves having different polarization states propagate the same power, when they encounter a reflective medium the amount of reflected power changes according to the polarization state. For this reason, in optical circuits, it is often important to control the polarization.

2.1.4 Power and losses

In the analysis of fiber optic elements, we rarely consider electric and magnetic fields as they are hard to measure and characterize. Typically, we study the power of the waves that propagate into media, instead; this information is measured with standard protodetectors, spectrometers, or other optical hardware. We define the Poynting vector **S**, always directed in the direction of propagation of the wave, as

$$\boldsymbol{S} = \boldsymbol{E} \times \boldsymbol{H} \tag{2.12}$$

and the power of a wave is the integral of the intensity of the Poynting vector over the surface of the detector. It is important to state that for a wave propagating along direction z, both **E** and **H** are orthogonal to z while **S** is always along z; hence, the Poynting vector always points in the direction where the wave power propagates. When we discuss about the wave power, we will always refer to the average power of the wave, not the instantaneous value that is instead floating; we notice that for optical waves of interest operating at frequencies >100 THz, the periodicity of the waves is $<10^{-14}$ seconds, orders of magnitude below the resolution of any detector—and therefore the average power is what we measure on the instrument in our systems.

When the wave propagates in a real medium, we have to take into account the losses of the medium. Losses account for all different effects: absorption of light by the medium, and conversion of the energy to other effects (thermal effects, fluorescence, and frequency conversion); scattering, which guides the light into different directions; nonlinear frequency conversion; and other physical phenomena that reduce the power propagated in the medium. The power decreases exponentially along the direction of propagation: consider a wave having power P_0 at the initial location $z = 0$; at the location z the power is:

$$P(z) = P_0 e^{-\alpha z} \tag{2.13}$$

and we call the coefficient α as the *attenuation coefficient*, or simply the attenuation of the medium. The attenuation coefficient is measured in m^{-1}: for lossless media, in the ideal case, we have that $\alpha = 0$, while for low-loss media α is negligible with respect to the distance traveled by the wave; instead lossy media have a non-negligible value of the attenuation coefficient, and we have also to account for the propagation losses.

In fiber-optic systems, we prefer to convert Eq. (2.13) into logarithmic units, since the exponential term would convert to a linear term. To do so, we introduce the *decibel* (dB) unit; given a generic unitless number A, its corresponding value in dB is:

$$A \quad [\text{dB}] = 10 log_{10}(A) \tag{2.14}$$

The dB units simplify calculations: 1 corresponds to 0 dB, while 10 corresponds to 10 dB and 100 is 20 dB; similarly 0.1 is −10 dB and 0.01 is −20 dB. Since $10\log_{10}(2) = 3$, then 2 corresponds to 3 dB, 4 corresponds to 6 dB, 0.5 corresponds to −3 dB and so on. In short, any increase of 10 dB corresponds to a 10× multiplication, and an increase of 3 dB corresponds to a 2× multiplication, and subtractions of 10 dB and 3 dB corresponds to division of 10 and 2, respectively. Logarithmic units facilitate the operations on light propagation, particularly when it comes to detect power that varies by large amounts and to account for all the devices that compose an optical system. A common way to describe power units in logarithmic terms is to use the dBm unit:

$$P \quad [\text{dBm}] = 10 log_{10}\left(\frac{P}{1\text{mW}}\right) \tag{2.15}$$

where P is a power term. We can then rewrite Eq. (2.13) in logarithmic units:

$$P(z) = P_0 - \alpha z \tag{2.16}$$

where both P and P_0 are in dBm units, and the attenuation α is expressed in dB/m units. For example, the datasheet of optical fibers always reports the attenuation in logarithmic units. The conversion of α between dB/m and m^{-1} units is: α [dB/m] $= \alpha$ [m^{-1}] × 4.343. Fig. 2.3 shows the power propagation of waves, in linear units where power decreases exponentially along z, and in logarithmic units where the power decreases linearly. By measuring the power in dBm, the power drops linearly with distance, and the attenuation coefficient is the slope of the curve.

2.1.5 Reflection and transmission of waves

We now consider the case of a wave traveling at the interface between two media, as shown in Fig. 2.5. The incident wave has electric field E_{in}, carries the power P_{in}, travels in a medium having RI n_1 at the interface between a medium with RI n_2; the incident wave travels at an incidence angle θ_{in}, measured between the direction of propagation of the wave and the normal to the plane at the boundary between the two media. A special case is observed for normal incidence ($\theta_{in} = 0$), but we are interested in the general case as it also underlines the condition of propagation of light into optical fibers. As shown in the figure, two waves are generated when the incidence light travels at the

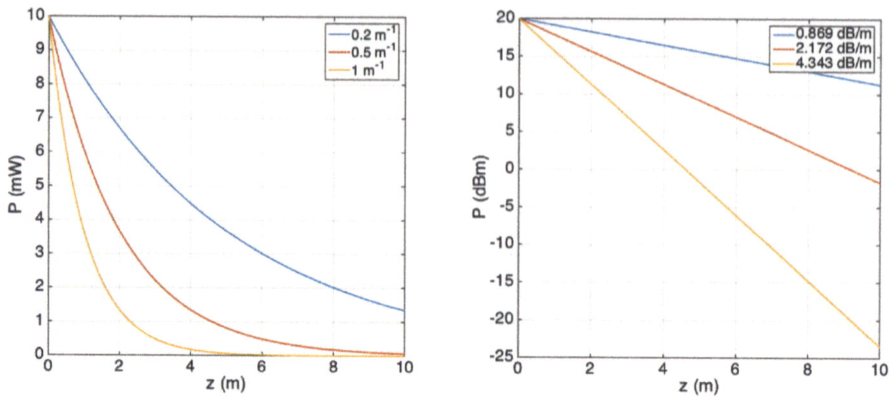

Figure 2.3 Attenuation of waves in media. The charts show the power of a wave having 100 mW over 10 m propagation along *z*, for three media having attenuation 0.2 m^{-1}, 0.5 m^{-1}, and 1 m^{-1}. The left chart reports the power in linear units; the right part reports the same chart in logarithmic units, with powers in dBm and attenuations in dB/m.

boundary between the two media: (1) a reflected wave, which is reflected from the incidence point backwards into the first medium and traveling along the opposite direction and (2) a transmitted (or refracted) wave that propagates into the second medium.

We now focus on the angles of each wave. The Snell's laws determine the relationships between angles and RIs:

$$\theta_r = \theta_{\text{in}} \tag{2.17}$$
$$n_1 \sin\theta_{\text{in}} = n_2 \sin\theta_t$$

The first equation shows that, for whatever RI and θ_{in} values, the reflected wave is symmetrical to the input wave, having the same propagation angle. The second equation relates the transmitted wave to the incident wave through the respective RI values. When $n_1 < n_2$ we always have that $\sin(\theta_{\text{in}}) > \sin(\theta_{\text{t}})$ and therefore $\theta_{\text{t}} < \theta_{\text{in}}$: in this case, the transmitted wave travels at a lower angle with respect to the incidence angle; this case is shown in Fig. 2.4. In this condition, we always observe the presence of a transmitted and a reflected wave, and the incidence power gets split between the two waves traveling in the opposite directions.

A more interesting case holds when $n_1 > n_2$: in this case, since $n_1/n_2 > 1$, there are cases for which $\sin(\theta_t) > 1$, which would be impossible. In this case, *there is no transmission* into the second medium, and the light is entirely reflected into the first medium. The limit case is occurs when $\sin(\theta_t) = 1$; in this case, we would have $\theta_t = 90°$ and the transmitted wave would travel exactly at the boundary between the media. Hence, we have here a split condition: for cases when $\sin(\theta_t) < 1$, we have a reflected and a refracted wave but for $\sin(\theta_t) > 1$,

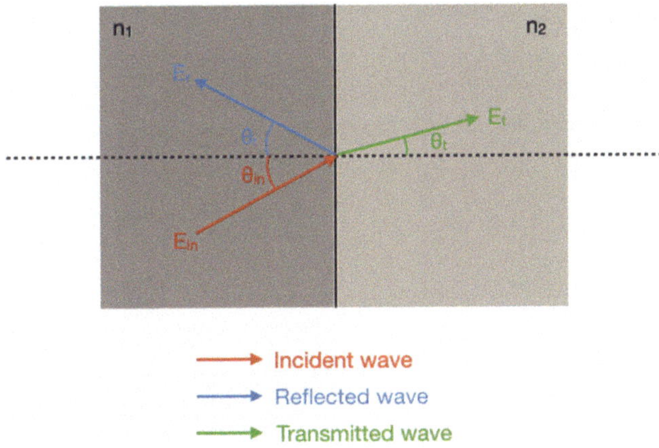

Figure 2.4 Schematic of the reflection and transmission of waves at the interface between two media having refractive index values n_1 and n_2.

we only have a reflected wave, with no transmission. We define as *critical angle* (θ_c) the incidence angle at which we observe $\sin(\theta_t) = 1$, and therefore the angle that satisfies the no-transmission condition: by solving the second Snell's law for this condition, we obtain:

$$\theta_c = \sin^{-1}\left(\frac{n_2}{n_1}\right) \tag{2.18}$$

The critical angle condition is essential for the light propagation over long distances and is at the base of all the optical waveguides, including the optical fibers. Consider the case shown in Fig. 2.5: for $\theta_{in} > \theta_c$, we have both a reflected wave and a transmitted wave, and if $n_1 > n_2$ we have an outward looking refracted wave. The limit case is observed for $\theta_{in} = \theta_c$ where the refracted wave would be bent at the 90° limit, and then for $\theta_{in} > \theta_c$ we have no transmission, and the light is entirely reflected.

We define this condition as the *total internal reflection* (TIR). Consider now the case of a waveguide having an inner layer n_1 sandwiched between two layers having RI n_2. If $n_1 < n_2$, there is no critical angle, and every time the waves would rebound at the interface, we would observe a transmitted wave. The generation of refracted waves at every interface would rapidly attenuate the power in the inner part of the waveguide: hence, $n_1 < n_2$ is not a condition for which we can guide light over long distances. A similar case holds for $n_1 > n_2$ but $\theta_{in} < \theta_c$, as shown in Fig. 2.5E: light continuously splits between reflected and refracted waves, constantly attenuating along the propagation direction.

When however we realize $\theta_{in} > \theta_c$, we are in TIR condition. The light incident on the boundary gets reflected entirely, with no transmission; then, the reflected wave maintains the same incidence angle (first Snell's law) when it rebounds a second time, and therefore satisfies once again the TIR condition. All the rebounding at the n_1/n_2 interface hold the TIR and maintain the

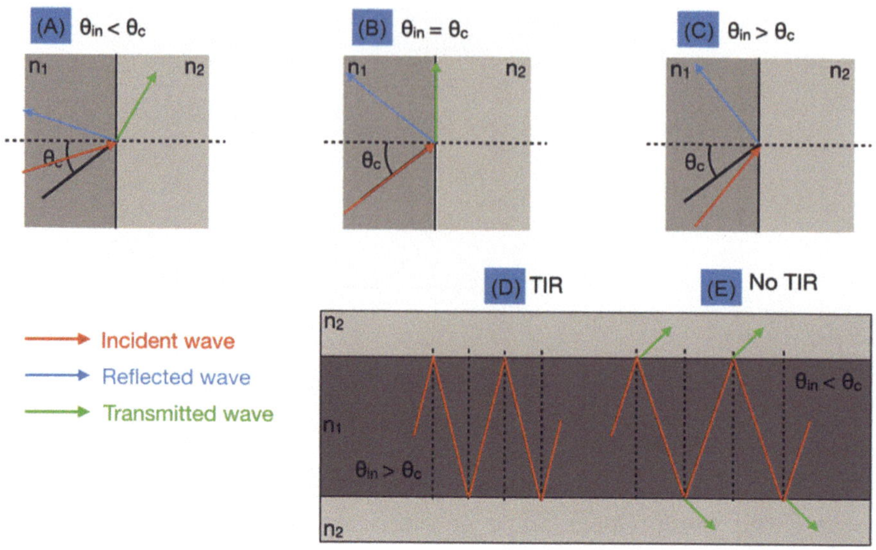

Figure 2.5 Conditions of propagation of light with respect to the critical angle θ_c. (A) Outward refraction, $n_1/n_2 > 1$ and $\theta_{in} < \theta_c$. (B) Limit case for $\theta_{in} = \theta_c$. (C) No transmission case, for $\theta_{in} > \theta_c$ and total reflection at the interface. (D) Design of a waveguide through reflection mechanism: $\theta_{in} > \theta_c$ which yields total internal reflection (TIR) at any interface; (E) $\theta_{in} < \theta_c$ and no TIR condition, which generates continuous transmissions into the n_2 medium.

incidence/reflection angle, and this condition allows propagating light over a very long distance, limited only by the attenuation of the medium. Therefore the TIR is the principle that we adopt for optical fibers and for all sorts of waveguides.

We now focus on calculating the amount of light that is reflected and transmitted at the interface between the two media. We introduce two parameters: the *reflection coefficient* Γ is defined as the ratio between the reflected wave E_r and the incident wave E_{in}; the *transmission coefficient* τ is the ratio between the transmitted wave E_t and the input E_{in}.

In the general case, when the light is incident at an angle θ_{in}, we observe that the transmission and reflection coefficients depend on the polarization. It can be shown (Ulaby et al., 2010) that in this condition, we can decompose the input wave into two states of polarization, each having a different polarization state:

1. The *parallel* (or *p*) polarization: this is the polarization that is parallel to the plane of incidence;
2. The *perpendicular* (or *s*) polarization: this is the polarization that is perpendicular to the plane of incidence.

For any problem of light incidence onto a surface, we can decompose the input wave into its two *s* and *p* polarization states, and calculate the reflection coefficients separately. Fresnel's formulas (Saleh & Teich, 2019) provide the expressions for the reflection and transmission coefficients for parallel and perpendicular polarizations:

$$\begin{aligned}\Gamma_p &= \frac{n_2\cos\theta_{\text{in}} - n_1\cos\theta_t}{n_2\cos\theta_{\text{in}} + n_1\cos\theta_t}\\ \Gamma_s &= \frac{n_1\cos\theta_{\text{in}} - n_2\cos\theta_t}{n_1\cos\theta_{\text{in}} + n_2\cos\theta_t}\\ \tau_p &= \frac{2n_1\cos\theta_{\text{in}}}{n_2\cos\theta_{\text{in}} + n_1\cos\theta_t}\\ \tau_s &= \frac{2n_1\cos\theta_{\text{in}}}{n_1\cos\theta_{\text{in}} + n_2\cos\theta_t}\end{aligned} \tag{2.19}$$

We have seen, however, that is easier and more intuitive to operate with power rather than field values, since the power is the actual parameter being measured. Since the power is proportional to the square of the magnitude of the field, we can now define the *reflectivity* (ratio between the reflected power and the input power), and the *transmittivity* or transmission (ratio between the transmitted power and the input power):

$$\begin{aligned}R_p &= |\Gamma_p|^2 = \left|\frac{n_2\cos\theta_{\text{in}} - n_1\cos\theta_t}{n_2\cos\theta_{\text{in}} + n_1\cos\theta_t}\right|^2\\ R_s &= |\Gamma_s|^2 = \left|\frac{n_1\cos\theta_{\text{in}} - n_2\cos\theta_t}{n_1\cos\theta_{\text{in}} + n_2\cos\theta_t}\right|^2\\ T_p &= |\tau_p|^2 = \left|\frac{2n_1\cos\theta_{\text{in}}}{n_2\cos\theta_{\text{in}} + n_1\cos\theta_t}\right|^2\\ T_s &= |\tau_s|^2 = \left|\frac{2n_1\cos\theta_{\text{in}}}{n_1\cos\theta_{\text{in}} + n_2\cos\theta_t}\right|^2\end{aligned} \tag{2.20}$$

Since we must conserve the power, the amount of reflected and refracted power must equal the incident power, and therefore we always have $R + T = 1$.

In the case of normal incidence, $\cos\theta_{\text{in}} = \cos\theta_{\text{t}} = 1$, and the reflectivity and transmittivity have polarization-independent behavior: in this case, the Fresnel reflectivity depends only on the two values of RI:

$$R = \left(\frac{n_2 - n_1}{n_2 + n_1}\right)^2 \tag{2.21}$$

and $T = 1 - R$. The reflectivity at the interface between two media plays a significant role in the development of biosensors. For example, the Fresnel reflectivity at the interface between an optical fiber ($n = 1.454$) and air is 0.034, which means that about 3.4% of the light is reflected at the end of an optical fiber. At the boundary between the fiber and water ($n = 1.333$), the reflectivity is 0.0019 or 0.19%.

A very important condition occurs when the reflection coefficient is equal to zero for a specific incidence angle. We can obtain this condition by resolving the reflection coefficient equalities in Eqs. (2.19) or (2.20) and imposing the reflection coefficient to zero, hence determining the incidence angle that satisfies the equality.

Consider the case of a wave incident from air into media with different RI, as shown in Fig. 2.6. For waves having *s*-polarization, the reflectivity is always greater than zero and increases as the incident angle grows; hence, we never observe the condition $R_s = 0$. However, for *p*-polarized light, the reflectivity initially decreases until it reaches a zero value, and then rises again; for each value of n_2, there is one incidence angle for which $R_p = 0$. We define this incidence condition as the *Brewster angle* θ_B and it occurs for:

$$\theta_B = \tan^{-1}\left(\frac{n_2}{n_1}\right) \tag{2.22}$$

The Brewster angle plays a significant role in some of the biosensors, particularly those that make the use of polarization effects such as surface plasmon resonance or polarizing fibers because it is a polarizing angle: when light is incident at the Brewster angle, the reflected wave is entirely *s*-polarized, as the *p*-polarization has a null reflection coefficient.

2.2 Optical fiber fundamentals

Waves propagating in free space are unbounded and obey to the properties that we have described so far. However, we have seen that by operating on the Snell's law, we can propose optical structures that guide light over long distances through TIR principle: when the TIR condition is satisfied, and no light gets transmitted away from the inner layer, the main limiting factor for long-distance transmission is the loss of the material. We define as *waveguides* the structures that guide the light propagation into a small and effective device, capable of transmitting over a relatively long distance. The optical fiber is the most common optical waveguide, both in terms of manufacturing (fibers can

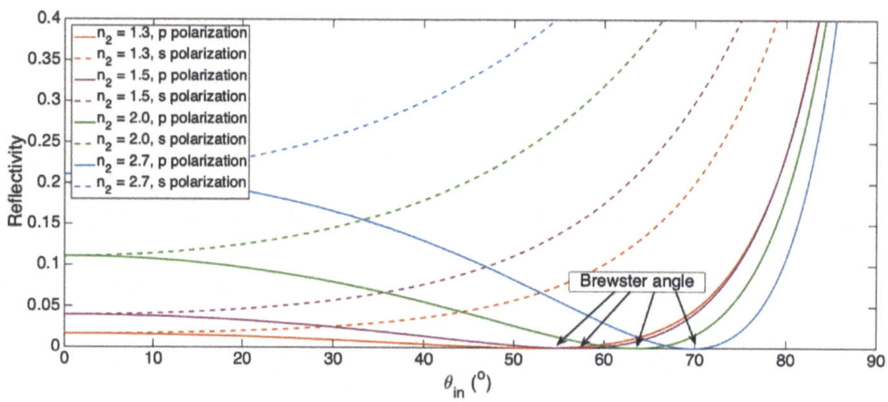

Figure 2.6 Reflectivity for a wave incident from air ($n_1 = 1$) into a medium with different values of RI ($n_2 = 1.3, 1.5, 2.0, 2.7$) for the parallel (solid lines) and perpendicular (dashed lines).

be drawn for thousands of kilometers) and performance; other geometries such as slab or channel waveguides are more common in optical devices such as lasers or integrated optical systems.

2.2.1 Structure of optical fibers

The structure of an optical fiber is shown in Fig. 2.7; the fiber has an inner layer called core, surrounded by an outer layer called cladding. The core is the inner medium where the light propagates, while the cladding around the fiber surrounds the core and provides the RI contrast necessary for the light propagation. The cross-section of the fiber is a cylinder, where core and cladding form concentrical layers. Usually, the cladding of the fiber is surrounded by a protective jacket; this external layer is only for protection, and its properties do not influence light propagation.

As seen in the previous section, to satisfy the TIR principle, the core of the fiber must have RI value higher than the cladding. Only in this condition, and satisfying the correct critical angle condition, we can obtain the TIR condition. Hence, if we consider z as the direction of light propagation, and the xy plane as the cross section, Fig. 2.7B shows the RI profile along the fiber section. The RI of the core is n_2, and the RI of the cladding is n_1, with $n_2 > n_1$. This type of structure is called *step-index* (SI) fiber, and it is by far the most common structure in current optical systems. Other profiles, called graded index, where the RI varies gradually with x,y, are not used in

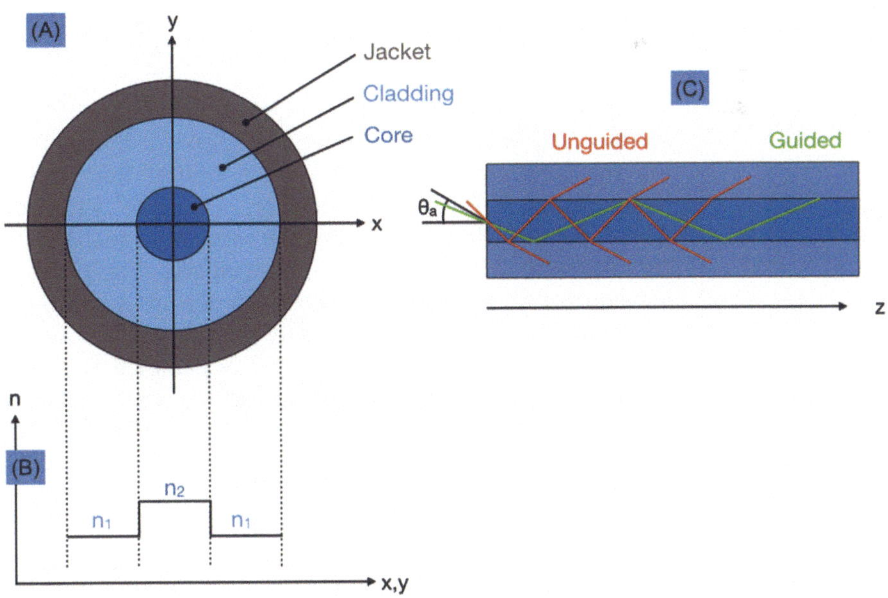

Figure 2.7
Structure of a step-index optical fiber. (A) Cross-section of the fiber. (B) Refractive index profile of the fiber. (C) Side view of the fiber, and its guided and unguided propagation.

biosensors. Weakly guiding fibers, such as those that we consider for most of the structures described in this book, have a small step or RI between core and cladding, that is, $(n_2 - n_1) << n_1$. Usually, the difference of RI between core and cladding is $\sim 10^{-2}$ for fibers having core and cladding made of glass. The weakly guiding condition might change in the exact location of the biosensor: for example, we may remove the fiber cladding and expose the core to the analyte, obtaining an RI change of 0.11 in the sensing point, but in general this change of weakly guiding condition occurs only in one sensing point, and not throughout the fiber propagation direction.

Fig. 2.7C shows the guiding propagation conditions for an optical fiber. We have seen that the condition that satisfies the TIR principle is that the angle of incidence at each core–cladding interface (which are reported for a two-dimensional structure in the figure for simplicity, but in a cylindrical fiber occur on a three-dimensional geometry) must be lower than the critical angle. In fiber optics, however, we prefer to report the *acceptance angle* θ_a, which is the angle at the fiber input that satisfies the TIR. As shown in the figure, light waves entering the core at input angle $<\theta_a$ are guided, while light waves entering at an angle $>\theta_a$ are not guided as they do not satisfy the TIR, and vanish rapidly (in few wavelengths) along the *z* axis.

We define the *numerical aperture* (NA) of an optical fiber the sine of the acceptance angle; the NA is a datasheet parameter of the fiber and depends only on the RI values of core and cladding:

$$\mathrm{NA} = \sin\theta_a = \sqrt{n_2^2 - n_1^2} \tag{2.23}$$

2.2.2 Light propagation and modes

As for in any waveguide, we need to solve the Maxwell equations (2.3) imposing the boundary conditions; in the optical fiber, boundary conditions are related to the RI value (n_2 in the core, n_1 outside of the core assuming the cladding is infinitely thick) and solve the resulting equations in a cylindrical geometry (Agrawal, 2012). Unlike in free space, the propagation in the optical waveguides occurs through *modes*: modes are a specific solution of Maxwell's equations that satisfy the boundary conditions, and having spatial distribution (i.e., electric field shape around the *xy* plane) that does not change through the propagation. A full solution to the Maxwell equations in the optical fiber can be found in Agrawal (2012) and Saleh and Teich (2019).

We can identify three types of modes:

- *Guided modes* contribute to the light propagation, as they satisfy the wave equations; the light exciting guided modes propagates in the fiber over a long distance.

- *Radiation modes*, or cladding modes (in the optical fiber), having field intensity that is not confined in the fiber core but extends significantly to the cladding.
- *Leaky modes* have electric field that decays monotonically over distance, having an oscillatory behavior.

While cladding and leaky modes are often associated with biosensors structures and can often be found in biosensors having high performance (e.g., cladding modes are at the base of tilted fiber Bragg gratings and long-period gratings, while leaky modes are excited in plasmonic structures), only guided modes contribute to the fiber propagation. Cladding modes are indicated with the index LP_{lm}, where LP stands for linearly polarized, l is the azimuthal index, and m is the radial index.

The shape of LP modes is shown in Fig. 2.8 (image reproduced from (RP Photonics, 2020) with permission), which shows the electric field distribution on the fiber cross-section, centered around the fiber core. In the LP_{lm} modes, the index l starts from 0, while the index m starts from 1. The chart shows the electric field intensity with sign, red portions are positive values, blue portions have negative value. The m radial index describes the number of regions along the radial direction; in simple terms, m equals to the number of colors that we encounter if we move from the center of the fiber to its border. The azimuthal index l is equal to the number of transitions along the fiber circumference direction: in short, we can select a point on the x axis, and rotate all around the fiber until we reach the initial points, then $l=$ (number of colors that we encounter) − 1. The lowest order mode is LP_{01}, which is also known as the *fundamental mode*: its mode profile is similar to a Gaussian function in two dimensions, with a peak in the center of the fiber and rapidly decreasing on the side of the fiber. The *second order mode* is LP_{11} and it has a profile with one radial oscillation. In general, modes with even l (LP_{0x}, LP_{2x}, ...) have azimuthal symmetry, while LP_{1x}, LP_{3x}, ... are azimuthally asymmetrical.

We see that the field is not entirely confined in the fiber core, but rather decreases exponentially on the tails; hence, the power distribution on the fiber cross section is contained in the core by a large, but not total, amount, and a small part of it proceeds into the cladding. We define the *confinement factor* (CF) as the ratio between the power contained in the core and the total power carried by each mode:

$$CF = \frac{P_{core}}{P_{total}} = \frac{\int_{-r}^{r} \int_{-r}^{r} |E(x,y)|^2 dxdy]_{x^2+y^2 \le r^2}}{\int_{-\infty}^{\infty} \int_{-\infty}^{\infty} |E(x,y)|^2 dxdy} \tag{2.24}$$

where r is the radius of the core. Modes of lower order have a higher confinement factor, while higher order modes have lower CF as the electric field

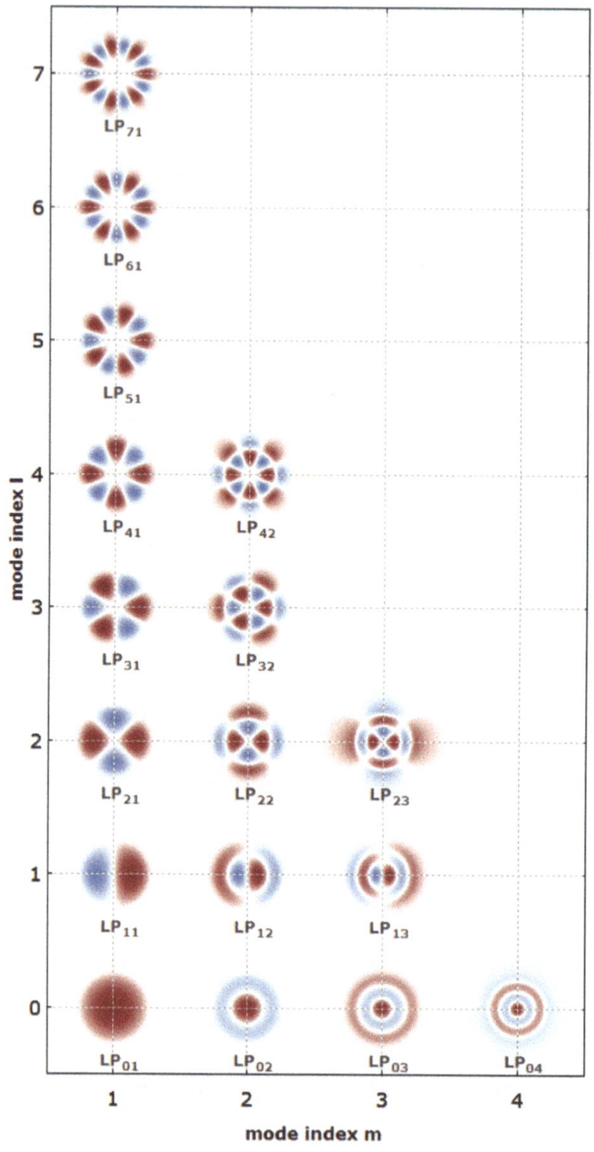

Figure 2.8 Electric field distribution of LP modes. Source: *Image reproduced from RP Photonics. (2020).* RP photonics encyclopedia. *https://www.rp-photonics.com, reproduced with permission.*

elongates closer to the edge of the fiber. The CF is a parameter of great interest in the design of biosensors, as well as for the light propagation. Efficient light propagation implies high CF values, hence modes that confine the energy primarily in the fiber core; however, modes with poor value of CF deliver significant amount of power in the neighborhood of the core, and therefore allow a better interaction of the light between the fiber core and the surrounding environment—and for this reason, this configuration finds great coverage in optical fiber biosensors.

Modal propagation, as from the electromagnetic theory (Ulaby et al., 2010), differs from free-space propagation as the number of supported modes depends on the frequency. For each mode, we can define a *cut-off wavelength*. For wavelengths longer than the cut-off wavelength, the mode is not supported; for wavelengths shorter than the propagation constant, the mode is a guided mode and therefore supports light propagation. To better understand the mode propagation, which is an essential concept also for optical fiber biosensors, we introduce the bV chart in Fig. 2.9.

The term b is the *normalized propagation constant*, defined as

$$b = \frac{n_{\mathrm{eff}} - n_1}{n_2 - n_1} \tag{2.25}$$

where n_{eff} is the effective RI of the mode. The term V is the *normalized frequency*, defined as

$$V = \frac{2\pi r}{\lambda} NA \tag{2.26}$$

Hence, given a certain fiber geometry (core radius and NA), the V number decreases with the wavelength as $\sim 1/\lambda$, and for this reason it has the resemblance of a frequency. The cut-off conditions, as seen in Fig. 2.9, correspond to

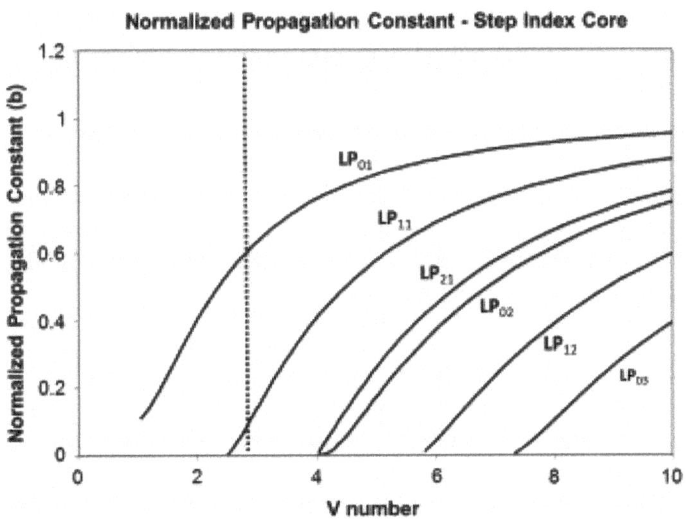

Figure 2.9 bV relationship for LP modes, reporting the normalized propagation constant b versus the normalized frequency V for modes of different index (Peckham et al., 2013). Source: *Image from Peckham, D. W., Sun, Y., McCurdy, A., Lingle Jr, R., Kaminow, I., Li, T., & Willner, A. E. (2013).* Few-mode fiber technology for spatial multiplexing. *Elsevier/Academic Press, reproduced with permission.*

the V values over which $b > 0$, and therefore $n_{eff} > n_1$. The term n_{eff} is different for every mode and increases with b. By focusing on the limit condition $b = 0$, we can identify how many modes can propagate: for example, at $V = 1$ there is only one mode (LP_{01}), while for $V = 6$ there are six modes (LP_{01}, LP_{11}, LP_{21}, LP_{02}, LP_{31}, LP_{12}).

We define *single-mode fiber* (SMF) a fiber having only one guided mode. This condition occurs for $V < 2.405$, which is the cut-off condition for the LP_{11} mode. Similarly, a *multimode fiber* (MMF) has more than one guided mode. It is important to recognize that the single-mode cut-off condition occurs at a specific wavelength; hence, a fiber is single-mode in a specific wavelength range. For example, a fiber having $r = 5\ \mu m$ and $NA = 0.1$ has the cut-off condition of the LP_{11} mode at the wavelength $\lambda = 2\pi r\ NA/V = 1306$ nm; this fiber is an SMF for $\lambda > 1306$ nm, while it is an MMF for $\lambda < 1306$ nm. For fibers having a large number of modes, a good approximation is

$$\#\text{modes} \approx \frac{V^2}{2} \tag{2.27}$$

2.2.3 Effective refractive index and single/multimode operation

The effective RI n_{eff} is a very important concept for optical fiber biosensors: most of the structures that we are going to analyze in the next chapters (such as all gratings and interferometers) are strongly based on changes of the n_{eff} term. The effective RI is the ratio between the propagation constant in the fiber along the propagation direction and the propagation constant in vacuum (Marcuse, 1991).

A ray-optics interpretation of the n_{eff} concept is shown in Fig. 2.10. In a single-mode fiber, the fundamental mode can only propagate. The light rebounds at the core–cladding interface. In a two-dimensional geometry, the light propagation appears as in the upper figure, with light propagating with a tilted pattern with respect to the axis z along the propagation. Similar to the RI definition, we can define n_{eff} as

$$n_{eff} = \frac{v_z}{c} \tag{2.28}$$

where v_z is the light propagation speed along the direction z. In the simple bidimensional geometry, v_z would simply be the light speed in the fiber core projected along z; similarly, in a cylindrical fiber, the light rays propagate with a tilted pattern, either with meridional rays (that touch the center of the core) or skew rays (that rebound on the side of the core, never touching the center). Clearly, $n_1 < n_{eff} < n_2$ to ensure the light propagation. As from the figure, a single-mode optical structure has only one mode, and therefore all the light propagates with the same n_{eff} value.

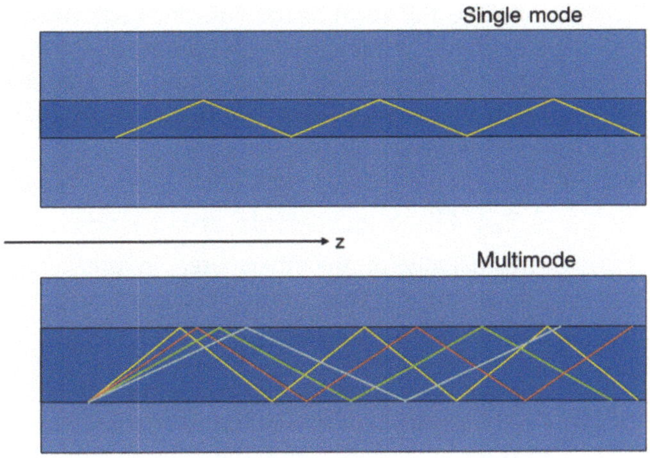

Figure 2.10 Ray-optics interpretation of the mode propagation in a single mode and a multimode fiber.

In a multimode fiber, instead, there are several modes that propagate with a different angle of approach into the fiber. As a result, each mode has a different effective RI: modes that propagate with a smaller angle, closer to the core, travel faster than modes with a steeper angle. Unlike in some microwave waveguides, in fiber optics we cannot control precisely the excitation of the modes, particularly when propagating over a long distance (considering that even few meters of fiber correspond to millions of wavelengths). Hence, we always assume that the power is carried by all the guided modes, with a mode coupling coefficient that we cannot control over the propagation.

The fact that each mode has a different n_{eff} has implications on the light propagation. An immediate consequence results from light pulses that propagate in the fiber that spread onto different modes, each traveling in the fiber at a different speed. This velocity differential gives rise to the mode dispersion, a detrimental effect in telecommunications but with limited impact on sensing. The main impact, however, is on the phase of the propagating field. Consider two modes having electric field E_0 at $z = 0$, as in Fig. 2.10 at the beginning of the fiber, and having $n_{eff,1}$ and $n_{eff,2}$ values of effective RI. At the coordinate $z = L$, the first electrical field would be $E_1(L) = E_0 \times \exp(-j\ 2\pi\ n_{eff,1}\ L/\lambda)$, while the second mode would be $E_2(L) = E_0 \times \exp(-j\ 2\pi\ n_{eff,2}\ L/\lambda)$, that is, introducing a phase difference between each mode that varies with length and wavelength. Since all propagation term always see the product $L \times n_{eff}$, the phase delay of each mode is always different from each other mode.

For this reason, the sensing structures based on resonant effects, such as interferometers or gratings, are most commonly implemented with single-mode fibers: different modes would see different resonant conditions, complicating the analysis of the light through the sensing region. Conversely, these structures typically aim at varying the n_{eff} term (e.g., removing the fiber cladding or shrinking the core) as the light interacts with the surrounding analyte. On the other hand, sensing principles based on the light intensity often use multimode fibers: they have a bigger core and NA that facilitates the light coupling in and out of the fiber, with a number of mode that varies as the fiber geometry is manipulated.

2.2.4 Fiber materials and losses

The majority of the fibers used in optical fiber biosensors derive from the devices used in telecommunications, thanks to the wide availability of components and the presence of standards that define the fiber material and geometry. While extensive research has been given to change the fiber materials, to impress additional properties on the fiber (e.g., biocompatibility, scattering, in vivo absorption), the presence of these fibers is limited to the sensing region. Instead, we will assemble the interrogation system using mostly fibers that are derived from telecommunications, and that have standards that allow us operating with them in an easy way. Commercially available fibers are based on two materials: glass, which results in the so-called glass optical fibers (GOFs), or plastic, which results in polymer optical fibers (POFs).

GOF fibers are made of silica (SiO_2) that have been optimized for long-haul transmission and, for this reason, have low losses. They have both core and cladding made of silica; the RI contrast between n_2 and n_1 is generated by doping the core or the cladding, hence lowering or increasing the RI to a contrast $n_2 - n_1 \sim 0.01$. Silica fibers are fabricated in two steps: at first, a fiber preform is fabricated, whereas a preform is a cigar-shaped piece of glass having the same material and core/cladding proportion of the fiber, but having thickness of few centimeters. Then, the fiber is drawn through a drawing tower which heats and pulls the preform, cooling it when it reaches the desired diameter. GOFs have several advantages in terms of sensing: they are based on a biocompatible material, which is also radiation immune and therefore it is compatible with magnetic resonance; they have very low losses in the IR wavelengths; they resist high temperatures and therefore are suitable for fabrication of coating up to $\sim$800°C; they are not hydroscopic; they can be easily fused and interconnected to other fibers; and they can be fabricated as SMF or MMF by choosing the core/cladding proportion as well as the amount of dopants.

The key characteristic of glass fibers is the low loss of silica at IR wavelengths, which makes it a perfect candidate for sensing and communications. Fig. 2.11, adapted from Agrawal (2012), shows the attenuation of silica fibers, which is the result of Rayleigh scattering (which has a λ^{-4} dependence), IR absorption that is very strong for wavelengths over 1700 nm, imperfections of the waveguide, and UV absorption. The peak around 1400 nm is due to OH^- absorption, surrounded by other smaller peaks that cause an increase of the attenuation.

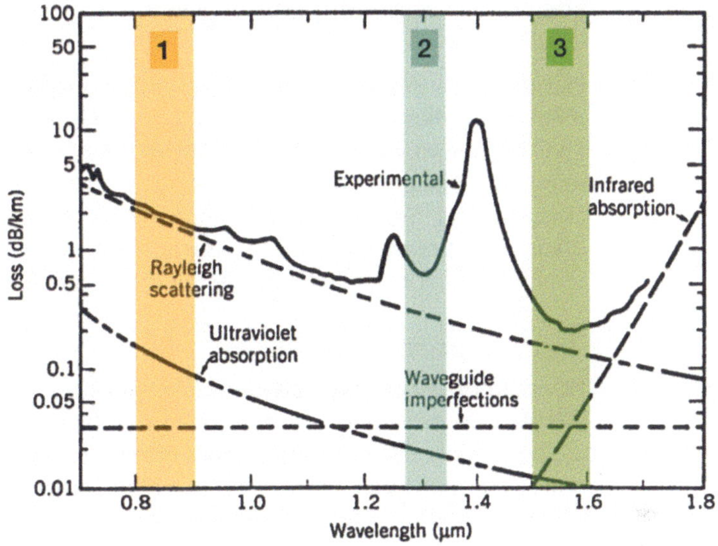

Figure 2.11 Attenuation of silica optical fibers, over the different wavelengths; the three highlighted regions indicate the optical windows. Source: *Image adapted from Agrawal, G. P. (2012).* Fiber-optic communication systems. *John Wiley & Sons, reproduced with permission.*

Historically, with few devices available operating over 1000 nm, the fibers operated in the so-called first optical window (800–900 nm), where the fiber attenuation is about 3–4 dB/km. The second generation of devices operated in the window centered at 1310 nm wavelength, where the fiber losses have a local minimum around 0.2 dB/km—this is also called the second optical window. Many biosensors, particularly those that have a large bandwidth, are operating in the second window around 1300 nm. The current generation of devices instead operates at the very minimum of the losses of the optical fibers, which occurs at 1550 nm and is 0.2 dB/km; this window, approximately 1500–1600 nm, is the third optical window and is characterized by the lowest losses. With such low loss, biosensing system can easily approximate the fiber as a lossless medium, since the attenuation over short spans are negligible. Instead, it is the broad availability of light sources and detectors that operate at 1550 nm that makes the difference in the selection of the wavelength of operation.

POF fibers instead are intended only for multimode operation, as they arise as a low-cost alternative to silica fibers. The reduction of cost is not to be intended for the price per meter of the fiber, but rather for all the components of the system (sources, detectors, hardware, sensing device). The main plastic fibers in use for telecom and sensing systems are based on polymethyl methacrylate (PMMA) material, and in general have a solid core that extends almost through the entire surface of the fiber. The cladding is a thin perfluorinated layer, with a process that slightly reduces the RI: as a result, POF fibers usually have a high NA that facilitates the light coupling and propagate millions of modes. POF fibers operate through the visible wavelength range, with 10–50 dB/km attenuation, which, however, rapidly rise to >>100 dB/km over the IR wavelength range.

Outside of the commercially available fibers, which benefit from material and geometrical optimization of their properties, fibers tend to have a very high attenuation; custom-made fibers, for example, designed to have customized in vivo resorbable operation (Ceci-Ginistrelli et al., 2016) or tailored Rayleigh scattering (Tosi, Molardi, Sypabekova, & Blanc, 2020) can easily achieve losses of tens/hundreds of dB per meter. It is recommended therefore to use these fibers only in the sensing point and assemble the rest of the system with other commercial fibers.

2.2.5 Commercial fibers

Having introduced the readers to the basics of optical fibers, we now focus our attention in providing a review of some of the fibers and their standards that are commonly used in the biosensor technologies. Table 2.2 shows a list of the most common fibers used in optical fiber biosensors, including both SMF and MMF for different operative wavelength ranges.

The most important SMF fibers are those operating in the third optical window: at this wavelength, we have the maximum availability of interrogators, light sources, detectors, and devices. The SMF-28 fiber, based on the ITU-T G.652.D telecom standard, is available at a low cost (about $0.08/m); the fiber has a cut-off wavelength around 1260 nm, and therefore is single-mode over both the second and third windows, which makes it effective also for broadband sensing devices (such as long period gratings or some interferometers) that require an SMF fiber but also a broad spectrum. Fiber losses are very low (0.18–0.35 dB/km), which makes attenuation negligible for biosensing system.

SMF fibers are available also at different wavelengths; in general, the core diameter gets smaller to reduce the V number and therefore the cut-off wavelength of the LP_{11} mode. Instead, the cladding is maintained at 125 μm diameter: by having a standard size for the cladding, identical to ITU-T G.652.D protocol, it is possible to use the same handling (fiber connectors, splicers, strippers) for all fibers, regardless of their core diameter. Similarly, all fibers have a similar coating diameter: the coating is a dual-acrylate layer with diameter of 250 μm, which can also have an additional protective jacket of 900 μm thickness; the 250 and 900 μm coating diameters are the two most common standards for glass fibers. In alternative, fibers with polyimide coating such as the SM1550P can be used for working at higher temperature ranges. SMF fibers can also be used at 980–1060 nm wavelength range, which is an important window because it is very popular in fiber lasers, and therefore it is possible to have availability of devices: popular fiber formats are the HI1060 and 980HP, with cut-off wavelength at 920 nm. Similarly, SM6XX (XX = wavelength) fibers are single mode at VIS wavelength; the most performing fiber is the S630XP, which can work through the upper part of the visible range.

Table 2.2 List of the most common commercial fibers and their characteristics for operation with optical fiber sensors and biosensors.

Fiber type	Material	Standard	Core/clad diameters	Jacket diameter	Attenuation	Cut-off	NA
SMF-28	Silica	ITU-T G.652.D	8.2/125 μm	250 or 900 μm	0.18–0.35 dB/km at 1310–1625 nm	1260 nm	0.14
1550 BHP	Silica		9/125 μm	250 μm	0.5 dB/km at 1550 nm	1400 nm	0.13
SM1550P	Silica, polyimide coating		9/125 μm	145 μm	0.7 dB/km at 1550 nm	1260 nm	0.12
HI1060	Silica		5.3/125 μm	250 μm	1.5–2.1 dB/km at 980–1060 nm	920 nm	0.14
980HP	Silica		3.6/125 μm	250 μm	3.5 dB/km at 980 nm	920 nm	0.20
S630HP	Silica		3.5/125 μm	250 μm	10 dB/km at 630 nm	590 nm	0.12
Panda PM1550	Silica, PM		–/125 μm	250 μm	0.5 dB/km at 1550 nm	1400 nm	
Bow-tie HB1500T	Silica, PM		–/125 μm	400 μm	2 dB/km at 1550 nm	1290–1520 nm	0.11–0.13
HB1550Z	Silica, polarizing		–/125 μm	250 μm	20 dB/km at 1550 nm	1150 nm	0.09–0.11
Infinicor 300	Silica	ISO 11801 OM1	62.5/125 μm	250 μm	0.6–2.9 dB/km at 850–1300 nm		0.275
Clearcurve OM2	Silica	ISO 11801 OM2	50/125 μm	250 μm	0.6–2.3 dB/km at 850–1300 nm		0.200
Clearcurve OM3	Silica	ISO 11801 OM3	50/125 μm	250 μm	0.6–2.3 dB/km at 850–1300 nm		0.200
Clearcurve OM4	Silica	ISO 11801 OM4	50/125 μm	250 μm	0.6–2.3 dB/km at 850–1300 nm		0.200
Core ϕ200 (FP200)	Silica		200/225 μm	500 μm	12 dB/km at 810 nm		0.50

(*Continued*)

Table 2.2 Continued

Fiber type	Material	Standard	Core/clad diameters	Jacket diameter	Attenuation	Cut-off	NA
Core ϕ400 (FP400)	Silica		400/425 μm	730 μm	12 dB/km at 810 nm		0.50
Core ϕ600 (FP600)	Silica		600/630 μm	1040 μm	12 dB/km at 810 nm		0.50
Core ϕ1000 (FP1000)	Silica		1000/1035 μm	1440 μm	12 dB/km at 810 nm		0.50
Core ϕ1500 (FP1000)	Silica		1500/1550 μm	2000 μm	12 dB/km at 810 nm		0.50
VIS-IR 0.22 NA	Silica		50/125, 105/125, or 200/220 μm	250 or 320 μm	8 dB/km at 810 nm		0.22
TECS-clad	Silica core, TECS cladding		200/225, 300/325, 400/425, 600/630, 800/830, 1000/1035, or 1500/1550 μm	500–2000 μm	10 dB/km at 810 nm		0.39
SK40	PMMA core, fluorinated cladding		980/1000 μm	2200 μm	0.3 dB/m at 660 nm		0.5

Optical fibers do not maintain the polarization state (Agrawal, 2012); that means that when light having a specific polarization state (e.g., linear or circular) is input into a fiber span, at the output of the span the polarization is random and it is not maintained throughout the fiber. PM fibers (PM = polarization maintaining) are used instead to maintain the polarization; the design of this fiber differs from Fig. 2.7 by having stress rods around the core. The most popular designs are Panda and Bow-tie, having different geometries of the stress rods that prevent the polarization changes. In general, it is recommended to use PM fibers only for detection schemes that rely on polarization control, as this type of fiber is more expensive and requires a special alignment of the stress rods. PM fibers exist almost only as single-mode fibers, and for the same wavelength range of the SMF fibers: for example, the PM1550 works around the third optical window, the PM1300 works in the second window, the PM980 works around the 980 nm range, and the PM630 in the visible wavelength. It is important to recall that PM fibers maintain the polarization but do not polarize a signal throughout the propagation. Instead, to generate a specific state of polarization, it is possible to use polarizing fibers (such as the HB1550Z) which work only on linear polarization states (horizontal or vertical, relative to the fiber axis); this approach, however, is rare on biosensors, where it is preferrable to use a polarization filter.

Multimode fibers instead have a broader selection in the marketplace: together with telecom fibers, which are mainly addressing short-length cabling (e.g., last mile communications), there is a strong offer for fibers specifically suited for sensing and imaging. Telecom fibers are mainly based on the ISO 11801 standard, which has four categories OM1, OM2, OM3, and OM4. All fibers have a cladding of 125 μm in diameter, and a core having diameter of 50 μm (NA = 0.2) or 62.5 μm (NA = 0.275). MMF silica fibers having these parameters are designed to operate at 850 and 1300 nm, but they can be easily extended to the 1550 nm maintaining a high number of modes ($V = 40-70$ at 1550 nm).

The so-called "core fibers" class is a set of fibers fabricated with two characteristics: a large core with respect to the cladding, so that the cladding appears as a thin crown surrounding the core; and a high NA obtained by having a steep contrast of RI between core ($n_2 = 1.4584$) and cladding ($n_1 = 1.3651$). This typology of fiber is gaining importance in biosensors based on surface plasmon resonance because the combination of a large core and a thin cladding allows an easy manipulation in plasmonic structures. They are designed to operate on the 300–1200 nm range, having a core that ranges from 200 to 1500 μm, with a cladding up to 50 μm in thickness. The NA of the core fibers is 0.50, which implies an acceptance angle of 30°, which makes it easy to couple light into the fiber even from low-cost LED sources or even smartphone flashlights. Core fibers are intended as heavily multimode fibers: they propagate around 75,000 (ϕ200 fiber) to 4.2 million (ϕ1500) modes at 810 nm.

Other glass MMF fibers of importance are designed to work in visible and IR range, having NA = 0.22 or 0.39; TECS-clad (Technology Enhanced Clad Silica) fibers have the cladding made of a Hard Fluoropolymer to increase its resistance and are used in medical diagnostic and imaging.

POF fibers instead have almost one unique design that has been consolidated for short communications and for sensing (Abrate, Gaudino, & Perrone, 2013); other designs, particularly involving graded-index fibers, are not used in sensing. The POF fiber has a 980 μm PMMA core with a thin crown serving as cladding (1000 μm diameter) made of fluorinated material. Unlike silica, PMMA shows its best transparency at visible wavelengths; as such, POF sensors work almost entirely in the visible wavelength range, with best attenuation around 0.3 dB/m at red wavelength. POF fibers have a polymer coating of 2.2 mm diameter. PMMA fibers are designed with a large NA (0.5), which ensures a large V number ($V = 2330$ at 660 nm, corresponding to 2.7 million modes).

2.2.6 Fiber connectors, splicing, and general handling

To facilitate the interconnection of devices and the assembling of sensing networks, fiber cables can be either terminated with connectors, which are terminals mounted at the end of the fiber, or fused together. Connectors are used in commercial instruments, and in fiber devices such as light sources, detectors, splitters, and polarizers. They provide an efficient method to align the core of the fibers, so that light can pass through with almost no losses. The connectors are fabricated using a subassembly, with a spring-based crimp that holds the fiber in position. The fiber is hosted in a terminal cylindrical ferrule and polished on the top.

Fig. 2.12 shows the main standards for fiber connectors that are used in current systems, with different performance and interconnections. Connectors are typically identified by the standard and by the type of fiber termination. The output fiber can either be terminated on a flat surface, or with a tilt angle; a flat surface minimizes the fiber losses, and for this reason it is preferred in telecommunications particularly those channels limited by the optical power budget, while angled surface termination is preferred in sensing and imaging because it minimizes the backreflections. Angled terminations are labeled APC (angled physical contact), and APC connectors are fabricated with green color; flat terminations are labeled UPC (ultra physical contact) or simply PC, and have blue color. The FC connector is the most popular in research because of its performance; the fiber is locked in position through a slot, and then screwed to fix the connector. LC and E2000 connectors are locked in position with a spring mechanism, they are simpler to insert and remove also for the unfamiliar user; similarly, the SC connector is housed in a mount that holds in position through a side slot. Generally, FC/APC connectors are used for most of the works presented in research and they are the go-to standard for most research laboratories, but

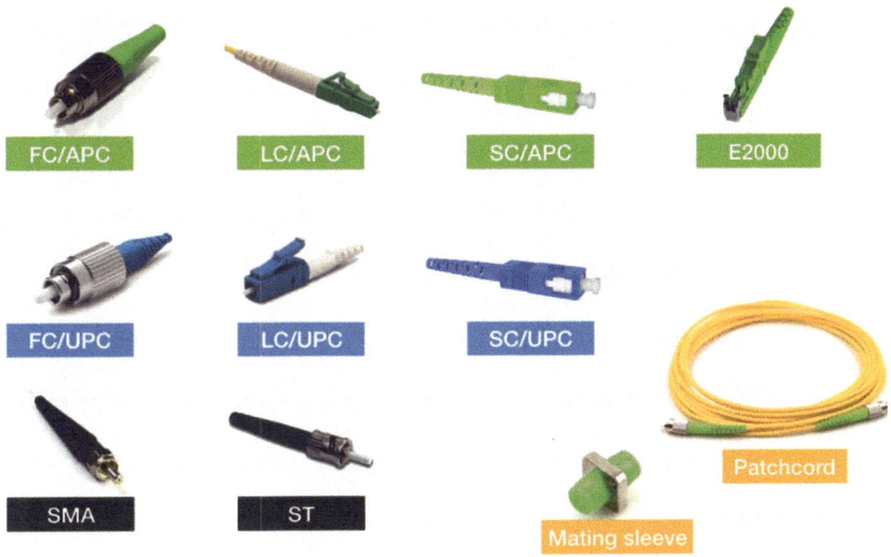

Figure 2.12 Image of optical fiber connector standards.

other APC connectors are often used on commercial instruments as they have simpler implementation. To interconnect two fibers, we use mating sleeves that are double-sided holders in which two connectors of the same type can be inserted. Mating sleeves can work either with APC or UPC connectors, but the user must insert always two connectors of the same type; for example, Fig. 2.12 shows an FC mating sleeves, suited for FC/APC-FC/APC or FC/UPC-FC/UPC connectors. SMA and ST connectors (black color) are not designed for fiber interconnection, but rather to facilitate fiber operations, for example, polishing.

To facilitate interconnections with the devices, it is possible to use *patchcords* that are short (1–10 m) spans of optical fiber, terminated with a connector on both sides; patchcords use SMF or MMF fiber, with an additional layer of protection of the fiber and an outer plastic cover, having labeled colors (SMF = yellow or blue; MMF = orange). It is also possible to have short patchcords with different connector terminals, to adapt one connector type to another one (e.g., FC/APC to LC/APC). Fibers terminated with the connector only on one side are labeled *pigtails*, and they are often used to interconnect the probe fabricated for sensing to an interrogator. As a note for users, it is important to use connector cleaners to remove the dust from the connector tips; these cleaners use lint-free paper and isopropyl alcohol to remove the dust particles, which can damage the quality of the connectors.

The alternative to connectors is to fuse two optical fibers together; this fusion is called *splice*, and the machine that performs this operation is called splicer. The simplest splicer is an arc-fusion splicer that has two micropositioners (left and right) where two fibers are set in position and two electrodes that heat the fiber tips in a controlled way. The fiber fusion is realized by simultaneously applying a current to the electrodes to heat up and melt the fiber tip, while pushing the fibers at both sides with the micropositioner. Both left and right positioners have an alignment system that allows matching either the core (core-aligning splicers, usually more expensive and performing) or the cladding (cladding-aligning splicers, usually more portable and cheaper). Commercial splicers usually have a set of splicing recipes already preloaded, which define the set of parameters (speed of positioning, type of alignment, number and power of the electrical arcs) of the splice for each type of fiber, for example, SMF–SMF, MMF–MMF, etc. Several splicers are also portable and battery operated and can be used in the field. An alternative to arc-fusion splicers is laser-based splicers that use a laser source (usually a CO_2 laser) to fuse the fibers. Laser splicers are only available as benchtop instruments and have cost largely superior to electrical splicers; they are not used for general fiber handling but rather for the fabrication of devices—including several of the sensors included in this book.

The other general fiber handling operations include stripping a cleaving. A stripper is a fiber tool resembling a cable stripper that is used to remove the fiber protective jacket from the fiber cladding. Before manipulating the fibers in any operation such as splicing, cleaving, or etching, it is always necessary to remove the outer jacket. The cleaver is an instrument with a sharp cutting blade that cuts the fiber with a high precision flat angle (or, in some cleavers, performing a tilted cleave). Stripping and cleaving the fibers should always be performed before splicing, as all splicers require the fibers to have a perfectly flat end-surface to fuse the fibers. Cleavers and splicers have holders that should match the size of the fibers: in general, the most popular standards are 250 and 900 μm, matching the most popular fiber jacket dimensions; it is important to match the dimension of the fibers to the holders and size of the splicers, strippers, and cleavers used to build the devices.

2.3 Light sources and detectors

We now focus our attention on assembling optical fiber systems that use the fiber as a transmission medium. We describe now the main optical fiber sources and detectors that represent the front- and back-end of the optical fiber systems.

Fig. 2.13 shows the underlying principles of optical sources and detectors, and their role in fiber optic systems. Broadband sources, based on light emitting diode (LED) principle, have a power spectral distribution that covers a broad range of wavelengths, usually tens or hundreds of nanometers; hence, LED sources illuminate wide portions of the optical spectrum (e.g., the entire third optical window or the entire visible range) and therefore can be used to measure the spectral response of devices. A laser source, on the other hand, has a very narrow spectral emission, no larger than few picometers; its emission spectrum resemble an infinitely narrow line, and therefore it can be used to measure the response at one specific wavelength. A tunable laser has the spectral properties of a laser, but it can scan spectral portions (usually several tens of nanometers); hence, tunable lasers can detect broad spectra, scanning wavelength-by-wavelength. Light detectors also work on two different principles. Photodiodes detect the optical power integrated over a wide bandwidth: when a wide spectrum is incident on a photodiode, it returns the integration of the spectrum over the photodiode bandwidth, which is proportional to the light intensity. Spectrometers, or optical spectrum analyzers, instead resolve the whole spectrum wavelength-by-wavelength and return the light intensity at each wavelength.

The principle of operation of light sources and detectors, from an optoelectronic standpoint, is reproduced in Fig. 2.14. The three different mechanisms are spontaneous emission, stimulated emission, and absorption (Rosencher & Vinter, 2002):

- *Spontaneous emission* is the process at the base of LEDs: at the atomic level, the light source is at the excited energy level e_2, which is higher than the

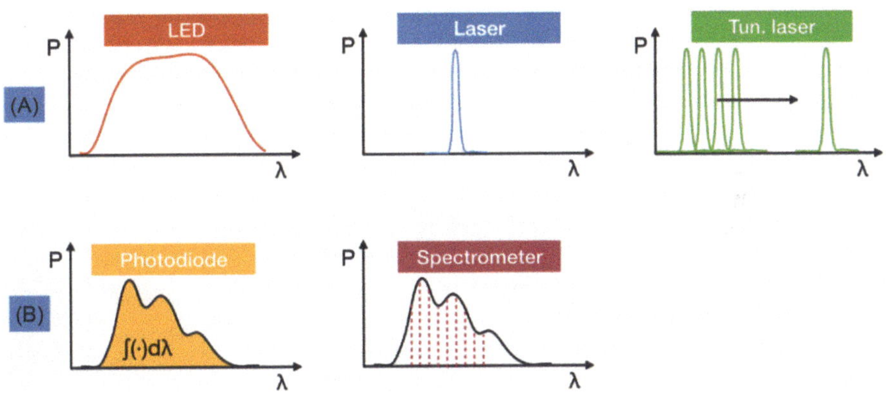

Figure 2.13 Spectral properties and response of light sources (A) and detectors (B) used in optical fiber sensing networks.

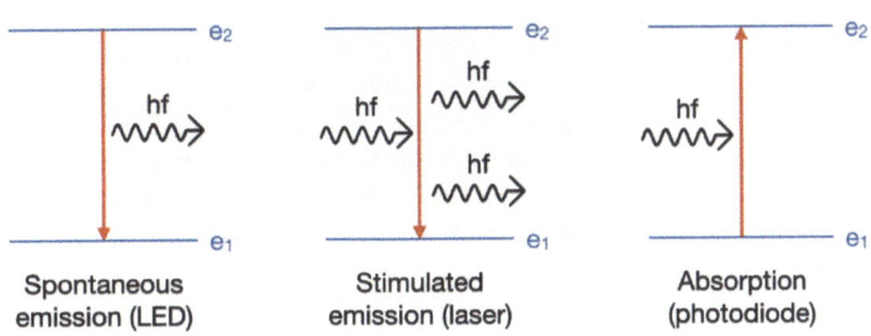

Figure 2.14 Working principles of spontaneous emission, stimulated emission, and absorption of photons having energy level *hf*.

ground level e_1. Spontaneously, the atoms at excited state can decay to the ground level, causing the emission of a photon having energy $hf = e_2 - e_1$ where $h = 6.626 \times 10^{-34}$ J s is the Planck constant.

- *Stimulated emission* is similar to the spontaneous emission but involves the presence of a photon. In the presence of photons having energy *hf*, and atoms at the excited state e_2, stimulated emission results in the generation of a new photon having the same properties (frequency, direction, and polarization) of the incoming photon. Hence, stimulated emission implies some form of feedback, which is the working principles of laser cavities.
- *Absorption* is the principle of operation of light detectors and is the reversal of emission: an incoming photon of energy *hf* is absorbed, increasing the energy from the ground state to the excited state.

2.3.1 Light emitting diodes

An LED is a semiconductor light source that converts the current driving the LED into the emission of light through spontaneous emission. The working principle of an LED is shown in Fig. 2.15. An LED is derived from a pn junction, which is a structure popular in electronic diodes; a solid-state pn junction is formed by combining an n-doped region (n = negative), which is doped with an excess of electrons, with a p-doped (p = positive) region, with an excess of holes. The spontaneous emission occurs when the junction is forward biased as

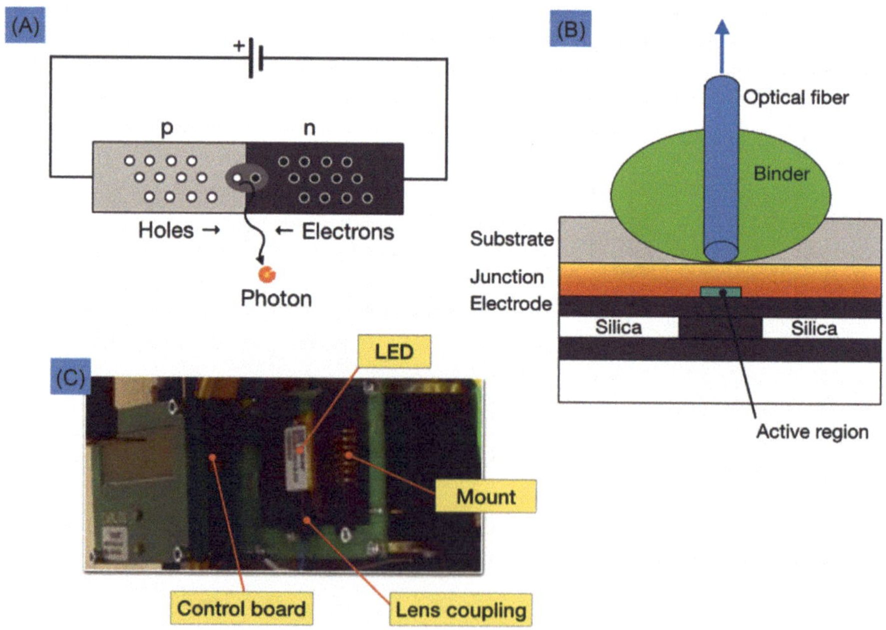

Figure 2.15 Schematic and operation of an LED source. (A) Schematic of a pn semiconductor junction, under forward bias; (B) schematic of a surface-emitting LED diode coupled to a large fiber; and (c) photograph of a commercial SLED source with single-mode fiber output.

in Fig. 2.15A, when a positive voltage is applied to the circuit. The spontaneous occurrence of electron–hole recombination that occurs for each unit time generates photons having energy level equal to the energy gap between the excited and ground state. The power emitted by an LED is proportional to the driving current.

The characteristics of spontaneous emission result in an incoherent optical spectrum; coherency, in this case, refers both to the bandwidth of the spectrum and to its spatial distribution. The emission spectrum of LED is has a range of several tens, or even hundreds of nanometers. At the IR, LED usually cover the entire third optical window, with spectra that have 60–120 nm width centered at 1550 nm, or ~100 nm width at 1300 nm to cover the entire second window. At visible wavelengths, LED spectra usually cover 50–100 nm corresponding to one color, although it is possible to combine multiple LEDs to cover the entire visible wavelength range. Because of their wide emission spectrum, we often refer to LED as broadband source or white light source (even when they operate in the IR). In optical fiber biosensors, therefore, LED sources play a fundamental role as they allow illuminating a wide portion of the optical spectrum and therefore allow measuring unknown spectra corresponding to the sensors under investigation. Similarly, the light emitted from an LED is not collimated but it is rather spread around a wide angle; this effect prevents from efficiently coupling the light of the LED into a fiber, and therefore the technological complexity of LED sources for fiber-optic sensors is mainly sitting into the efficient and stable coupling of the source into the fiber.

Large-core multimode fibers are mainly designed to propagate a large number of modes and therefore have a high NA that facilitates light coupling. For example, large-core silica and POF fibers have an acceptance angle of 30°, while smaller silica MMF fibers have acceptance angle of 10°–20° and operate at visible and near-IR wavelength. For these applications, it is common to use a surface LED design, shown in Fig. 2.15B, which allows a direct coupling of the LED into the output fiber. A surface LED emits from a surface parallel to the plane of the junction, with an active region placed in close proximity to the fiber core to maximize the radiation efficiency. The schematic shows a typical design of a silicon LED for visible light emission, with the fiber fixed into the substrate of the LED with a binder (usually a thermally stable epoxy). This design is proposed for low-cost sources, coupled directly into the fiber, with high thermal stability and sustain high current; it is also possible to use a design where the fiber is fixed in place through a slot, to give users the possibility to replace the launch fiber.

The operation of LED with single-mode fibers, usually at 1550 or 1300 nm, is hampered by the low NA of the fibers, which prevents an easy coupling of the light emitted by the source into the fiber. The solution used in most systems is to use a lens-coupled superluminescent LED (SLED), with a control board, as shown in the photograph of Fig. 2.15C. We can consider an SLED as a half-way source between an LED and a laser because it is based on amplified spontaneous emission (ASE): the source has a gain medium, like a laser, but no optical feedback, and therefore its emission properties have a largely incoherent behavior, very similar to an LED with a higher emission power. The coupling between the SLED and the SMF fiber is performed through a beam expander and a collimating lens, usually embedded on the mount of the source. Unlike an LED–MMF pairing, an SLED–SMF pairing requires a control board that stabilizes the driving current and, most importantly, the temperature of operation of the device, which controls the gain medium properties and therefore the transmitted power. For this reason, the SLED is not a low-cost light source, but rather it requires the use of a control board; the figure shows a commercial SLED with a "butterfly" mount, very common in miniaturized system, with a control board that drives current and thermal control to the light source. Since a SMF fiber has a small acceptance angle, and the alignment between the fiber and lens coupling is critical, the operation of an SLED into an SMF fiber often results in slight power fluctuations over time, which might need to be compensated or accounted during the operation; however, this arrangement allows operating SMF fiber biosensors with a relatively miniaturized optical source.

An alternative to LED, SLED, or other ASE sources, is given by supercontinuum sources, which are based on a nonlinear fiber medium fed by a pulsed laser. Supercontinuum light source can span spectra much broader than LED; most sources span 450–2000 nm, with the possibility extend this range over the UV or toward 2400 nm. The output fiber is usually an endlessly single-mode microstructured fiber. In general, supercontinuum sources are more expensive and bulkier than SLED sources, and have a more delicate power coupling and thermal stability; however, they can be an important resource for the analysis of very broad spectra that exceed the bandwidth of LEDs, particularly at IR wavelengths.

2.3.2 Laser sources

The word laser stands for "light amplification by stimulated emission of radiation," which is the optical working principle behind its operation. Stimulated emission differs from the spontaneous emission in terms of coherence. Spontaneous emission is a random effect that generates an *incoherent* photon, which has random frequency, direction, and polarization; however, stimulated emission occurs when an incoming photon interacts with the excited electron, causing the electron to drop the energy and the emission of a *coherent* photon that is the "carbon copy" of the incoming photon, that is, having same frequency, polarization, and direction. In a weakly excited structure, stimulated emission and spontaneous emission coexist, and therefore the emission spectrum would be similar to an LED with an overlapping narrow linewidth. However, in a laser, we can optimize the structure to improve the efficacy of the stimulated emission, and therefore obtain the emission of light having a very narrow bandwidth and a very collimated directionality.

To exploit stimulated emission to obtain a laser source, we need two elements: (1) a gain (or amplifying) medium, which inverts the population and allows the rate of stimulated emission to be higher than the rate of absorption—this condition ensures that the rate of photons amplified by stimulated emission exceeds by a far amount the rate of photons absorbed in the device and (2) a feedback element, which ensures that a fraction of the photons generated by stimulated emission travels back into the laser structure and allows the generation of numerous coherent photons.

The simplest form of a laser is shown in Fig. 2.16A and is a Fabry-Perot laser. This device is formed by a cavity, made of two optical mirrors on each side of the amplifying medium. The left mirror has a total reflectivity, close to 100%, while the right mirror reflectivity controls the amount of feedback. By setting the right mirror to a low reflectivity, we reduce the amount of feedback (and therefore the quality of the laser coherency) but increase the transmitted power; with a high reflectivity, the laser feedback is strong causing more photons to be amplified, but the transmitted power is lower. Fig. 2.16B shows the oscillator, which is the electrical equivalence of the laser: the amplifier is constituted by the gain medium, while the feedback consists in the amount of optical reflectivity that sets the number of photons available for stimulated emission.

The Fabry-Perot (FP) laser is formed by a cavity of two mirrors and has a simple implementation. Commercially, the two most popular implementation of lasers improve the quality of the cavity by controlling the emission directionality and the amount of reflectivity are the distributed feedback (DFB) laser and the vertical-cavity surface-emitting laser (VCSEL). DFB lasers are used mainly at IR and they ensure a very narrow optical spectrum at low optical power. In a DFB device, rather than having two mirrors at the side of the structure, a continuous reflective element is integrated in the laser cavity—for example, a Bragg reflector that continuously reflects a small portion of the light at each part of the amplifier. DFB have usually an improved performance with respect to FP in

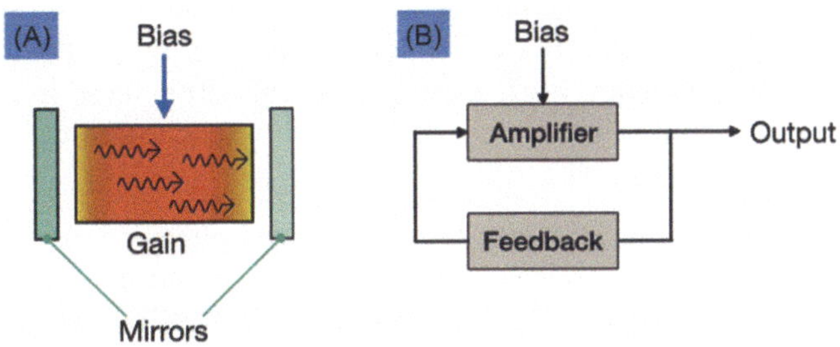

Figure 2.16 Laser diode working principle: (A) schematic of a Fabry-Perot laser and (B) its electrical oscillator equivalent.

terms of coherency, since they prevent the photons to travel longer distances between the mirrors (which results in a partial loss of coherence) and can efficiently integrate the amplifier and the feedback on a single, more compact element. The VCSEL emits the light perpendicularly to the direction of the light propagation in the cavity, in a structure optimized for low cost and ease of testing process (VCSEL lasers can be tested directly on the semiconductor wafer where they are grown).

The optical spectrum of a good laser is characterized by a very narrow linewidth; commercial lasers operating at 1550 nm for telecommunication purposes can launch up to 10–100 mW power with linewidth of ~1 MHz, which is equivalent to 0.008 pm. With such narrow spectra, we can approximate the laser spectrum to a Dirac's delta at the emission wavelength. Also, lasers have a very focused emission beam; VCSELs have a circular emission, launching an omnidirectional beam that can be easily coupled into a fiber; DFB lasers instead have an astigmatic beam, characterized by an elliptic beam that polarizes the light when launched into a fiber. Another important factor to consider is that, given the oscillatory behavior of a laser, we must ensure that the amplification occurring in the cavity is larger than the amount of photons absorbed in the structure. For this reason, the emission power is not proportional to the driving current, but we need to take into account the *threshold current* I_{th} that defines the regime of the laser. Below the threshold current, the emitted power is zero as the rate of stimulated emission is not sufficient to sustain the loss of photons due to absorption. Over the threshold current, the power emitted by the laser is proportional to the injected current (subtracting the I_{th} term), and we define as slope efficiency the ratio between the output power and the input current.

A typical packaging for lasers is shown in Tosi et al. (2020) and requires several elements around the laser diode (LD) for thermal control, isolation, and fiber coupling. The LD is mounted on a Peltier cell, which stabilizes the temperature: by changing the current input to the cell, it is possible to tune the temperature of operation of the laser diode which result in a slight (<1 nm) wavelength tuning and power control. A thermistor is mounted on the cell to detect the surface temperature, which is used by the temperature control to stabilize the temperature of operation. The laser is terminated with a collimating lens that focused the light into the fiber output of the diode. The transmission side is terminated with an isolator, which allows light forward (from the laser to the fiber) and prevents any backreflection to travel back into the laser, preserving the feedback from outer reflections. The laser is controlled by a thermo-electric controller, which drives both the current to the LD and the current to the Peltier cell.

Scanning lasers allow use an optical source with narrow spectral linewidth to scan spectra for several tens of nanometers at a high speed. A wavelength-swept tunable laser combines a VCSEL-type laser coupled in the fiber with a scanning interferometer, which allows rapid scanning of the emission wavelengths. The resulting spectrum, as shown in Fig. 2.13A, is a <1 pm wide spectral line rapidly scanning the spectrum. Wavelength-swept lasers coupled to a single-mode fiber are used in many optical fiber interrogators, as they allow scanning the spectrum of an unknown sensor at a rapid rate, wavelength-by-wavelength. IR wavelength-swept laser sources are typically coupled to an SMF as they are used for the interrogation of sensors inherently operating on single-mode fiber optics, and operate at 1550 or 1300 nm. The scanning range typically ranges from 2 to 20,000 nm/s over 100 nm (1520–1620 nm) with a resolution of 10 pm.

2.3.3 Photodiodes

Photodiodes exploit the principle of a reversely biased pn junction, whereas an incoming photon is converted into a photocurrent; its principle of operation appears similar to a reversed LED. The most common implementation of photodetectors, as shown in Fig. 2.17, is a *pin* photodiode, where the i stands for intrinsic (depletion) region spacing between the p/n regions. By adding a depletion layer, it is possible to increase the efficiency of the photodetector. Incident photons having energy higher than the bandgap, that is, $> (e_2 - e_1)$, are absorbed: the optical energy is converted into the formation of an

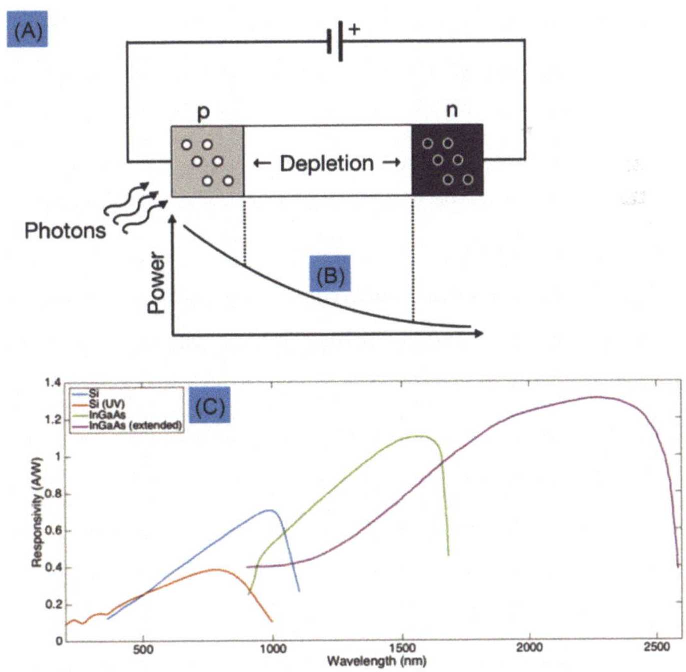

Figure 2.17
Principle of operation of *pin* photodetectors. (A) Schematic of a pin junction; (B) diagram of the optical power trend over the photodetector region; and (C) responsivity of Si and InGaAs photodetectors.

electron–hole pair through the promotion of an electron from ground to excited state. Photons absorbed in the intrinsic region, electrons move toward the cathode and holes toward the anode, resulting in a current flowing through the circuit called *photocurrent*. In general, optical detectors return an output voltage, and therefore the output of the photodetector is amplified through a transimpedance amplifier that converts the photocurrent into an output voltage.

The responsivity of the photodiode, measured in A/W, is the most important figure for the photodiode as it shows the amount of photocurrent as a function of the detected optical power. The bandgap of the semiconductor material defines the responsivity of the photodiode; hence, different materials operate in different wavelength ranges. The two most common pin photodetectors are made of silicon (Si) and indium gallium arsenide (InGaAs). As shown in Fig. 2.17C, Si photodetectors have a responsivity that increases from 0.2 A/W at 400 nm to 0.7 A/W at 1100 nm, and span the visible wavelengths as well as the IR portion up to 1100 nm. Extended Si photodetectors can also cover the UV spectral range, from 190 nm onwards, although they have a smaller responsivity. InGaAs photodiodes have a responsivity that rises from 1000 nm (0.5 A/W) to 1600 nm (1.1 A/W), and rapidly decay at 1650 nm. Hence, they are suitable to work in the 1550 and 1310 nm windows and can span the entire second and third optical windows. Extended InGaAs photodiodes can shift the responsivity curve up to 2400 nm.

Given that the spectral characteristics of the photodiodes are broad (broader than the bandwidth of LED sources), and that they are polarization-insensitive devices, a photodetector integrates the optical power incident on the intrinsic region: the photocurrent is therefore proportional to the total amount of detected power, without any spectral analysis. In sensing networks, it is common to use photodiodes as detectors for intensity-based sensors, in which the optical power level changes as a function of the analyte under investigation. In alternative, photodiodes can be used for spectral analysis when a scanning laser is used as a source: the laser sweeps the spectrum wavelength-by-wavelength, and the photodiode detects the optical power intensity at each wavelength.

Photodiodes are packaged into miniature form factor with a 3-pin output, while the active area is mounted on the top surface of the detector and usually has a square size. Since a *pin* detector is a reverse-biased junction, photodiodes operate with a typical bias voltage of −3 to −5 V. Often, the photodiode and the transimpedance amplifier are embedded in the same device that returns the output in V/W. When selecting the photodiode in sensing networks, two main factors need to be taken into account: the coupling of the light from the fiber to the active area and the size of the active area. SMF fibers have a low NA and a small core, and therefore the fiber-detector coupling is simply done by aligning the active surface to the fiber, without external elements. For MMF fibers instead it is possible to use lenses that focus light onto the active surface or choose photodiodes with a large active size. On the other hand, a large active surface means higher parasitic capacitance, which limits the response time of the photodiode—although biosensors in general are not affected by this limitation as they have a slow response.

2.3.4 Spectrometers and optical spectrum analyzers

As a stand-alone device, photodiodes cannot resolve an optical spectrum since they integrate the power of a wide spectral range, without distinguishing photons having different frequency. However, most optical fiber biosensors require the detection of the spectral response of a sensing unit over a wide range of wavelengths; to accomplish this task, we introduce the use of spectrometers and optical spectrum analyzers, which have the capability to resolve the spectrum if incoming light over a broad range of wavelength.

To resolve the intensity of light at each wavelength, spectrometers employ the working principle of chromatic dispersion as shown in Fig. 2.18A. The input light is filtered through a slit to focus the beam, which is incident into an optical prism. The prism is a polygonal (usually triangular)-shaped transparent glass element having RI dependent on the wavelength, $n = n(\lambda)$. When the input beam has a broad wavelength range, the Snell's law applied on the facet of the prism results in spreading each wavelength component of the beam, since the

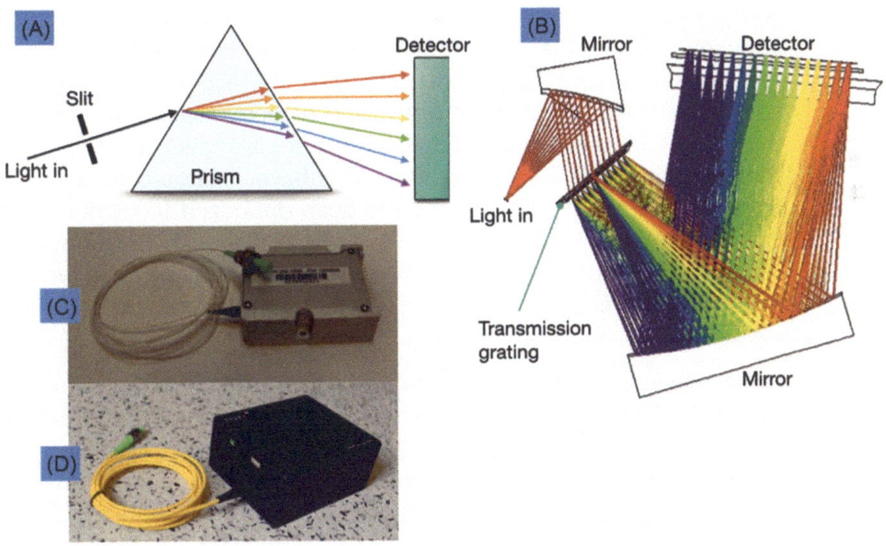

Figure 2.18 Working principle and implementation of optical fiber spectrometers. (A) Prism-based spectrometer architecture; (B) implementation of a grating-based spectrometer in compact detecting devices; (C and D) photographs of commercial single-mode infrared fiber spectrometers with (C) OEM package and (D) USB interface, with input FC/APC SMF fiber. Source: *Images (B–D) courtesy of Ibsen Photonics.*

transmission angle θ_t is different for each wavelength. A similar pattern is occurring at the output facet of the prism: since each wavelength has a different incidence angle, the transmission angle in air is different for each wavelength component. The result of this dispersion mechanism is the spatial spreading of each wavelength component at the output of the prism. After decomposing the wavelength of the input beam, the light is received by an array of photodetectors, which is constituted by an linear set of Si or InGaAs photodetectors (typically, 256 or 512 elements also called pixels). The figure shows the schematic of a visible light spectrometer, but commercial devices can operate also on the IR range, on the third optical window, or on the UV–VIS range.

The prism-based spectrometer is used for bulky devices but is not practical since the prism and its alignment system have a considerable size, and the chromatic dispersion of glass is quite small, which means that the light must travel long distances to separate adjacent wavelengths. To compress the size of the spectrometer to a portable, and even handheld, form factor several arrangements can be taken, and the schematic is shown in Fig. 2.18B. At first, the spectrometer is replaced by a grating (a transmission grating in the figure); a diffraction grating is a compact element characterized by a periodic structure that diffracts the incoming light into different directions, depending on the wavelength. It serves the same function of the prism, but at a much more compact size and enhancing the spreading angles. In addition, rather than having a straight path from the input light to the array of photodetectors, it is possible to fold the light propagation using mirrors. Fig. 2.18B shows the working principle of a VIS compact spectrometer having an input slit, two mirrors between a transmission grating, and an array of Si photodetectors; the second convex mirror collimates each wavelength component onto each detector. Spectrometers can be either packaged with a free-space slit, requiring a collimation of the input light from the fiber through the slit, or they can have a large-core multimode fibers. Recently, several spectrometers have been optimized to work on SMF fibers at the third optical window; Fig. 2.18C and D shows IR 1550-nm spectrometers with an input SMF fiber, with OEM (original equipment manufacturer) packaging, or with an encasing package with an USB interface; photographs and schematic courtesy of Ibsen Photonics.

Three main factors determine the main performance of spectrometers. At first, the spectral resolution determines the wavelength span between two adjacent wavelengths; this depends on the number of photodetectors and on the bandwidth of the incoming signal, and therefore on the grating or prism characteristics—considering that light out of bandwidth is spread outside of the photodetector array, and therefore goes undetected. In general, spectrometers imply a trade-off between bandwidth of analysis and resolution: the detection of a large wavelength range comes at the price of a coarser resolution, while a precision wavelength resolution can be implemented only on a narrow bandwidth. A second element determining the performance is the optical power conversion, since the spectrometer makes use of an analog-to-digital converted for the photodiodes. The exposure time defines the time used by the detectors to integrate the light, which is the same for each element of the array; therefore, the exposure time must be set to have a detectable signal but at the same time avoid saturation effect, whereas the spectral intensity reaches or surpasses the maximum detectable value. This implies that spectrometers are not very efficient in detecting signals having a wide power difference between the maximum and minimum values. Another factor that determines the performance is the thermal stability: temperature changes affect the pixel-to-wavelength conversion, and therefore it is important to ensure that the spectrometer is not exposed to large temperature variations, particularly when operating over a long time.

A more accurate spectral analysis can be performed using an OSA (optical spectrum analyzer); the OSA differs from the spectrometer as the wavelength separation is obtained through a monochromator formed by a grating that mechanically rotates. As opposite to a photodetector where there is an array of detector, an OSA in general has only one detector and the wavelength separation occurs as the grating mechanically scans the spectrum over a wide wavelength range. OSA devices can achieve spectral detection with better resolution and over a wider wavelength range, but the detection is slow due to the mechanical rotation of the monochromator, and the instrument is benchtop and much more expensive, with no portability option.

2.4 Optical fiber components

To assemble optical fiber sensing networks, in addition to the optical fiber and the light source and detector, we employ additional components that compose the optical circuitry of the system. Optical devices are therefore used in the optical circuits for light splitting or routing, separating wavelengths, handle polarization, or perform other tasks. In this section, we describe the principal optical fiber components and their implication on light propagation (Agrawal, 2012).

2.4.1 Splitter, combiner

Splitters and combiners are used in optical fiber sensing networks to manage the power propagation between multiple fibers; for this reason, they are all multiport devices. Schematics of the main splitters and combiners are shown in Fig. 2.19. Splitters are always labeled as $1 \times N$, having one input channel and N output channels; the power from the input channel is split between the multiple outputs, therefore performing the task of delivering the input fiber to multiple power channels. Ideally, the splitter is a lossless device, so the input power is perfectly split between the sum of all outputs; however, in practical devices, there are minimal power losses, usually reported as *excess loss* in datasheets and limited to 0.2–0.5 dB. Balanced splitters divide the power equally on each

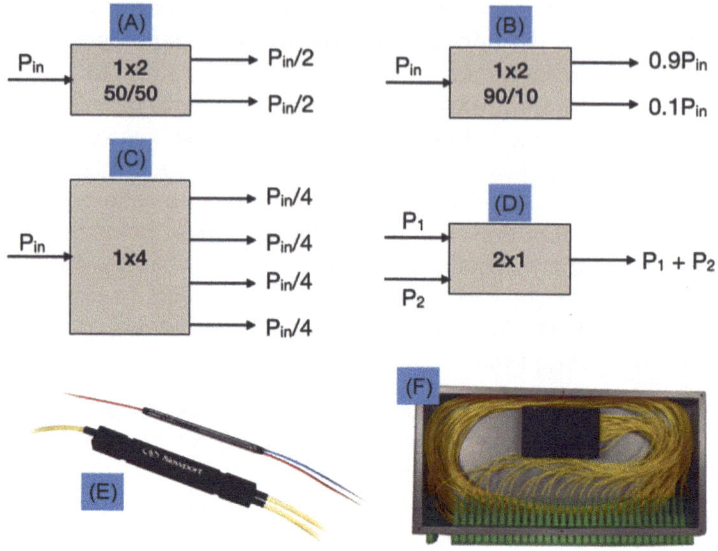

Figure 2.19 Working principle of splitters and combiners. (A) 1 × 2 splitter 50/50; (B) 1 × 2 splitter 90/10; (C) 1 × 4 splitter; (D) 2 × 1 combiner; (E) packaging of 1 × 2 splitters with SMF fibers; and (F) packaging of a 1 × 32 splitter with SMF fibers.

channel: the simplest case is the 50/50 splitter (Fig. 2.19A), which divides evenly the input power between the two output ports. Unbalanced splitters perform an uneven power division: for example, a 90/10 splitter sends 90% of the input power to the first port, and 10% to the second port. Commercially, 1 × 2 splitters are found in 50/50, 80/20, 90/10, 95/5, and 99/1 formats; balanced splitters are the most common form factor because they can route light more efficiently, but 90/10 or similar form factors are often used in fiber optic sensors for creating "monitor ports," subtracting a few percent of the optical power from the main propagating channel to monitor the signal in a specific key point. Larger splitter formats include 1 × 4, 1 × 8, 1 × 16, 1 × 32, up to 1 × 64; these devices are typically fabricated as balanced splitters. Combiners are the reciprocal of splitters, as they combine the power from multiple input channels into one output. They are usually labeled $N \times 1$, with N inputs and one output. Again, the ideal combiner has output power equal to the sum of all inputs.

Multiport fiber splitters are fabricated as fused fiber Y-shaped devices; for a device with N inputs/outputs, N fibers are aligned and twisted together, forming an inner knot. The portion of the overlapping fibers is then fused with a splicer or melted with the help of a flame, tapering the inner portion. This technology allows fabricating a $N \times N$ device (e.g., 2 × 2, 4 × 4), which is rarely used in sensing networks; a 1 × N device in general is fabricated by terminating the additional ports. This fabrication process allows fabricating compact and inline devices as shown in Fig. 2.19E; large splitter formats, for example, 1 × 32 or 1 × 64, are usually packed in a box for the use in large sensing networks.

The process of fabrication of couplers is optimized for the nominal wavelength, for which the splitting ratio has the nominal value; outside of the central wavelength, the splitting ratio progressively differs from the nominal value. The bandwidth of splitters is defined as the wavelength range in which the splitting percentage deviates by a value usually of 3% from the nominal value: for example, a 50/50 splitter with a bandwidth of 100 nm has splitting percentage ranging from 47% to 53% over the 100-nm range, for each channel. The bandwidth of the splitters has to be taken into account when operating with sensors having large bandwidths, while sensors operating in a single optical window are usually not significantly affected by the splitting ratio inequalities.

Splitters and combiners, similar to any optical coupler, are reciprocal devices: properties of light traveling from the Xth port to the Yth port are the same when traveling from the Yth to Xth port. Hence, splitters and combiners can be implemented with the same device, flipping input and output ports.

2.4.2 Circulator, isolator

A circulator is a device with three or four ports, in which light is routed according to a specific direction. Consider the three-port circulator in Fig. 2.20A; the routing direction of the circulator is represented by the arrow, in this case clockwise. When the light is input in the first (left) port, the light is entirely routed to the second (upper) port, following the routing direction; no light is instead directed on the third (right) port. Similarly, when light enters from the second port, it entirely travels to the third port, with no transmission to the first port; light is also routed from port 3 to port 1, with no transmission to port 2. Circulators are particularly important in sensing networks working in reflection, as they allow decoupling the light from the source to the sensor and the reflection from the sensor to the detector; most networks use a three-port device, but a four-port device can use in some wavelength filters.

A special case is a two-port device, which is represented with an arrow as in Fig. 2.20B; this device is called isolator and is used to protect lasers from spurious backreflections as well as to block specific transmissions in optical networks. The circulator allows the power to travel through the direction of the arrow (left to right in the figure) but blocks the transmission in the opposite direction (right to left). The isolation defines the amount of power attenuation of the

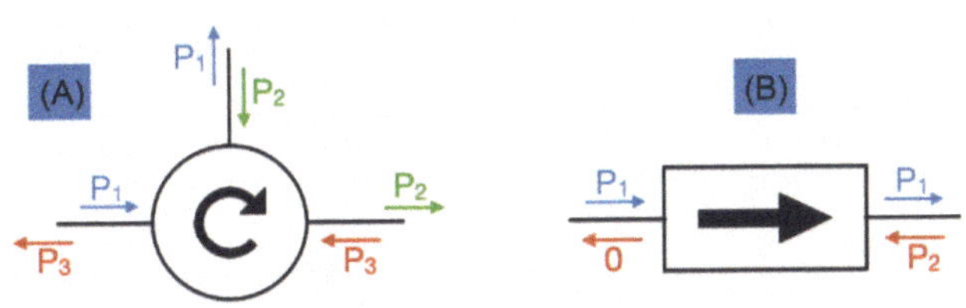

Figure 2.20
Light routing in (A) three-port circulator and (B) two-port isolator.

signals traveling against the direction of the isolator; devices with 20–30 dB isolation are the standard of most devices in the IR.

Unlike splitters or combiners, circulators and isolators are nonreciprocal devices. To break the symmetry and implement a device that selectively allows or blocks transmission of light, a magneto-optic device is used such as a Faraday rotator. In a Faraday rotator, a magneto-optic material is used, capable of polarizing light into a preferential direction according to the field line direction; light is then filtered through a polarization filter. On the reverse side, light is polarized on the opposite direction to the filter, blocking the transmission.

2.4.3 Switch

An optical switch serves the same function of the electrical counterpart: it is a device with one input and multiple outputs, and by selecting the position of the switch, it is possible to transmit all the light to the selected channel. The switch is a programmable device, with the user that can select one permanent output, switch between multiple channel at a preset time, or rapid switching all the channels to interrogate multiple sensors; for this reason, switches are very common in the interrogation of multiple sensors with a single interrogator, alternating between all the channels to interrogate one sensor at a time. Most commonly, switches are $1 \times N$ (one input, N output channels), but it is also possible to have multiple inputs.

The most common implementation of an optical fiber switch is through an MEMS (micro electro-mechanical system): the device has N optical fiber outputs, one optical fiber input, and an electrical input that encodes the switch position. Fig. 2.21 shows the implementation of an MEMS switch, through a pair of mirrors. Light from the input fiber is collimated onto the first rotating

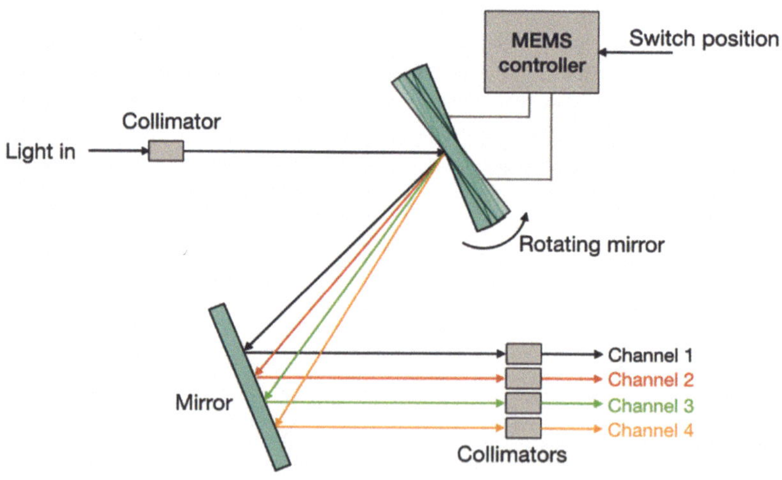

Figure 2.21 Schematic of an optical fiber MEMS switch.

mirror. By selecting the angle of the first mirror, the light is then transmitted onto the second mirror in different configurations, each traveling in a different direction according to the tilt angle. The outputs are then collimated again into the fiber, at each output channel. The mirror is controlled by the MEMS microcontroller that mechanically tilts the mirror according to the switch position set by the user.

MEMS switch devices commute between different positions with speed of few milliseconds, which is compatible with interrogation time of biosensors. In general, biochemical sensors detect at a speed slower than the switching time. However, rapid sensors that work at 10–100 Hz speed (e.g., breathing rate detection) need to take into account the switching time.

2.4.4 Wavelength-selective couplers

Wavelength division multiplexing (WDM) splitters or combiners allow combining signals having different frequency components; they are the electronic equivalent of bandpass filters that allow extracting frequency bands from a signal. WDM devices are usually fabricated through the arrayed waveguide grating principle, using a wavelength-selective interferometer that separates each wavelength component into separate channels.

The scheme of WDM devices is shown in Fig. 2.22. The first chart shows the combiner or multiplexer, which combines signals having different spectral bands into one output channels. The WDM is a reciprocal device and it can be reversed into a splitter or demultiplexer; this configuration is often used in fiber optic sensors to separate different wavelength ranges, particularly at visible wavelengths. In this case, the input signal has a broad bandwidth, and it is split into each output component.

2.4.5 Polarization optics

In sensing networks that control the polarization of light, it is common to use polarization controllers to define a polarization state. In general, optical fibers do not maintain the polarization, which implies that the polarization state at

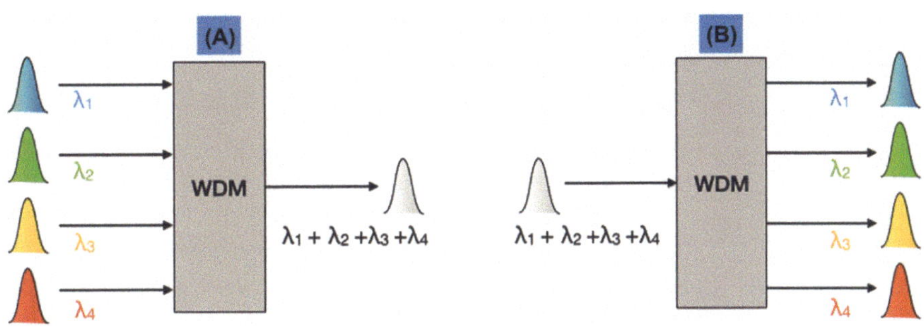

Figure 2.22 Schematic of WDM devices: (A) combiner and (B) splitter.

a given point of the fiber is random and not arbitrarily selected by the user. To set a well-defined polarization state, we can use polarizers that take light with random polarization as input, and return light with a set polarization state on the output. In general, the polarization control is performed with linear (horizontal or vertical) polarization states, and seldom with circular polarizations.

A polarizer is a device with two ports that lets the light waves aligned with the defined polarization state pass, while blocking the light of the opposite polarization state. For example, a horizontal polarizer allows only the portion of light horizontally polarized to pass, while blocking (ideally, in a complete way) the vertical polarization; circularly polarized light entering a horizontal polarizer would be half blocked. Linear polarizers can be fabricated according to two principles. Absorbing polarizers are more common in free space, whereas the polarization orthogonal to the polarizer experiences high propagation losses, while the principal polarization experiences a low optical loss. Beam-splitting polarizers are more common in fiber devices and resemble Fig. 2.18A replacing the prism with a birefringent device having RI dependent on the polarization state: therefore, light having orthogonal polarization gets deflected to a different location, while only polarized light reaches the output. The most important parameter defining the polarizers is the *extinction ratio*, which defines the ratio (in dB) between light the allowed polarization and the blocked polarization.

An alternative mechanism, very common in fiber optics, is the inline polarization controller; unlike the polarizer, which introduces losses to the rejected polarization, the goal of the polarization controller is to rotate the input polarization until it matches the desired output. With a polarization controller, it is possible to select any arbitrary polarization state (e.g., elliptical). This process is implemented by wrapping a fiber span into three loops, and rotating or stretching the fiber into each of the loop independently. Inline polarizers can be manual, where users manually rotate each loop, or automated in which the user stretches the fiber through a micropositioner. The main drawback of the polarizer is that the output polarization is referred to the input polarization; hence, a rotation of the input polarization results in a change on the output, which requires repositioning the fiber loops. However, it is not a lossy device because it does not block any incoming light.

2.5 Optical fiber sensors

In the previous chapter, we have described each element of a fiber optic system (Del Villar & Matias, 2020): the optical fiber constitutes the medium in which light propagates, we have then added the light sources and detectors that constitute the front-end of the system, and then we have added the other circuitry elements that allow handling power, wavelength, and polarization of light. As such, we have now all the elements to assemble a generic fiber optic system, from the transmitter to the receiver. In this section, we will describe how we can use the fiber and components to build optical fiber sensors that have the capability of measuring one or more generic parameters along the fiber, and how we can define their performance and characteristics.

2.5.1 Principles and properties of fiber optic sensors

A measurement instrument is a generic system that detects the change of a physical, chemical, biological, or electrical parameter, called measurand; this detection implies that the variation of the parameter under investigation is translated into a measurable change of another parameter. A transducer is a device that converts a signal of one form into a signal into another form; clearly, a transducer is an important element of a measurement instrument because it converts a parameter that is usually hard to measure (e.g., the concentration of a specific analyte) into a parameter that we can handle with electrical or optical common system (e.g., a voltage or the intensity of light). Sensors are a subset of measurement instruments. Although there is not a specific definition in this terms, we usually define a sensor as a miniature and localized device in which the transducing effect takes place, connected to a hardware system that sends the input to the sensor and detects the output of the sensor. While this is not always the case, we usually imply a certain physical separation between the sensor and the hardware used to interrogate it.

Optical fiber sensors (OFSs), also called fiber optic sensors (FOSs), are a class of sensors that use optical fiber technology for the detection. The optical fiber accomplishes two functions in OFS systems: it is an integral part of the sensor, transducing the measurand into an optical variation of the light propagating in the fiber; and it is also the cable that connects the light source to the detector, and through all the other elements needed to implement the sensing principle. Having now discussed in details the properties of the fiber, we can now see that OFSs have some advantages in comparison with electrical, chemical, electrochemical, or mechanical sensors:

- *Form factor*: the form factor of OFS is, substantially, the form factor of optical fibers; and since fibers have a size of few hundreds micrometers, the size of sensors is small, with a lightweight footprint. We can assemble sensors that have percutaneous operation, or size comparable with human cells, with small invasiveness.
- *Biocompatibility*: silica fibers have advantageous properties in terms of biocompatibility, as glass is not harmful for the body or for the analytes that we want to detect.
- *Electromagnetic immunity*: Since the light propagates well confined in the fiber core, it does not interact with the surrounding medium and with surrounding waves: as such, it is immune to the magnetic fields or magnetic resonance imaging machines, or to the acoustic fields emitted by ultrasound

imaging machines, or to the radiated particles emitted by tomography or chemotherapy machines. Clearly, in medicine, this is a clear advantage.

- *Passivity*: FOSs manipulate the light but do not amplify it and do not trigger electrical phenomena along the fiber, even in case of malfunctioning. That means that if we control the amount of light running into the fiber, we cannot damage tissues or ignite electrical sparks in any form, guaranteeing safety.

The minimal building blocks of any OFS system are: a light source that transmits light into the fiber link; an optical fiber link that delivers the light to the sensing point and from the sensing point to the detector; an optical fiber sensor that transduces the measurand into a variation of the light properties; a light detector that receives the output light; and a technique (usually a software) that takes the signal at the detector and converts it into a displayed signal, estimating the measurand from the sensor output.

In OFS, the sensor transduces the variations of the physical or biological parameter under analysis into one or more of the properties of the light traveling through the link. Fig. 2.23 shows a schematic of the most popular ways, we can implement to convert measurands into well-measurable optical parameters, each exploiting a different property of the light waves. The simplest sensing forms are *intensity-based sensors*: here we consider as key information the power of the light transmitted through, and the sensor modulates the optical power when the measurand changes. Intensity-based sensors, in short, attenuate the light traveling through the sensor by an amount that varies with the parameter under test. This is a simple yet effective form of sensing because we can introduce several simple devices (e.g., bending or stretching the fibers)

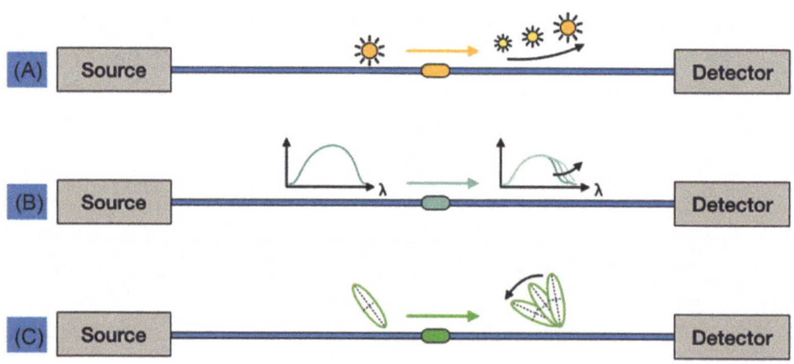

Figure 2.23 Sketch of the three main working principles of optical fiber sensors, in which the sensing device modulates the properties of light traveling through the fiber link. (A) Intensity-based sensors: the input power varies traveling through the sensing region and is measured by a photodetector. (B) Spectral sensors, in which the transmission or reflection spectra of the sensor vary according to the measured parameter; the detector resolves the optical spectrum of incoming light. (C) Polarization-based sensors: the sensing device alters the polarization state of incoming light, for example, rotating the input polarization as in the figure.

that have repercussions on the intensity of the light waves. Intensity-based sensors do not resolve the other properties of light, and for this reason, they can use photodiodes as detectors, with the benefit of a lower cost but the requirement of a stable light propagation though the whole link.

The most important type of OFS, and the one that we will mostly discuss in the next chapters, is represented by spectral sensors. We have seen that LED/SLED sources can illuminate large portions of the optical spectrum at visible and IR wavelengths, and that spectrometers or OSAs can resolve the spectrum, measuring the intensity at each wavelength. Therefore spectral sensors represent all those working principles in which the measurand affects the spectral response of light traveling through the sensing point. For example, sensors can filter a specific wavelength band or allow a specific wavelength band to pass through the fiber; other sensors have periodical spectral patterns or can introduce distortions to the input light at specific wavelengths. The common denominator of spectral sensors is that they encode the sensing mechanism in a variation of the optical spectrum, which is detected by a wavelength-resolved analyzer.

We have also seen that another property of light, as for any electromagnetic wave, is the polarization state. Polarization-based sensors vary the polarization of light as it travels through the sensor; for example, in Fig. 2.23C, the sensor rotates the polarization of input light by an amount that depends on the measurand. Polarization sensors can be also implemented with intensity or spectral characteristics: since polarization detectors are not very common, we can convert the changes of polarization into an easier parameter to measure (such as the optical power or spectrum). Similarly, there are sensors that operate on the number of modes traveling in the fiber, as this is another key property of the waveguide; clearly, these sensors operate with multimode fibers, and since the number of modes is not a parameter that we can directly inspect the sensors operate with power or spectrum detection.

2.5.2 Transmission and reflection sensors

It is very important, from a sensing system standpoint, to define whether the optical fiber sensor modulates the light traveling through the sensing point, or the sensor is intended to reflect light backwards in the fiber. Fig. 2.24 shows the schematic of transmission and reflection sensors, regardless of the optical parameter that the system detects.

For sensors working in transmission, the light emitted by an optical source travels through the sensing point, and then reaches a detector placed at the opposite end. In this case, we disregard the light that is reflected from the sensor or that vanishes out in its surrounding, and analyze the transmission through the sensing zone. Transmission-based sensors are very common for laboratory analysis because they minimize the amount of optical hardware involved in the optical fiber link; in addition, this approach works well with all

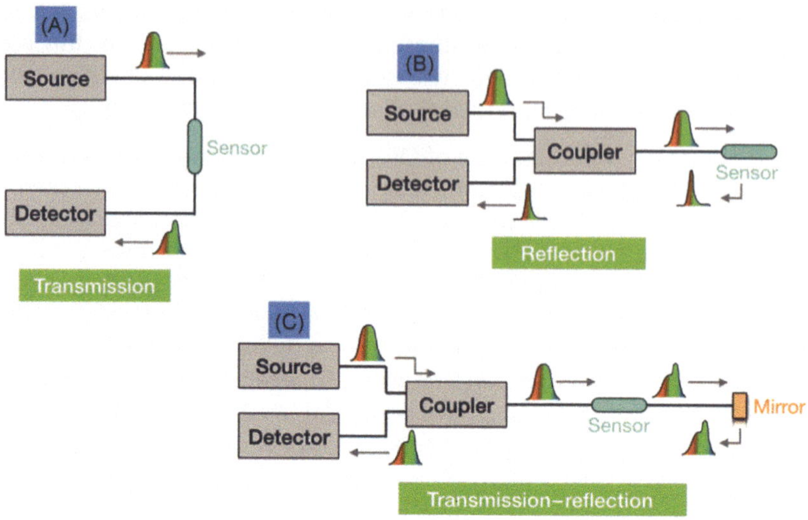

Figure 2.24 Schematic of (A) transmission, (B) reflection, and (C) transmission–reflection optical fiber sensors.

the sensing devices that will be introduced in the next chapters, since optical fiber biosensors modulate the light propagating in the forward direction. In practical applications, the light source and detectors (as well as the other circuit elements) are usually mounted in the same device, called *interrogator.* Experimentally, transmission-based sensors suffer from issues related to the fiber link, particularly when we intend to position the sensor in a human tissue (e.g., through a medical device), or in the slot of an analyzer, or in a compact assay. In fact, since the fiber must enter and exit the sensor, it is required that the fiber loops around the sensing element; this is not practical when the fiber is tightly positioned—also considering that fibers cannot be bent on a very tight radius without introducing high losses or breaking the structure. Therefore this architecture is applied in laboratory, and less practical in the final sensing prototypes.

A step forward in terms of practicality is the operation in reflection, as shown in Fig. 2.24B. In this case, the sensor reflects part of the light backwards into the fiber, while the transmission component is disregarded. In the simplest implementation, a coupler (combiner) or a circulator (clockwise direction) is needed for the correct operation. The light from the source travels within the combiner into the fiber link, reaching the sensor: the light reflected propagates in the same fiber, entering the coupler from the opposite side, that splits it between the source (where it has no effect) and the detector, which then picks up the reflection component only. Clearly, this architecture is more practical for positioning the sensor in situ, as the same fiber that carries light to sensor collects its reflection; effectively, the fiber link terminates in the sensing region, with no need to collect and propagate light on the opposite side. Often, we define as *probe* a sensor that terminates the fiber link, with a definition similar to electrical probes. This approach increases the complexity of the network, as it requires an additional coupler; moreover, when using lasers, it is necessary to insure that the source is protected by an isolator from the backreflection (or, in alternative, a circulator can be used). The main aspect of OFS operating in reflection is that this arrangement does work with every type of sensor. In fact, several types of sensors that we will describe (e.g., etched fiber Bragg gratings and interferometers) reflect light at specific wavelengths and allow passing light at other wavelengths, and therefore they are well compatible with the operation in reflection. On the other hand, some of the most performing biosensors (e.g., surface plasmon resonance, long period gratings, and tilted gratings) have working principles that do not reflect any light, or at least the reflection is not a parameter of interest, but rather vary only the light transmitted through the sensors. These principles are therefore not compatible with a reflection operation.

The transmission–reflection configuration has been designed for some types of sensors that require the analysis of transmission spectra, but they are required to have a reflective probe for miniaturization purposes (Guo, Liu, Guan, & Albert, 2016). The optical hardware is similar to the reflection configuration, with a coupler routing the light to from the source and to the receiver. To flip the transmission spectra backwards to the input fiber, the far end of the fiber is coated with a mirror. To this end, it is possible either to use a gold-tip fiber termination for the maximum reflectivity or to cleave the fiber and exploit the Fresnel reflectivity at the fiber end; in some systems, a gold coating is deposited on the fiber surface to improve the reflectivity, coating the metallic layer during the process of functionalization of the biosensor. The mirror can be fabricated in proximity of the sensor, which then works as a terminated probe. In this transmission–reflection configuration, we observe a combination of the reflection spectrum and transmission spectrum at the receive, and high-reflectivity components might rebound several times between the sensor and the mirror.

2.5.3 Types of sensors

FOSs are divided into two class: intrinsic and extrinsic sensors as shown in Fig. 2.25. Intrinsic sensors hold the entire transducing mechanism within the optical fiber itself. The fiber can be manipulated, for example through the inscription of a reflective device or changing the fiber thickness; however, the sensing mechanism remains confined in the fiber itself—whether the operation is in reflection or in transmission. The sensor sketched in Fig. 2.25 is an etched grating biosensors, with a reflective element inscribed in the fiber core, and the fiber subsequently etched to deplete the whole cladding in the central part: this is an extrinsic sensor because the light that interacts with the surrounding

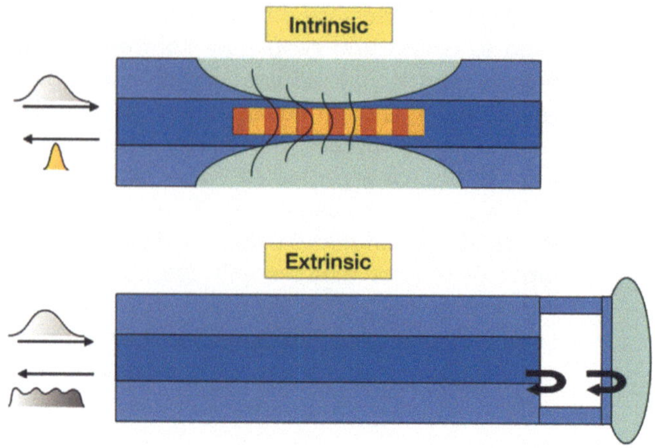

Figure 2.25 Examples of intrinsic and extrinsic sensors.

medium, that is, the analyte that we detect, travels through the fiber itself. Intrinsic sensors are often referred to as *inline* when operated in transmission because the light passes through the fiber. Extrinsic sensors, on the other hand, require external elements to the fiber to implement the detection system. The example of Fig. 2.25 is an extrinsic interferometer, formed by terminating a fiber with an external cavity positioned in the analyte; since the sensing mechanism is external to the fiber, in general, extrinsic sensors are fabricated at the fiber end, and therefore suitable for reflective probes.

Another important aspect of fiber optic sensors is that we can build networks that incorporate multiple sensors within the same network, often having one light source and one detector. Several sensors that we will describe in the next chapters are suitable to operate in sensing networks. A common rationale of FOS is to use multiple sensors for the simultaneous detection of a plurality of parameters. This can be designed if we aim at detecting more than one analyte or measurand, and also to compensate for other parameters that might affect the measurement; an example is the compensation of temperature variations, which can affect the biological measurement. Optical switches are often used in multisensor networks, as they allow switching to different sensors, interrogating one device at a time.

2.5.4 Input–output relations

We now aim at defining the main parameters and characteristics of sensors, which include also optical fiber biosensors. A full analysis of all the metrological terminology of sensors can be found in a white paper from National Instrument (National Instruments, 2013); here, we limit to the fundamentals, which are the common definitions and characteristics of all FOS.

The most important characteristic of any sensor is the relationship between the sensor input (the measurand that we want to estimate) and the output (the parameter that we detect on the interrogator). This relationship defines the operation of the sensor because it displays in a quantitative format the conversion from a biological or physical parameter into an optical value that we can detect through the sensing network. For a refractometer, the horizontal (input) axis is the RI of the medium; for a biosensor that selectively detects an analyte, the *x* axis displays the concentration of the analyte. The vertical axis shows the output that is the parameter detected at the end of the system; for sensors that detect an optical intensity as in Fig. 2.23A, the output is usually the power or voltage output of a photodetector, while for sensors detecting a spectrum this usually reports the wavelength or intensity level of a specific spectral feature (e.g., the wavelength of a specific spectra peak).

The *calibration* procedure defines the process of obtaining the input–output relation, building up the input–output relation for every point of the horizontal axis (within a reasonable range). Often, the input–output relation is defined as the calibration curve or calibration function.

The shape of the calibration function defines in a very significant way the performance figures of the sensor. As shown in Fig. 2.26, we can identify four main types of calibration function. An important case occurs when the calibration function is linear, as shown in the first chart; in this case, every increment of the measurand results in a proportional variation of the output, with a constant rate. The *sensitivity* defines the rate of change of the output versus the rate of change of the input; analytically, the sensitivity is the derivative of the calibration function—i.e., the slope of the curve. Clearly, for a linear calibration function, the sensitivity is constant. It is important that the sensitivity is always measured in a unit equal to the units of the output divided by the units of the input.

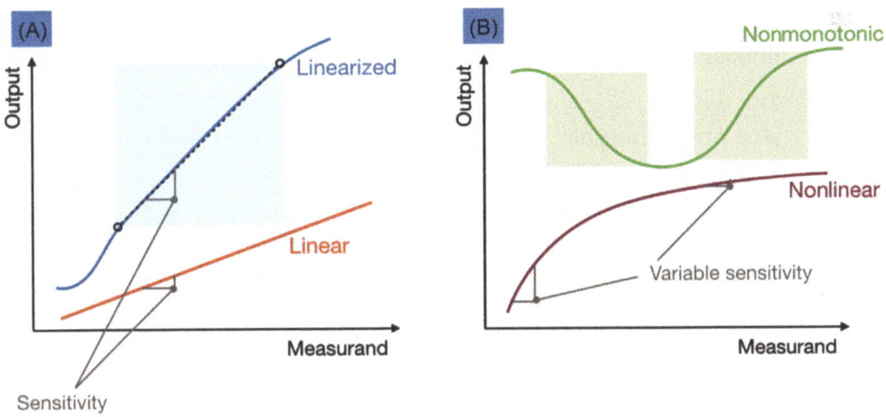

Figure 2.26 Examples of input–output relations of generic sensors that report the output (measured parameter) as a function of the input (measurand parameter). (A) Linear or quasilinear relationships and (B) nonlinear relationships.

Linear calibration curves are an ideal behavior but many sensors are characterized by an almost linear function, at least for a range of values. This is the example shown in the upper curve of Fig. 2.26A. In this case, while the function is not perfectly linear, we can clearly identify a range of input values for which the linear function is a very good approximation; we can then conclude that in the considered range, the calibration function can be linearized, and here it shows a constant sensitivity.

The sensitivity is an important factor because if quantifies the amount of response of the sensor for a given small input change. If we consider the curves of Fig. 2.26A, the lower function has a smaller sensitivity than the upper function, which means that for a given change of the input (e.g., a change of the concentration of the analyte that we detect), the upper sensor has a much larger response. While we cannot conclude that the sensitivity itself defines the performance metrics of the sensor because they also depend on many other factors, it is frequently true that a sensor with high sensitivity performs better than a sensor with a lower sensitivity—at least for the range of operation. So, it is important to design sensors having in mind to optimize the sensitivity as a key performance indicator.

The cases in Fig. 2.26B show a typical one that occurs when the calibration function is not linear; this is a common event in biosensors, particularly for sensors that detect analytes in a wide range of concentrations. The lower curve shows a nonlinear calibration function, and we can immediately see that the sensitivity is not constant; this implies that for some range of inputs the sensor is more responsive, while for other intervals the response to the same input variation is inferior. This curve has a monotonic trend through the whole horizontal axis: it means that for each output there is only one input without ambiguity. Therefore nonlinear but monotonic calibration functions still return an unambiguous input–output relation, but with a nonconstant sensitivity that implies that some range of input values show a greater response than others.

The worst case scenario occurs when the calibration function is nonlinear, and also nonmonotonic; in this case, the detection is ambiguous, since (as it can easily be seen from the upper curve in Fig. 2.26B) there are at least two input values that generate the same output. In this case, besides the nonconstant trend of the sensitivity, the sensor cannot work on the whole range of input values, but we have to narrow down the range of measurand values until we obtain a monotonic relationship, which removes the ambiguity. The figure shows two possible working ranges that show a monotonic trend.

The calibration process is usually performed step-by-step, hence the calibration function is inferred from a finite set of datapoints rather than from one continuous measurement. When performing the calibration, it is important to ensure that the uncertainty of the input values should be smaller (ideally, much smaller) than the estimated uncertainty of the sensor.

2.5.5 Performance metrics

Besides the calibration function and the sensitivity that provide in a nutshell the blueprint of the sensing mechanism, a few other parameters of interest are needed to define the basic properties of a sensing system. Some of the main characteristics are graphically shown in Fig. 2.27.

- *Uncertainty*: it is a metric the accuracy of the sensor, quantifying how much the detected output differs from the nominal value. The definition of uncertainty is not straightforward, as it depends on the number of calibration experiments performed as well as on the quality of the method to estimate the reference values. Typically, the uncertainty is estimated statistically from a set of measurements, for example as three times the standard deviation of a sufficiently large dataset. As in Fig. 2.27, uncertainty is usually reported with error bars for each datapoint, each defining the range of detected output for the same input value; in this case, users need to specific the method chosen to estimate the accuracy.
- *Resolution*: the resolution is the minimum variation of the input that can be clearly detected on the output, that is, produces a change of the output that can be detected by the receiver.
- *Repeatability*: the repeatability defines how the properties of the sensor reproduce over different measurements. The repeatability can be inferred by plotting the calibration functions of different measurements, and evaluating the range of values. Depending on the type of sensor and its utilization, the repeatability can be intended for repeated measurements with the same probe or with the same measurement over time (e.g., evaluating aging effects or degradation through multiple runs of measurements) or evaluating the calibration curves of different sensors fabricated with the same method (for the evaluation of how reliable is the manufacturing of a type of sensor).
- *Hysteresis*: while an ideal sensor has the same calibration curve regardless of how rapidly and reversibly the measurand changes, in a real sensor we might observe a deviation from the ideal curve. In particular, sensors suffering from hysteresis exhibit a different calibration curve between increasing and decreasing value of the calibration curve; this effect is particularly detrimental in sensors having a slow response.

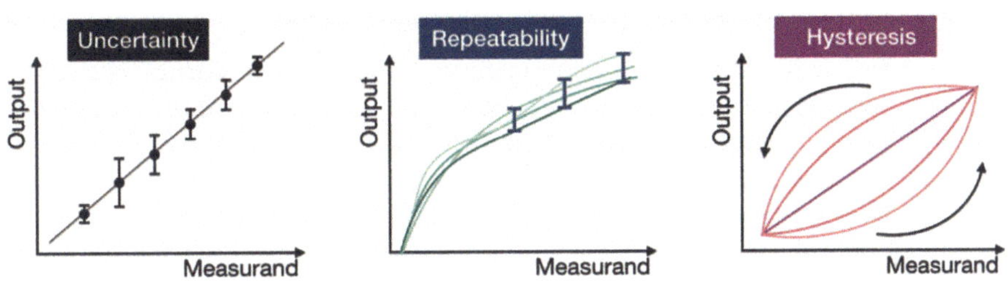

Figure 2.27 Graphic representation of the main performance metrics of sensors: uncertainty, repeatability, and hysteresis.

2.6 Optical fiber biosensors

Fiber optic biosensors have been designed and implemented for a broad range of measurand parameters, including in medical applications. Most of the proposed methods rely on the measurement of physical parameters such as pressure, temperature, strain, acceleration, or bending. These sensors encode a physical deformation of the fiber, for example, a compression of the fiber core due to a bending applied to the fiber or an expansion of the fiber due to temperature increase.

Optical fiber biosensors represent another subset of the FOS landscape, and they aim at the detection of biological analytes. While there is not a specific definition that separates biological sensors (which detect proteins, cells, biomarkers, antibodies, and other biological analytes of interest) from biophysical sensors (that detect physical parameters in medicine, such as body temperature, breathing pattern, blood pressure, or other similar markers), in recent years the terminology of optical fiber biosensors has restrained to include all those sensors, intrinsic and extrinsic, that selectively detect a biological analyte through a functionalization process (Chiavaioli, Gouveia, Jorge, & Baldini, 2017). In this book, we refer to this specific terminology and describe the techniques that allow detecting biological analytes with optical fibers. In other contexts, biosensors embrace all types of environmental or chemical sensors including those that do not specific sense biological analytes; for example, sensors for water quality analysis, for agriculture, or for gas sensing. While environmental sensors have several points of contact with biosensors, as both require optical structures capable of probing the environment around the fiber, the lack of specificity of environmental sensors (at least, for binding to some form of biomarker) makes the difference; in the following, we will define as biosensors only those sensor that achieve a specific sensing, and implement this through a specific biological process.

The first step toward designing an optical fiber biosensor is to generate a sensing element that probes the environment around the fiber. The surrounding environment is usually a liquid analyte (e.g., water, saliva, urine, blood) or a solid medium (e.g., solid tissues or cells), and in a first step we need to be able to detect it through an appropriate system. Detecting an analyte means that we can define a reliable and sensitive phenomenon that allows light traveling in the fiber core to interact with the surrounding, and this process requires modifying the fiber structure.

Fig. 2.28 shows the main concepts behind the design of optical fiber biosensors. At first, the fiber itself is not an advantageous biosensing device: since the fiber is designed with the purpose of confining the light into the core, it negates any interaction with the surrounding analytes; hence, to consider the fiber for biosensing, we need to change the type of light propagation into the fiber, as TIR-based propagation does not lead to efficient biosensors. However, one possibility that is shown in Fig. 2.28B is to modify significantly the fiber geometry, for example, removing a portion or the totality of the cladding or

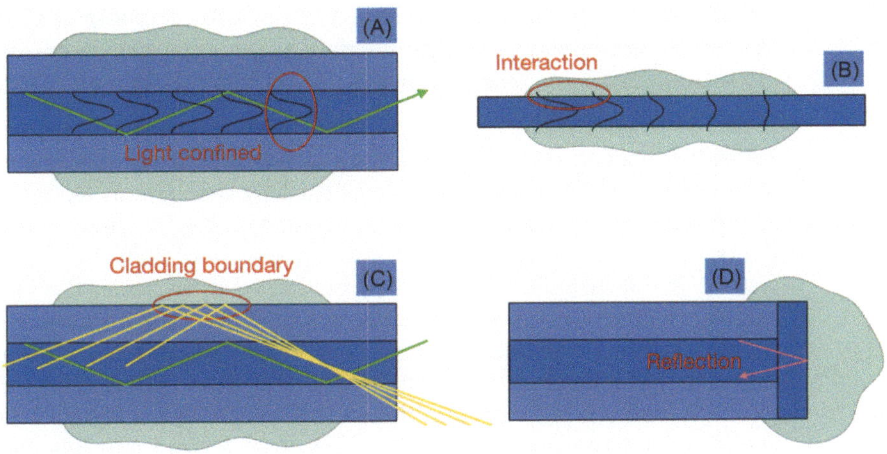

Figure 2.28 Visualization of the main concepts behind optical fiber devices capable of interrogating a surrounding analyte. (A) A stand-alone fiber confines the light in the core, preventing interactions with the surrounding medium. (B) Removing or reducing the fiber cladding, or altering the fiber geometry allows incoming wave to interact with the outer medium. (C) Structures that excite light traveling in the cladding allow the interaction of waves at the cladding-surrounding medium interface. (D) A device fabricated in-line or on the fiber tip can exploit the reflection at the glass-outer medium boundary.

shrinking the fiber side to a much smaller format. In this case, the light propagating is subjected to additional losses and changes of the effective RI, which can then be incorporated in the spectral changes. This is the working principle behind etched fiber Bragg gratings and fiber tapers—all based on different geometrical modifications of the fiber.

Another technique that we can employ, shown in Fig. 2.28C, involves modifying the propagation properties of the fiber. The idea is to excite light traveling in the cladding, and therefore satisfying the TIR condition between the cladding and the outer analyte. Since the cladding is much larger than the core, the cladding-propagating modes (or simply cladding modes) transmit in a multimode format even when the core is single mode. Since the cladding modes interact with the outer medium, we have then a sensitivity to the surrounding environment. The key idea then is to design a device that can excite cladding modes from the light that is propagating in the core; the most popular sensors that implement this concept are the long period grating (where core and cladding light propagates in the same direction) and the tilted Bragg grating (where the cladding modes counterpropagate).

Finally, another possible design that incorporates the detection of an unknown analyte is to make use of Fresnel's equations in Eq. (2.19): at the boundary between the fiber made of glass and the outer analyte, light is both transmitted through and reflected with reflection and transmission coefficient that depend on the RI values of the fiber and analyte. We can then engineer sensing structures that make use of the glass/analyte interface as sensing information—usually building structures with multiple reflections. This common sensing mechanism is at the base of optical interferometers.

For all the working principles underlying optical fiber biosensors, the capability of sensing the surrounding medium is evaluated by changing its RI. So, the first task is to explore the RI sensitivity of the sensor, measuring the effect of RI changes to the optical power or reflection/transmission spectra of light through the sensing system. The RI measurement is usually performed by exposing the sensor to analytes with different RI values, for example, water with mixtures of sucrose or ethanol at different concentrations; hence, the RI sensitivity does not return a selective detection, but it rather quantifies the response of the sensor to changes of the surrounding medium. This effect is shown in Fig. 2.29A: as the waves travel at the fiber/RI boundary, light vanish in the analyte at a rapid rate due to evanescent wave losses, while the reflected light encodes the sensing parameter.

This information is usually shown in the RI sensitivity chart, shown in Fig. 2.29B; here, we report for each sensor the output (usually a wavelength or power change) as a function of the surrounding RI. Sensors are usually

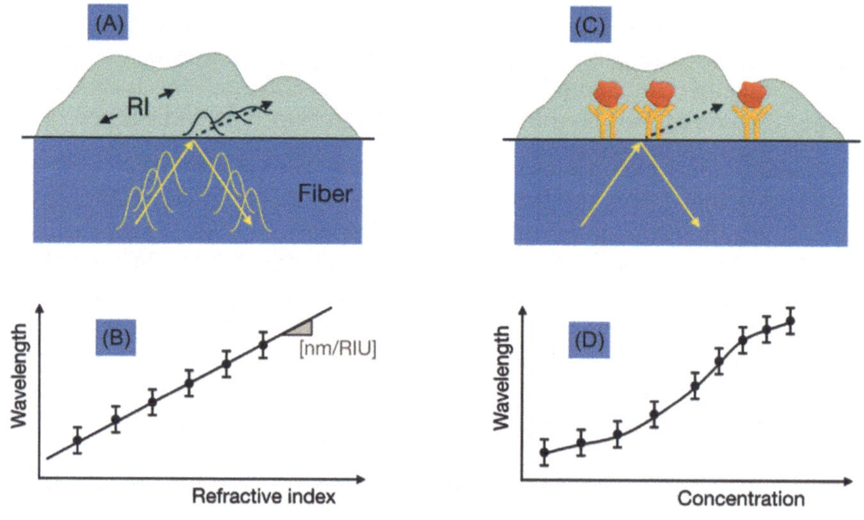

Figure 2.29 Sketch of the optical fiber biosensors layout. (A) The working principle is an RI sensor, which senses the light at the boundary between the fiber and the surrounding RI. (B) The sensitivity is then expressed by evaluating the sensor output, usually a wavelength or a power level, as a function of the RI changes; the sensitivity is evaluated in nm/RIU figure for wavelength changes. (C) The sensor is then functionalized for a specific analyte detection: bioreceptors (yellow, y-shaped) are deposited on the fiber surface, usually through an additional layer; the sensor then can detect the analyte (red, o-shaped) that binds to the receptor, on the fiber surface. (D) The sensor then responds to the concentration of the analyte, with the sensor output that varies as the concentration rises.

characterized for small variations of RI, usually 10^{-3}–10^{-2} to mimic the small environmental changes occurring on the fiber surface. Although the RI is a unitless number, the RI changes are usually reported with refractive index unit (RIU) figure; for example, a change of RI from 1.33 to 1.34 corresponds to 10^{-2} RIU, and this allows expressing the RI change in an intuitive form. The sensitivity is therefore estimated in nm/RIU for wavelength-changing sensors, or in mW/RIU or dB/RIU for sensors that operate by detecting power changes.

In this arrangement, the sensor is detecting analytes changes but not selectively. We need therefore to engineer the fiber surface to introduce the specificity. The bioreceptors and analytes have size that is much smaller than the wavelength, and therefore they have an optical function that we can approximate as the RI change; for this reason, we can consider the biosensor as a "selective RI sensor." This surface modifications, usually labeled *functionalization*, are shown in Fig. 2.29C: bioreceptors lay on the fiber surface, and chemically bind the analyte while rejecting other types of substances.

The process for converting an RI change into a biosensor, therefore, requires several chemical functionalization steps, such as silanization or metallic layer deposition followed by immobilization of the bioreceptors. The better chemical bonds tie the analyte to the receptors, the more selective is the sensor. This usually is evaluated with the concentration chart shown in Fig. 2.29D, whereas the sensor output is reported as a function of the concentration change (usually reported in molar units or in g/mL in flowing sensors).

Ultimately, the selectivity of the sensor is estimated by measuring the wavelength or power changes occurring with one analyte concentration, and the output changes corresponding to a control analyte at the same concentration; an ideal sensor, with perfect selectivity, would respond only to the analyte under investigation, while showing no response to the control analytes.

2.7 Conclusions

As a concluding remark, this chapter guides readers from the basic principles of optics down through the underlying principles of optical fiber biosensors. Here we have described the whole sensing networks, pairing the optical fiber to light sources and detectors and the other hardware, and evaluating how the sensing network respond to external parameters. In the next chapters, we will begin the discussion of each type of optical fiber biosensor.

References

Abrate, S., Gaudino, R., & Perrone, G. (2013). Step-index PMMA fibers and their applications. *Current Developments in Optical Fiber Technology.*, 177–202. Available from https://doi.org/10.5772/52746.

Agrawal, G. P. (2012). *Fiber-optic communication systems*. John Wiley & Sons.
Ceci-Ginistrelli, E., Pugliese, D., Boetti, N. G., Novajra, G., Ambrosone, A., Lousteau, J., ... Milanese, D. (2016). Novel biocompatible and resorbable UV-transparent phosphate glass based optical fiber. *Optical Materials Express, 6*(6), 2040–2051.
Chiavaioli, F., Gouveia, C. A., Jorge, P. A., & Baldini, F. (2017). Towards a uniform metrological assessment of grating-based optical fiber sensors: From refractometers to biosensors. *Biosensors, 7*(2), 23.
Danciu, M., Alexa-Stratulat, T., Stefanescu, C., Dodi, G., Tamba, B. I., Mihai, C. T., ... Ianole, V. (2019). Terahertz spectroscopy and imaging: A cutting-edge method for diagnosing digestive cancers. *Materials., 12*(9), 1519.
Del Villar, I., & Matias, I. R. (Eds.), (2020). *Optical fibre sensors: Fundamentals for development of optimized devices*. John Wiley & Sons.
Guo, T., Liu, F., Guan, B. O., & Albert, J. (2016). Tilted fiber grating mechanical and biochemical sensors. *Optics & Laser Technology, 78*, 19–33.
Marcuse, D. (1991). *Theory of dielectric optical waveguides* (2nd ed.). Academic Press.
National Instruments. (2013, September). *Sensors terminology, white paper*. http://www.ni.com/white-paper/14860/en/
Peckham, D. W., Sun, Y., McCurdy, A., Lingle, R., Jr, Kaminow, I., Li, T., & Willner, A. E. (2013). *Few-mode fiber technology for spatial multiplexing*. Elsevier/Academic Press, May.
Refractometer. (2020). *PL refractive index database*. http://www.refractometer.pl/refraction-datasheet-basic
Rosencher, E., & Vinter, B. (2002). *Optoelectronics*. Cambridge University Press.
RP Photonics. (2020). *RP photonics encyclopedia*. https://www.rp-photonics.com.
Saleh, B. E., & Teich, M. C. (2019). *Fundamentals of photonics*. John Wiley & Sons.
Tosi, D., Molardi, C., Sypabekova, M., & Blanc, W. (2020). Enhanced backscattering optical fiber distributed sensors: Tutorial and review. *IEEE Sensors Journal, 21*(11), 12667–12678.
Ulaby, F. T., Michielssen, E., & Ravaioli, U. (2010). *Fundamentals of applied electromagnetics* (6th ed). Boston, Massachussetts: Prentice Hall.

3

Grating-based sensors

3.1 Fiber Bragg gratings: concept and working principle

Fiber Bragg grating (FBG) is defined as a periodic modulation of the refractive index, within the core of an optical fiber (Othonos and Kalli, 1999). After the discoveries from Hill et al. (1993), Meltz, Morey, and Glenn (1989), which gave the first experimental evidences of the formation of Bragg resonators in the optical fibers, FBGs have been significantly consolidated as an optical element, and find extensive applications in sensing.

The FBG is a narrow-band, reflective optical filter, which resembles its electronic counterpart, the notch filter, or the microwave resonators, having a large quality factor in the order of >5000. When a broadband light enters an FBG, as sketched in Fig. 3.1, a narrow set of wavelengths centered at the Bragg wavelength (λ_B) is reflected backward, and guided into the same fiber, while the remaining signal is transmitted through the FBG; therefore, the FBG is transparent to all wavelengths, except for the narrow resonance occurring in proximity of the Bragg wavelength.

The Bragg wavelength λ_B is dependent upon the grating pitch Λ, that is, the spatial periodicity of the refractive index modulation, and by the effective refractive index of the optical fiber n_{eff} according to the Bragg relationship:

$$\lambda_B = 2n_{eff}\Lambda \tag{3.1}$$

In order to have an accurate model of the spectrum of the FBG, Erdogan's coupled mode theory (CMT) (Erdogan, 1997) can be used. In the CMT, the interactions between the waves propagating forward and backward in the grating sections are studied, evaluating the local interactions between the waves. The result is a closed form expression for the FBG spectrum, which is quite accurate for most of the commercial gratings having length within 1 and 20 mm. According to the CMT, the reflection coefficient of the FBG [hereby labeled $\rho(\lambda)$, where λ is the wavelength) can be expressed as:

$$\rho(\lambda) = \frac{-\,k sinh\left(L\sqrt{k^2-\sigma^2}\right)}{\sigma sinh\left(L\sqrt{k^2-\sigma^2}\right) + j\sqrt{k^2-\sigma^2} cosh\left(L\sqrt{k^2-\sigma^2}\right)} \tag{3.2}$$

Optical Fiber Biosensors.
DOI: https://doi.org/10.1016/B978-0-12-819467-6.00004-4

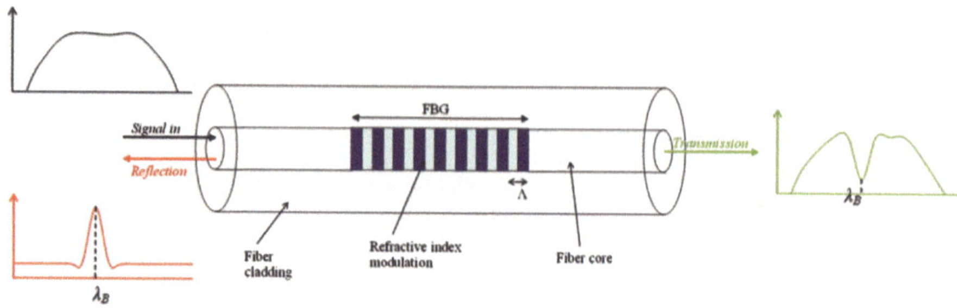

Figure 3.1 Schematic of the principle of operation of an FBG. *FBG*, Fiber Bragg grating.

where L is the length of the grating, and kL is a unitless number that defines the grating strength coefficient, and typically ranges from $kL = 0.1$ for very weak gratings to $kL = 4$ for very strong gratings. For most of the gratings described in this chapter, we can assume that kL is within 0.5–1.5, as biosensors in general do not require FBGs to be highly reflective.

The parameter σ encodes the dependence on the amplitude of the FBG modulation δn_{eff}, that is, the difference between the maximum and the minimum values of refractive index in the FBG, and the Bragg wavelength. Its formal definition, for a uniform FBG, is:

$$\sigma(\lambda) = \frac{\pi}{\lambda}\delta n_{eff} + 2\pi n_{eff}\left(\frac{1}{\lambda} - \frac{1}{\lambda_B}\right) \tag{3.3}$$

Usually, the interrogation of the FBG involves the detection of the reflectivity of the grating R, which corresponds to the amount of power reflected backward at each wavelength:

$$R(\lambda) = |\rho(\lambda)|^2 = \frac{sinh^2\left(L\sqrt{k^2 - \sigma^2}\right)}{cosh^2\left(L\sqrt{k^2 - \sigma^2}\right) - \frac{\sigma^2}{k^2}} \tag{3.4}$$

In this sense, the maximum reflectivity is observed at the Bragg wavelength, and depends on the grating strength:

$$R_{max} = max[R(\lambda)] = atanh^2(kL) \tag{3.5}$$

Fig. 3.2 shows the reflection spectra of an FBG having the following parameters, which are typical for an FBG operating in the third optical window: L = 5 mm, n_{eff} = 1.464, δn_{eff} = 10^{-6}, λ_B = 1550 nm; kL values are varied from 0.7 to 2. The spectrum is narrow and centered around the Bragg wavelength, having bandwidth in the order of 0.3 nm (measured as FWHM, full-width half-maximum of the reflectivity). In comparison to a resonator, the quality factor is ~5200, defined as the ratio between the Bragg wavelength and the grating bandwidth. The reflectivity grows from 36% for kL = 0.7 to 58% for kL = 1, and to 93% for kL = 2. These are typical values, as in most applications, depending on the

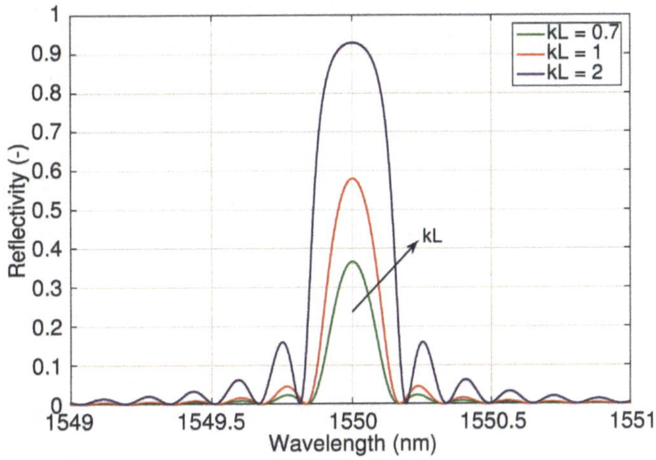

Figure 3.2 Reflectivity spectrum of an FBG having Bragg wavelength 1550 nm, for different values of *kL*, simulated according to the CMT model. *FBG*, Fiber Bragg grating; *CMT*, coupled mode theory.

setup for FBG inscription, the reflectivity of FBGs used in biosensors is typically within

10%–90%. Adjacently to the main lobes, the FBG exhibits side lobes that progressively fade, occupying a bandwidth of about 2 nm. The effect of side lobes grows with the increase of *kL* coefficient. In order to partially mitigate the effect of side lobes, it is possible to inscribe apodized gratings, in which the modulation of the refractive index has a constant periodicity, but a varying amplitude (Othonos and Kalli, 1999); the apodization pattern, often present in commercial gratings, has the effect to reduce the reflectivity of side lobes, making the FBG spectrum more compact.

A useful note for researchers is that the CMT model is currently applied in the grating simulators (either in-fiber FBGs, but also gratings in other optical waveguides) that are commercially available. The main CMT-based simulators are RSoft (BeamPROP and GratingMOD tools) and OptiGrating, which resolve the coupling of waves in each section of the grating. A CMT-based code that reproduces several types of FBGs in MatLab has been provided in Tosi and Perrone (2017).

FBGs are used in physical sensing, particularly for strain and/or temperature sensing, since the Bragg wavelength can shift when either n_{eff} or Λ change in Eq. (3.1). For example, when a strain is applied on the FBG, the pitch of the grating enlarges causing the Bragg wavelength to shift from the original position, toward longer wavelength for extension of the FBG or toward shorter wavelengths when the FBG is compressed. Similarly, both n_{eff} and Λ are sensitive to temperature, as the thermo-optic coefficient and the thermal expansion coefficient of the silica are functions of temperature (Kersey et al., 1997). The sensitivity coefficients to strain and temperature for a grating having Bragg wavelength around 1550 nm are, approximately, 1 pm/$\mu\varepsilon$ and 10 pm/°C (whereas 1 $\mu\varepsilon$ is one microstrain, i.e., an extension of 1 μm applied to a length of 1 m). Thus the sensing mechanism applied to FBG relies on monitoring the change of the Bragg wavelength:

$$\lambda_B = \lambda_{B,0} + \Delta\lambda \tag{3.6}$$

The Bragg wavelength in reference condition, usually at the start of the experiment, is referenced as $\lambda_{B,0}$, while we monitor the amount of wavelength shift $\Delta\lambda$ (positive or negative) from the original value of the Bragg wavelength.

3.2 Etched FBG sensors

3.2.1 Etched FBG fabrication

Uniform FBGs are unsuitable for refractive index sensing, because both n_{eff} and Λ do not have an adequate sensitivity to the refractive index surrounding the grating: while the pitch is clearly unaffected by the change of surrounding refractive index (SRI), in a standard single-mode fiber the propagating mode is well confined inside the fiber core even when perturbed by the grating, and thus the n_{eff} term is not altered cy SRI changes. The simplest solution to turn an FBG into a SRI sensor is therefore to etch the fiber cladding, removing almost entirely the cladding and exposing the fiber core to the outer changes of refractive index. This configuration is labeled as etched FBG (EFBG) (Ayupova et al., 2019; Bekmurzayeva et al., 2018; Iadicicco, Cusano, Campopiano, Cutolo, & Giordano, 2005; Iadicicco, Cusano, Cutolo, Bernini, & Giordano, 2004), and in literature it can be also referred as thinned FBG, or cladding-depleted FBG.

The EFBG is fabricated by depleting the cladding of the fiber, shrinking the thickness until the fundamental mode is affected (Bekmurzayeva et al., 2018): in this case, we can obtain the Bragg wavelength to be dependent on the SRI, and therefore use the EFBG for biosensing. The most common method for etching the FBG is to use wet-etching, in hydrofluoric acid (HF) concentration ranging from 24% (Iadicicco et al., 2004, 2005), to 48% (Ayupova et al., 2019; Bekmurzayeva et al., 2018), up to 52% (Liang, Huang, Xu, Lee, & Yariv, 2005); an alternative solution makes use of ammonium fluoride and sulfuric acid, which acts with a slower etching rate. The HF etches the fiber cladding in a progressive rate, and the etching rate depends on the concentration of the acid and on the temperature. The process reported in Bekmurzayeva et al. (2018) makes use of 48% acid, which is the highest concentration commercially available for research laboratories equipped with fume hoods that are required to ventilate the area used for etching. The high HF concentration allows a rapid etching, which lasts several minutes. In Fig. 3.3, we show the chart that displays the fiber diameter as a function of the time elapsed during etching in ammonium fluoride and sulfuric acid. In this chart, the fiber size has been estimated using an optical microscope at each etching time. We can see that over the course of the process, the diameter decreases faster when the fiber has

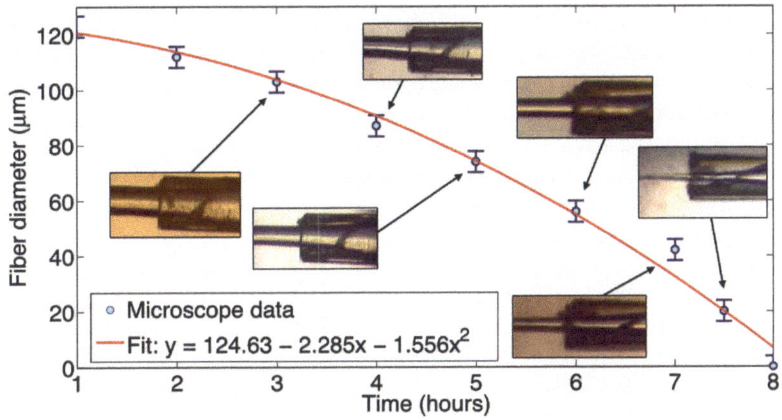

Figure 3.3 Etching of an optical fiber in ammonium fluoride and sulfuric acid; the chart reports the fiber diameter (estimated through an optical microscope with $\pm 4\ \mu m$ accuracy), as a function of time elapsed during etching. Photographs show the progressive reduction of the fiber thickness.

already been thinned by half of its original diameter. The polynomial fit shows an etching rate decreasing with the etching time, from the initial 125 μm until even the core is etched after 8 hours into the solution. A similar solution has been obtained for 48% HF, with etching time of 30 minutes to completely deplete the fiber.

The measurement of the thickness by optical microscopy is not efficient for EFBG fabrication, because the fiber is fragile; besides, the etching rate is not very repeatable (Iadicicco et al., 2005), particularly since the HF is diluted with deionized water, and the HF evaporates at room temperature while water does not, thus the HF concentration keeps reducing as the HF is exposed to the open environment. To circumvent this, a viable option is to measure the spectrum of the EFBG in real time during etching, as this is a repeatable information and does not require manipulating the fiber (such as moving it in and out of the etching chamber). During the etching process, we can observe two changes affecting the spectrum of the grating: (1) Due to the evanescent waves, the spectral level that is observed on the analyzer reduces over time; this is not a direct effect on the grating reflectivity, but it is rather an effect of the increase of the light propagation losses through and back from the EFBG. (2) As the grating becomes sensitive to the surrounding RI, specifically the HF refractive index, we observe a change of the Bragg wavelength toward the shorter values, which is directly related to the increase of sensitivity to the SRI.

In Fig. 3.4, we report the evolution of the spectrum of the EFBG, through the etching process, as recorded in real time by an optical spectrometer (I-MON-USB-512, Ibsen Photonics) having 156 pm wavelength resolution. During the first 7.27 hours, the etching depletes the outer part of the cladding, but as the mode remains well confined, no effect on the Bragg wavelength is recorded. As the etching progresses, we observe a progressive deviation of the Bragg wavelength as well as a reduction of the peak reflectivity detected on the spectrometer: from the initial signal level, the peak of the spectrum decreases by 3.8 times from 7.27 to 8.06 hours, and the wavelength shifts by −1.3 nm as effect of the cladding depletion. The FBG reported in Fig. 3.4 has length 10 mm, initial reflectivity ~90%, and Bragg wavelength 1566.7 nm, and the spectral plot shows how etching significantly affects the reflected signal and the central part of the spectrum.

This evolution can also be shown in Fig. 3.5, which shows how the Bragg wavelength of the FBG and the peak value of the FBG spectrum evolve over the etching process. As expected, no significant change is observed for the first 7.3 hours: after this, we observe an abrupt change as the Bragg wavelength and the spectral amplitude both rapidly decrease, until the reflection spectrum of the FBG becomes undetectable (8.06 hours), and subsequently the core is also depleted.

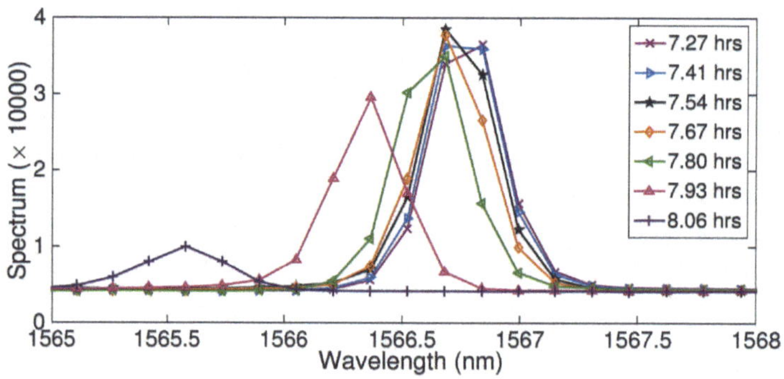

Figure 3.4 Spectrum of an FBG during etching in ammonium fluoride and sulfuric acid: the chart reports the spectrum, measured through an optical spectrometer, for each etching time. *FBG*, Fiber Bragg grating.

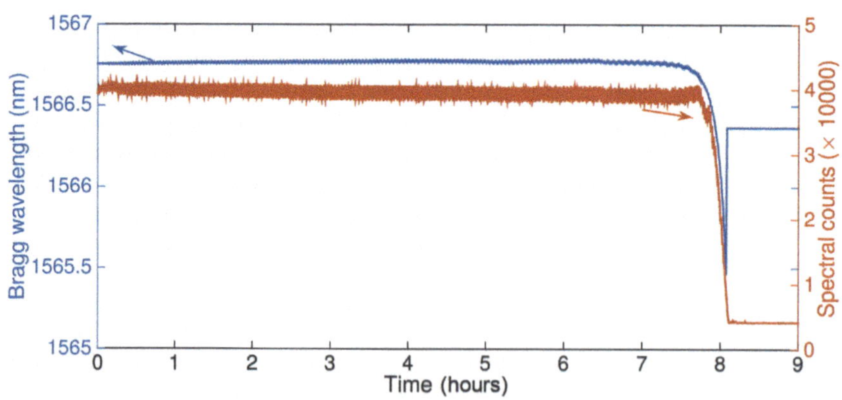

Figure 3.5 Evolution of the Bragg wavelength (left axis (*blue*)) and of the peak reflectivity (right axis (*red*)) for the EFBG in Fig. 3.4 during the etching process.

This chart, obtained in real time by simply connecting the EFBG to its interrogator, is valid for every type of etching solution, by simply accelerating or slowing the time axis to take into account the appropriate etching rate, based on the etching solution and its concentration. Thus this information is valuable for optimizing the EFBG fabrication: higher values of negative wavelength shifts correspond to a more sensitive grating element, but also imply working with poor reflected signals and therefore with a worse signal/noise ratio figure at the detector.

We can also combine the real-time wavelength and spectral data in Fig. 3.5 with the diameter of the fiber estimated by microscopy in Fig. 3.3, and thus provide a chart that displays the wavelength shift and spectral reduction as a function of the fiber diameter. This chart is shown in Fig. 3.6, displaying an exponential trend for both spectral level and wavelength shift $\Delta\lambda$ as a function of the fiber diameter. As shown in Fig. 3.3, the fiber diameter estimate is more accurate when the diameter is thicker, and less accurate for smaller diameters; however, this chart can provide a quantitative indicator of the fiber diameter directly from the change of Bragg wavelength.

The Bragg wavelength tracking is more robust than the spectral amplitude detection, due to insensitivity to the power fluctuations; we can approximate the relationship between the wavelength shift $\Delta\lambda$ and the fiber diameter d_F with an exponential:

$$\Delta\lambda = -(5.432\ \text{nm}) \times \exp\left[-(0.307\ \mu\text{m}^{-1}) \cdot d_F\right] \tag{3.6}$$

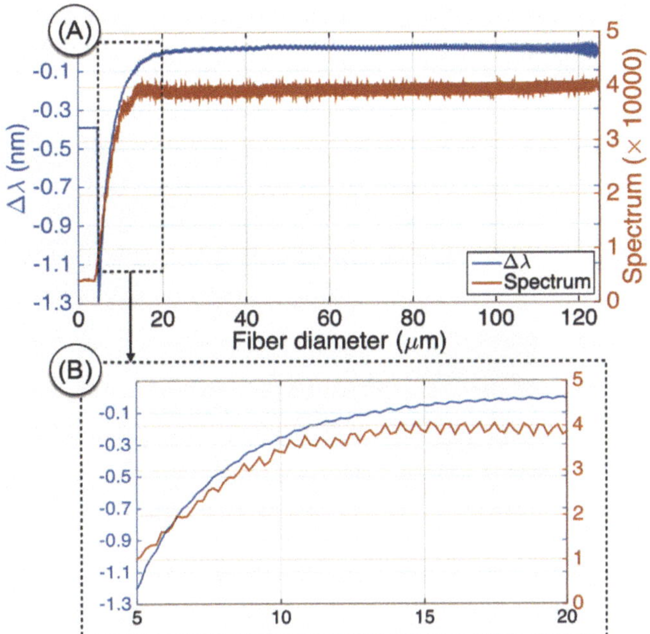

Figure 3.6 Relationship between the wavelength shift $\Delta\lambda$ observed by the EFBG during the etching process (left axis (*blue*)), and the spectral level (right axis (*red*)), as a function of the fiber diameter estimated by a microscope. (A) Data reported for the whole 8-hour process; (B) inset on the region displaying the sensitivity.

which provides a direct relationship between the wavelength shift measured on the interrogator and the estimated fiber diameter:

$$d_F = \frac{1}{0.307\ \mu m^{-1}} \times \ln\left(\frac{-5.432\ nm}{\Delta\lambda}\right) \tag{3.7}$$

The relationship in Eq. (3.7) is an important function as it allows monitoring in real time the fiber diameter without any microscopy analysis, and can be used to find the trade-off between the sensitivity and the requirement to preserve the fiber diameter to maintain the mechanical stability of the fiber. It has been obtained empirically for ammonium fluoride etchant, but it can be obtained for other etching fluids such as HF as it does not contain the etching speed. Fig. 3.7 (Ayupova et al., 2019) shows the photograph of a chemically EFBG, resulting from the etching process.

3.2.2 EFBG sensitivity

The sensitivity of an EFBG relies on the variation of effective refractive index of the fiber, as a function of the SRI (Liang et al., 2005). When the fiber becomes thinner, and the cladding is partially replaced by the outer medium having a different refractive index, we observe an alteration of the fundamental mode propagating in the fiber, and an increase of the evanescent power due to the lower confinement of the mode within the fiber core. This phenomenon, explained in Ayupova et al. (2019), results on the alteration of the Bragg wavelength and of the spectral level, explained in the previous subsection, but also on the dependence of these two terms of the SRI. Thus the EFBG working principle relies on the change of Bragg wavelength due to the change of SRI.

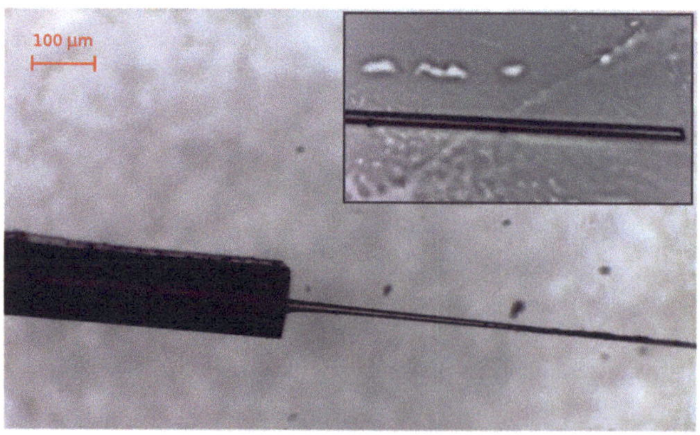

Figure 3.7 Photograph of a chemically etched FBG, obtained from a fiber having initial cladding diameter 125 μm. Source:*Image from Ayupova, T., Sypabekova, M., Molardi, C., Bekmurzayeva, A., Shaimerdenova, M., Dukenbayev, K., & Tosi D. (2019). Wavelet-based demodulation of multimode etched fiber Bragg grating refractive index sensor.* Sensors, *19(1), 39.*

If we consider that the effective refractive index n_{eff} changes by a quantity Δn_{eff}, then the Bragg wavelength changes by a quantity $\Delta\lambda$, according to Eq. (3.1):

$$\Delta\lambda = 2\Delta n_{eff}\Lambda \tag{3.8}$$

In an EFBG, the relationship between Δn_{eff} and the surrounding refractive index change Δn_s has been derived in Ayupova et al. (2019), by means of resolving Maxwell's equations in a glass fiber with depleted cladding, for different values of cladding thickness and SRI.

The result is shown in Fig. 3.8. We observe an exponential relationship between Δn_{eff} and the cladding thickness, defined as the thickness of the cylindrical crown wrapping the fiber core, which confirms the exponential variation of the Bragg wavelength during the etching of the grating observed in Fig. 3.6. The variation of the outer SRI induces a further differential deviation of the Δn_{eff} from the baseline value, which becomes more significant as the cladding reduces its thickness, thus increasing the sensitivity to SRI. In Fig. 3.8, the change of SRI is reproduced, as explained in Chapter 8, Interrogation of sensors, by varying the sucrose concentration in a water–sucrose mixture, from 0% to 50%.

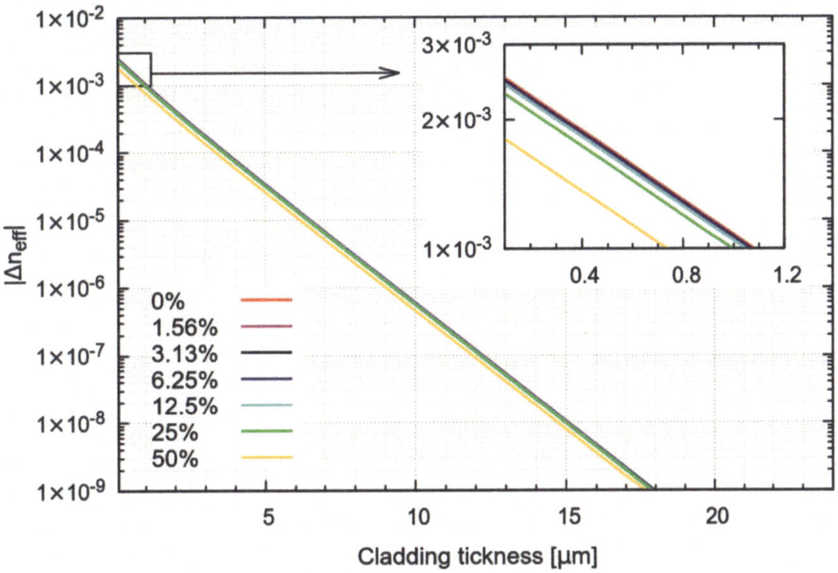

Figure 3.8 Relationship between the variation of effective refractive index Δn_{eff} of an optical fiber and the cladding thickness, for different values of surrounding refractive index (simulated by changing the sucrose concentration in water from 0% to 50%). Source: *Image from Ayupova, T., Sypabekova, M., Molardi, C., Bekmurzayeva, A., Shaimerdenova, M., Dukenbayev, K., & Tosi D. (2019). Wavelet-based demodulation of multimode etched fiber Bragg grating refractive index sensor.* Sensors, *19(1), 39.*

The sensitivity s_n of an EFBG is defined as the variation of the Bragg wavelength as a function of the change of SRI:

$$s_n = \frac{\Delta\lambda}{\Delta n_s} \tag{3.9}$$

The sensitivity depends on the thickness of the fiber after the cladding, which can be estimated by the Bragg wavelength change during etching. Fig. 3.9 shows the result presented in Bekmurzayeva et al. (2018). Fig. 3.9A shows the effect of etching on the initial grating, which causes a wavelength shift of −2.1 nm and a reduction of the peak reflectivity signal of 11.6 dB. As a consequence, the grating becomes sensitive to SRI change, which has been highlighted in Fig. 3.9B: the sensitivity is not linear through the whole range of operation, but can be approximated with a 17.4 nm/RIU linear fit, which is sufficient to detect 5.7×10^{-6} RIU considering that the interrogator has an accuracy of 1 pm.

The limit of detection (LoD) is defined as the lowest variation of SRI that can be unambiguously detected by the setup. Most setups have an accuracy in the order of 0.1−10 pm (depending on whether signal processing is used to refine the Bragg peak estimation), and the sensitivity also plays a significant role; the LoD is equal to $\Delta\lambda_{min}/s_n$ (where $\Delta\lambda_{min}$ corresponds to the lowest detectable wavelength shift on the interrogator); thus the sensitivity is inversely proportional to the LoD. It is, however, to be noticed that both the interrogator accuracy and the sensitivity play a significant role in the LoD determination: while the increase of sensitivity corresponds to a thinner grating, which implies that the fiber is thinner and more fragile, and also a lower amount of surface usable for hosting bioreceptors, it is possible to obtain an equivalent increment of performance by acting on the quality of the interrogator, and particularly to the signal processing used for FBG

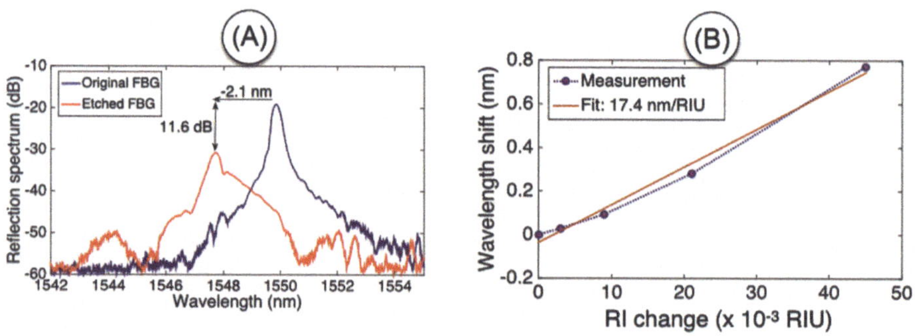

Figure 3.9 Sensitivity of an EFBG to the change of SRI, as exposed in Bekmurzayeva et al. (2018); (A) comparison of the original FBG spectrum and the etched FBG spectrum; (B) sensitivity of the EFBG, measured as the wavelength shift observed for each RIU change, with linear fit equal to 17.4 nm/RIU. Source: *Image taken from Ayupova, T., Sypabekova, M., Molardi, C., Bekmurzayeva, A., Shaimerdenova, M., Dukenbayev, K., & Tosi D. (2019). Wavelet-based demodulation of multimode etched fiber Bragg grating refractive index sensor.* Sensors, *19(1), 39.*

tracking. Chapter 8, Interrogation of sensors, will discuss interrogation techniques and peak-tracking methods, which can guarantee an improvement of LoD that does not require a further reduction of the fiber thickness.

In this regard, results obtained with a thicker fiber such as Bekmurzayeva et al. (2018) are particularly interesting for biosensing, because they maintain a relatively resistant fiber and do not compromise the operation of the fiber probe. This work achieves a good LoD, estimated around 5×10^{-6} RIU, by using accurate peak tracking methods.

Table 3.1 shows a comparison between the main works on EFBG reported by University of Sannio, Italy (Iadicicco et al., 2004; Iadicicco et al., 2005), University of Maryland, United States (Chryssis, Lee, Lee, Saini, & Dagenais, 2005), California Institute of Technology, United States (Liang et al., 2005), and Nazarbayev University, Kazakhstan (Ayupova et al., 2019; Bekmurzayeva et al., 2018).

One important note concerns the number of modes propagating in the etched portion of the fiber, as the cladding thickness reduces. The theoretical considerations made so far assume the fiber to maintain its single-mode feature even when the cladding shrinks significantly. The evidence reported in Ayupova et al. (2019) and in Fig. 3.10, which shows the number of modes propagating in the etched fiber as a function of the cladding thickness, suggests that the number of modes appear to increase as the cladding gets thinner, and that the

Table 3.1 Comparison of EFBG sensors presented in recent literature for refractive index sensing and biosensing.

Reference	Fiber thickness	Initial FBG parameters	Etching method	Sensitivity @ $n_s = 1.33$	Limit of detection	Interrogation method	Application
Iadicicco et al. (2004)	10–12 μm	$L = 4$ mm, $\lambda_B = 1550$ nm	24% HF	~2 nm/RIU	10^{-4} RIU (estimated)	Spectral detection	SRI detection
Iadicicco et al. (2005)	10–12 μm	$L = 4$ mm, $\lambda_B = 1550$ nm	24% HF	0.9–2.3 nm/RIU	10^{-4} RIU (estimated)	Spectral detection	SRI detection
Liang et al. (2005)	6 μm	SMF-28 fiber, $\lambda_B = 1515$ nm	Etching of FBG to form cavity	71.2 nm/RIU	1.4×10^{-5} RIU (estimated)	Detection of resonant wavelength	SRI detection
Chryssis et al. (2005)	3–7 μm	$\lambda_B = 1560$ nm	Wet etching	20–90 nm/RIU (approx.)	7.2×10^{-6} RIU	Optical spectrum analyzer	SRI detection, glucose measurement
Bekmurzayeva et al. (2018)	~12 μm	$\lambda_B = 1550$ nm, $L = 1$ cm, SMF fiber, 95% reflectivity	48% HF	17.4 nm/RIU	5×10^{-6} RIU (estimated)	Swept laser interrogator, FBG peak tracking	Thrombin sensing
Ayupova et al. (2019)	8 μm (approx.)	$\lambda_B = 1550$ nm, $L = 1$ cm, SMF fiber, 95% reflectivity	48% HF	–	~5×10^{-4} RIU	Swept laser interrogator, wavelet analysis	SRI detection

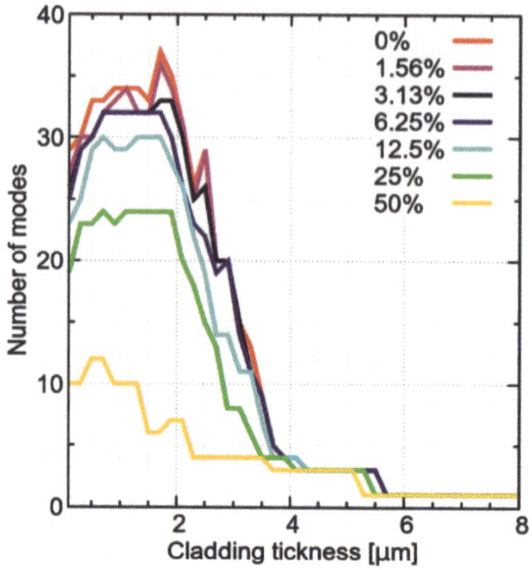

Figure 3.10 Number of modes for an optical fiber as a function of cladding thickness, for different values of sucrose/water % concentration. Source: *Image from Ayupova, T., Sypabekova, M., Molardi, C., Bekmurzayeva, A., Shaimerdenova, M., Dukenbayev, K., & Tosi D. (2019). Wavelet-based demodulation of multimode etched fiber Bragg grating refractive index sensor.* Sensors, *19(1), 39.*

fiber becomes multimode for cladding thickness below 5.2 μm. In addition, as expected from Fig. 3.8, the number of modes is itself function of the SRI, as it changes the confinement factor of the fiber.

Since the effective refractive index is different for each mode, and therefore the Bragg wavelength has a different value for each mode, the spectrum of multimode EFBG appears as a broader spectrum, as some modes at various other wavelengths are partially excited. Most of the works reported in this section see the EFBG spectrum broaden from the original shape, while Ayupova et al. (2019) attempt at measuring the spectrum enlargement with a wavelet signal processing routine, rather than tracking the Bragg wavelength change.

3.3 Tilted FBGs

3.3.1 Working principle

A tilted FBG (TFBG) is similar to a uniform FBG, corresponding to the periodic modulation of the fiber effective refractive index with fixed periodicity Λ. However, rather than inscribing the grating perpendicularly to the fiber propagation direction, the modulation is spatially tilted by an angle θ (Dong, Zhang, Liu, & Miao, 2011; Guo, Liu, Guan, & Albert, 2016; Yu, Wu, Yang, Han, & Zhao, 2018).

The schematic of a TFBG is shown in Fig. 3.11. The modulation index, tilted by an angle θ with respect to the plane perpendicular to the fiber direction, affects

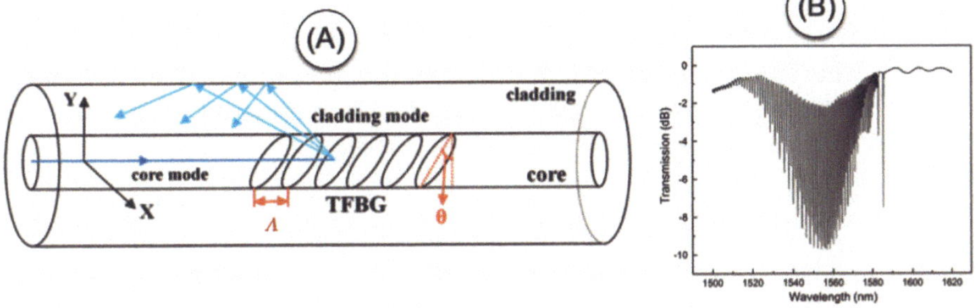

Figure 3.11 (A) Schematic of a TFBG; (B) transmission spectrum of a TFBG with tilt angle of 8 degrees. Source: *Image adapted from Yu, J., Wu, Z., Yang, X., Han, X., & Zhao, M. (2018). Tilted fiber Bragg grating sensor using chemical plating of a palladium membrane for the detection of hydrogen leakage.* Sensors, 18*(12), 4478.*

the light propagation in multiple ways. While the structure substantially behaves as a Bragg grating in reflection, by a suitable adjustment of the Bragg wavelength that takes into consideration the tilt angle, the image shows that the incoming light tends to excite cladding modes, which propagate in the fiber cladding and therefore also at the interface between the cladding and the outer medium. These modes do not propagate in the fiber core, and therefore do not appear into the reflection spectrum (Guo et al., 2016). However, when looking into the transmission spectrum of the TFBG, we observe a plurality of cladding modes, appearing as a hole into the spectrum. These modes correspond to all the cladding modes that are excited by the tilted grating structure: as the TFBG couples part of the incoming light into modes that do not propagate in the fiber, each hole corresponds to the "efficient" excitation of a cladding mode.

In a TFBG, the effective pitch wavelength Λ_e is adjusted by the tilt angle θ:

$$\Lambda_e = \frac{\Lambda}{cos\theta} \tag{3.10}$$

By replacing Λ_e in lieu of Λ, the Bragg condition for a TFBG is $\lambda_B = 2n_{eff}\Lambda_e$. For biosensing, it is essential to analyze the cladding modes as specific spectral features. While n_{eff} refers to the effective refractive index of the fiber core, we label n_m the effective refractive index of the *m*th cladding mode. The cladding mode effective refractive index has a similar definition than the core n_{eff}, that is, it corresponds to the ratio between the speed or propagation in vacuum and the longitudinal light speed of for the specific mode within the cladding. This way, the resonant wavelengths λ_m for each *m*th cladding mode correspond to:

$$\lambda_m = (n_{eff} + n_m)\Lambda_e \tag{3.11}$$

As suggested in Fig. 3.11, the n_m terms are lower than n_{eff}, thus the Bragg wavelength λ_B is longer than the resonant cladding wavelengths, which therefore appear on the leftmost part of the TFBG transmission spectrum.

3.3.2 Spectral characteristics

The spectral characteristics of the TFBG, often referred to as the spectral features, are the key metric for the interrogation of the TFBG as a biosensing unit. Referring to the spectrum in Fig. 3.11B, we identify the three main spectral components of a TFBG (Guo et al., 2016):

- Bragg mode: This corresponds to the longest resonant wavelength λ_B, and corresponds to the most confined mode for most gratings. The characteristics of the Bragg wavelength correspond to a standard FBG (upon adjusting the Bragg condition by the tilt angle), and its correspondent spectral feature is similar to a standard FBG. As such, the Bragg wavelength has a temperature sensitivity (the same $\sim$10 pm/°C coefficient of a uniform FBG), but does not sense the change of the surrounding refractive index. The Bragg mode is the only part of the spectrum that is visible in reflection, since it corresponds to a mode confined in the fiber core; as the other features correspond to modes not confined in the core, they are not visible in reflection (i.e., by terminating the fiber on an index-matching gel or fluid, no other feature than the Bragg mode would be visible).
- Ghost modes: The ghost modes are a cluster of modes, having wavelength adjacent to the Bragg wavelength, that are strongly coupled in the cladding. These modes have strong interaction at the core-cladding interface, hence to not reach and interact with the outer boundaries of the fiber. As such, the ghost modes have important in mechanical sensing since they respond to fiber strain and twists, but are less impactful in biosensing as they do not probe the surrounding of the fiber.
- Cladding modes: The cladding modes are the most important part of the TFBG spectral features of interest for biosensing, because they represent the modes that propagate at the boundary between the cladding and the outer medium. The analysis of cladding modes is the method used in biosensing to probe the SRI. Cladding modes appear as a sequence of valleys (or negative peaks) in the TFBG transmission spectrum, and are often referred to as a comb since their shape appears almost periodic (Erdogan, 1997). Since the effective refractive index of cladding modes becomes smaller as the mode order increases, the cladding modes of the highest order have the smallest wavelength. As explained in the previous chapter, however, in order to maintain guiding condition, we need to guarantee that the effective refractive index of the cladding mode is higher that the surrounding refractive index, otherwise the mode would become evanescent. Thus, the number of cladding modes is not constant, but depends on the SRI. Besides, since each resonant condition is also affected by the SRI, we observe that some of the cladding modes are subjected to a wavelength shift when the SRI is changed. Besides, the spectral properties of all features are also dependent on the temperature of the fiber, as the Bragg mode. Hence, for each value of SRI we have a cut-off condition, which we can label λ_{CO}: the cladding

modes having wavelength $\lambda_m > \lambda_{CO}$ (and therefore having effective refractive index higher than the outer refractive index, which is the essential condition to have total internal reflection) are excited and visible in the transmission spectrum; the modes having $\lambda_m > \lambda_{CO}$, on the other side, do not trigger TIR at the boundary between cladding and outer medium, and therefore do not appear on the transmission spectrum.

The higher order cladding modes are therefore of pivotal importance for biosensing, as they convey the dependence on the SRI. Fig. 3.12 shows the spectrum of a TFBG with $\theta = 6$ degrees, whereas the transmission spectrum is normalized. Looking at the first spectrum for SRI = 1.333, we observe a comb of cladding modes which occupy the wavelength range 1485–1535 nm. The cut-off wavelength is around 1485 nm; this condition, however, does not appear as a strong contrast between the modes below and over the cut-off, as a partial excitation of these modes might be present. Increasing the SRI results in both a wavelength shift of the modes at the same wavelengths, and an increase of the cut-off wavelength, which rises to 1490 nm for SRI = 1.3433. For higher values of SRI, less modes are over the cut-off; when SRI > 1.42, the comb appears depleted as no mode satisfies the cut-off condition.

The spectral properties of the TFBG are controlled also by the tilt angle, since the spatial periodicity between the modes in Eqs. (3.10) and (3.11) is controlled by θ, but also the capability to excite cladding modes varies with θ. Fig. 3.13 shows the spectrum of a TFBG for different values of the tilt angle. For smaller values of the tilt angle, the TFBG exhibits less cladding modes, and the

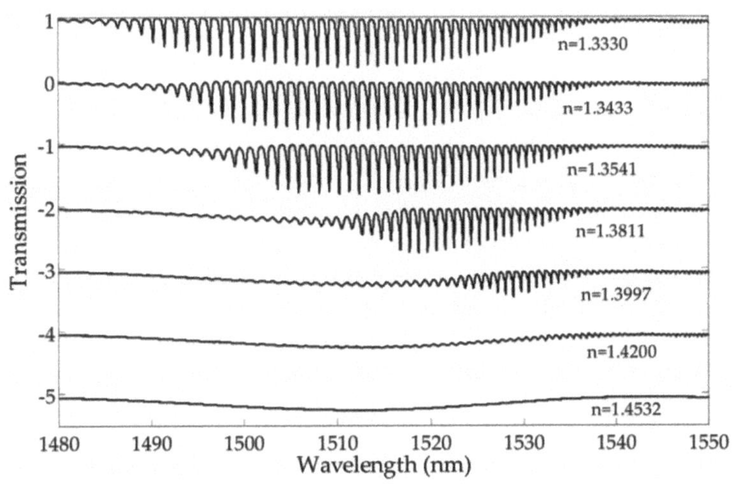

Figure 3.12 Spectrum of a TFBG with 6 degrees tilt angle, for different value of SRI ranging from 1.333 to 1.4532. Source: *Image from Cięszczyk, S., Kisała, P., & Mroczka, J. (2019). New parameters extracted from tilted fiber Bragg grating spectra for the determination of the refractive index and cut-off wavelength.* Sensors, 19(9), 1964.

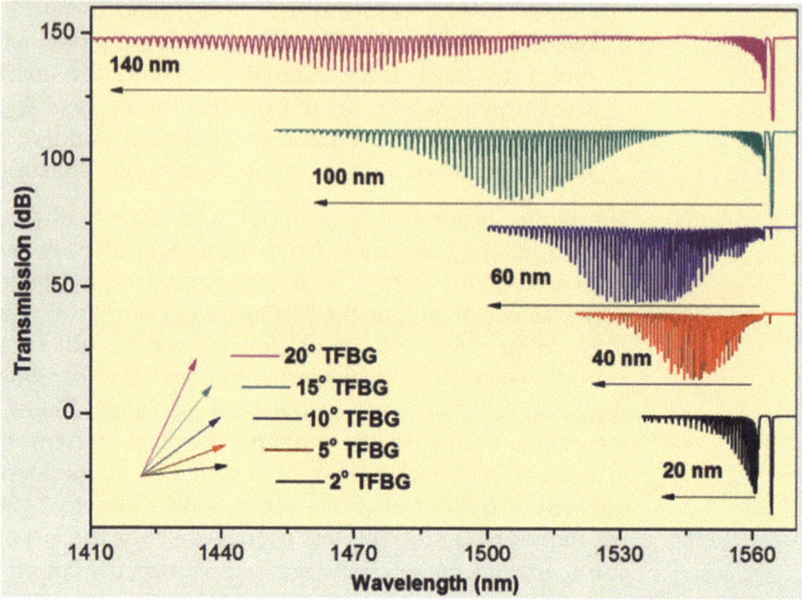

Figure 3.13 Transmission spectrum of a TFBG for different values of tilt angles ranging from 2 to 20 degrees. Source: *Image taken from Guo, T., Liu, F., Guan, B.O., & Albert, J. (2016). Tilted fiber grating mechanical and biochemical sensors.* Optics & Laser Technology, *78, 19–33 with permission.*

spectrum is more compact, with lower values of the spacing between each cladding mode composing the comb. As the tilt angle increases, the spectrum becomes broader, exciting more cladding modes at the shortest wavelengths. The overall extension of the TFBG can rise over 100 nm, for θ larger than 15 degrees, and reaches about 140 nm of extension for $\theta = 20$ degrees. For these range of tilt angles, the spacing between adjacent modes rises proportionally to $1/\cos\theta$.

3.3.3 Sensitivity and detection

Unlike in an EFBG, in the TFBG the detection method is not based on monitoring the Bragg wavelength shift, but rather on tracking the spectral features that characterize the TFBG as the refractive index change. The sensitivity therefore depends on which features can be detected. Simple detection methods are based on detecting a wavelength shift, or an amplitude change, in presence of a change of SRI. In this case, the sensitivity of a TFBG is expressed also in terms of nm/RIU for the wavelength shift, or in dB/RIU in case an amplitude change is detected (with the spectrum reported in dB)

The spectral features that are typically detected are the following:

- Change of wavelength of a cladding mode: This is the simplest and most immediate method for the detection of small SRI changes, because it focuses on a narrow portion of the spectrum. The key is to detect the change of wavelength of the most sensitive cladding mode, which is usually the mode just over the cut-off wavelength. With this method, Caucheteur et al. (Caucheteur, Loyez, González-Vila, & Wattiez, 2018) have reported sensitivity values of 21 nm/RIU for TFBG operating around 1550 nm of cut-off wavelength. It is noteworthy that such method can compensate temperature shifts by measuring the difference between the cladding mode under analysis and the Bragg wavelength.

- Change of amplitude of the cladding mode: This method has high sensitivity, as detectors measure power with a good precision, but might be unreliable for field operation as it is not easy to maintain the power levels in the optical setup. The technique consists of monitoring the change of amplitude of the most sensitive cladding mode, but measuring the spectral dip value, that is, the minimum reflectivity observed in proximity of the spectral resonance. The sensitivity shown in Caucheteur et al. (2018) is around 147 dB/RIU.
- Change of cut-off wavelength: This method has less accuracy than the analysis of one cladding mode, but it can interrogate larger changes of RI and therefore is compliant with applications in which RI changes are $>10^{-2}$ (Guo et al., 2016). The main obstacle to this technique is that, in real TFBG spectra as opposite to simulation works, there is no hard cut-off conditions as some modes around the cut-off might be slightly excited, as visible in Fig. 3.12. In this case, the sensitivity is also expressed as nm/RIU, referred to the wavelength shift of the cut-off condition.
- Signal processing: Several works applied signal processing techniques to the detection of TFBGs, treating the spectrum of the grating as a digital waveform and applying on it digital signal analysis techniques. Most notably, the work of Cięszczyk et al. (Cięszczyk et al., 2019) applies a low-pass filter on the grating spectrum, obtaining a Gaussian-shaped envelope that changes amplitude when the SRI changes. Shaimerdenova et al. (Shaimerdenova, Bekmurzayeva, Sypabekova, & Tosi, 2017) presented an advanced method based on KLT (Karhunen-Loeve Transform) that changes the domain of analysis applying a transformation on the TFBG spectrum; since this method is interesting also for low-cost interrogation, it will be reported in Chapter 8, Interrogation of sensors.

From the operational standpoint, the main advantages of a TFBG rely on the relatively high sensitivity, which can be either tied to wavelength shift or amplitude change, and to the fact that the TFBG can maintain the original size of the fiber cladding, hence allowing a better mechanical stability than all sensors in which the fiber is thinned (such as the EFBG). The two major drawbacks, however, are the fact that the TFBG works in transmission whereas users prefer to work in reflection, and the large bandwidth occupied by the cladding modes, which require a wideband interrogator and prevents multiplexing techniques, which can allow stacking multiple sensors on the same fiber. For this reason, when operating with TFBG sensors, it is a common method to terminate the fiber with a gold-tip reflector or with a perfect cleave, in order to visualize the cladding modes in the reflection spectrum (Guo et al., 2016).

3.4 Long-period gratings

The long-period grating (LPG) represents an alternative to the FBG structure, having a longer period and an inherent sensitivity to the SRI (Erdogan, 1997). The key difference between the FBG and all derived sensors, such as EFBG and TFBG, and the LPG concept is that, while FBGs look at resonances that occur at conditions that can be expressed as $(n_{eff} + n_m) \times \Lambda$, the LPG resonances occur at $(n_{eff} - n_m) \times \Lambda$. In other words, having a grating with pitch Λ, the resonances of an FBG occur at $(n_{eff} + n_{eff}) \times \Lambda = 2n_{eff}\Lambda$, the multiple resonances for each mth cladding mode of a TFBG occur at $(n_{eff} + n_m) \times \Lambda$, while the multiple resonances of a LPG occur at $(n_{eff} - n_m) \times \Lambda$. Given that $n_{eff} = 1.464$ for most optical fibers, and that the cladding modes have effective RI around 1.33–1.37 for interesting biosensors applications, in a TFBG the cladding resonances occur at wavelengths close to the Bragg grating equal to $2n_{eff}\Lambda$, usually designed to be around 1500–1600 nm and therefore detectable by most commercial interrogators. On the other hand, in order to obtain the mth resonance at a similar wavelength, the grating pitch Λ must be much longer, usually larger than 100 μm. For this reason, this type of grating is referred as long-period, as it takes a much longer length of the fiber pitch to generate a grating having a wavelength similar to an FBG, in the near infrared.

Erdogan's CMT (Erdogan, 1997) is also used to describe the wave propagation in a LPG; unlike FBGs, which study the interaction between the forward and backward coupled waves, an LPG is formed by the interaction between the forward core mode in the fiber, and the forward cladding modes. As the interactions appear between the two copropagating components, the LPG yields no reflection spectrum but the spectral features are all measured in transmission. The transmission spectrum of an LPG does not present a dominant (i.e., Bragg) mode in the spectrum, but is rather the combination of all the cladding/core modes that are excited in the structure; as for a TFBG, the spectrum can be visualized in reflection by adding a mirror on the fiber tip.

The spectral features of a LPG are more variable than for other types of grating, as they depend on the amount of interaction between the copropagating core and cladding mode, at the wavelengths of interactions and the modes chosen for operation, and also on the type of fiber. In general, a LPG presents multiple spectral peaks having a bandwidth much larger than a TFBG, and having a separation between adjacent peaks of tens of nanometers. For this reason, commercial interrogators usually visualize only a small set of spectral peaks, and the demodulation principle relies simply on detecting the shift of a spectral peak as a function of the RI change. We report in Fig. 3.14 the spectrum of two LPGs, designed for RI sensing and having operation in the near infrared. Fig. 3.14A reports the spectrum of a LPG inscribed on a hollow-core fiber and having two resonant peaks at 1495 and 1521 nm. Fig. 3.15B shows the spectrum of a LPG inscribed in a silica fiber and subsequently annealed. The figure shows the RI

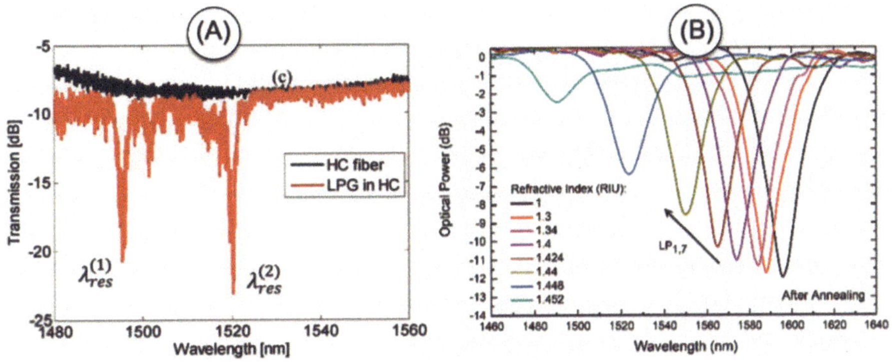

Figure 3.14 Transmission spectrum of LPG sensors. (A) Spectrum of a LPG inscribed into a hollow-core fiber. (B) Spectrum of a LPG inscribed on a silica fiber after thermal annealing. Source: *(A) Image from Iadicicco A., & Campopiano S. (2015). Sensing features of long period gratings in hollow core fibers.* Sensors, *Apr;15(4), 8009–8019. (B) Image from Viveiros, D., de Almeida, J.M., Coelho, L., Vasconcelos, H., Amorim, V.A., Maia, J.M., & Jorge, P.A. (2019). Spectral tuning of long period fiber gratings fabricated by femtosecond laser micromachining through thermal annealing.* Proceedings 2019, *15(1), 4.*

sensitivity of the LPG: as the refractive index of the external medium increases, the wavelength of resonance (initially around 1600 nm) starts to decrease, showing the opposite trend then EFBG and TFBG sensors. In this case, the wavelength shift observed with the increase of RI is toward the shorter values of wavelength, and this is due to the fact that EFBG and TFBG gratings couple counterpropagating modes, while the LPG couples forward modes hence its effect is different. We can notice that the spectrum of a LPG has a much wider bandwidth than the previous gratings; the FWHM of the spectrum reported in Fig. 3.14A is around 15 nm, while the TFBG and EFBG bandwidths are $<<$0.1 nm.

The sensitivity of the LPG, similarly than for the previous gratings, is estimated in nm/RIU units, by evaluating the wavelength shift as a function of the SRI change. Overall, the LPG operates for a broader RI window as the grating can operate from air to RI values similar to the silica; in biosensors, however, we rely on relatively small wavelength shift, and as a matter of fact the operation of a LPG is similar to the surface plasmon resonance spectra that will be described in the next chapter.

The sensitivity of a LPG is higher than the previous gratings by some orders of magnitude. Allsop et al. (Allsop et al., 2006) reported a LPG sensor having sensitivity of 560 nm/RIU in the near infrared, and several works reported recently have similar sensitivity (Socorro-Leranoz, Santano, Del Villar, & Matias, 2019). In order to increase the sensitivity, techniques that make use of thin-film deposition in order to tune the mode couplings have been employed. Smietana et al. reported in 2016 (Śmietana, Koba, Mikulic, & Bock, 2016) a record

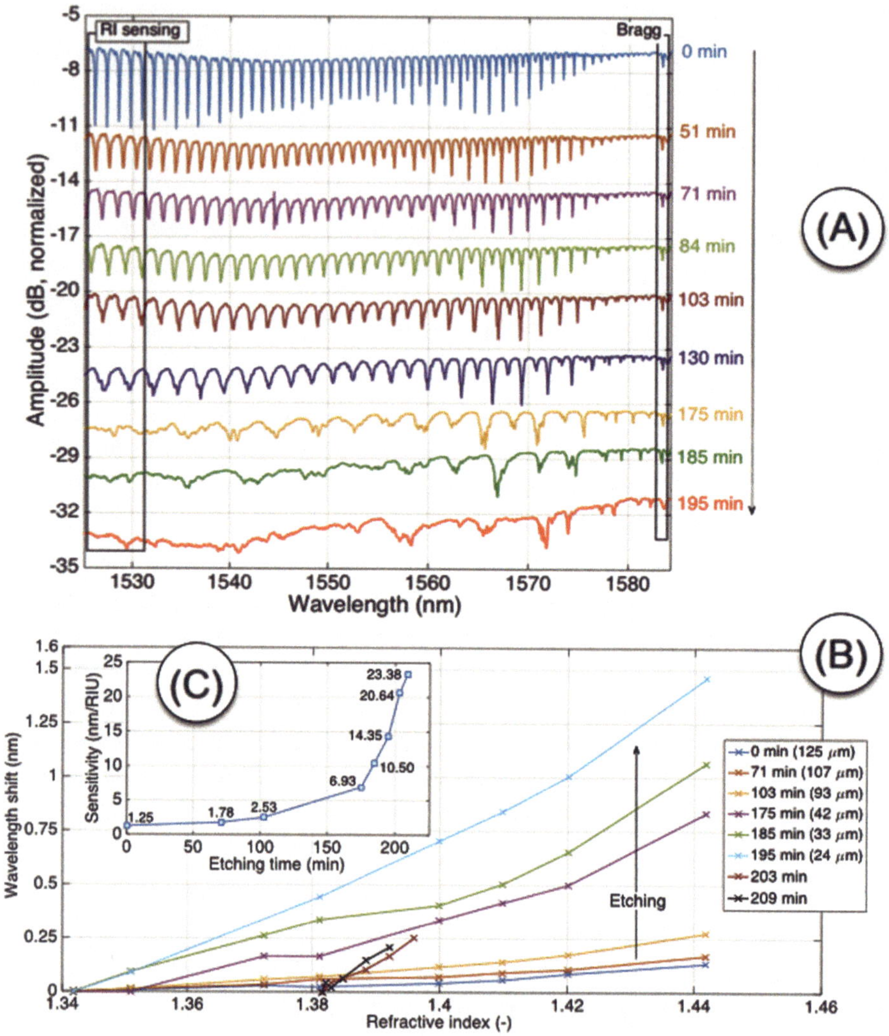

Figure 3.15 Sketch of an e-TFBG. (A) Spectral properties of the e-TFBG during 195-minute etching process, reporting the transmission reflection spectrum (normalized dB units) as the etching progresses; (B) wavelength shift as a function of surrounding RI for the e-TFBG, at different etching stages; (C) sensitivity of the e-TFBG, in nm/RIU units, evaluated at different etching times. Source: *Image adapted from Sypabekova, M., Korganbayev, S., González-Vila, Á., Caucheteur, C., Shaimerdenova, M., Ayupova T., ... & Tosi., D. (2019). Functionalized etched tilted fiber Bragg grating aptasensor for label-free protein detection.* Biosensors and Bioelectronics, *111765, with permission.*

sensitivity around 20,000 nm/RIU, obtained by etching the fiber and through a thin-film deposition of aluminum layer, which optimizes the transition of modes in RI sensing. Shen et al. reported (Shen, Zhou, Gordon, Zhang, & Shu, 2017) an LPG with a short pitch (15 μm) capable of obtaining a sensitivity of 504 nm/RIU.

Esposito et al. (Esposito, Ranjan, Campopiano, & Iadicicco, 2018) reported an efficient LPG fabrication method with sensitivity ranging from 5 to 70 nm/RIU depending on the typology of fiber used for inscription. From the operational standpoint, the fact that LPG yields broad transmission spectra covering a large portion of the infrared range, and the inherent working principle as a transmission device with no reflection makes the LPG device more similar to a surface plasmon resonance sensor rather than to a narrow-band grating, despite the similarities in mode coupling.

3.5 Advanced grating structures for refractive index sensing

3.5.1 Etched TFBG

Sypabekova et al. (Sypabekova et al., 2019) recently reported a structure for enhancing the sensitivity of a TFBG thrombin aptasensor, based on etching a TFBG sensor. This structure, labeled etched TFBG (e-TFBG), has been fabricated by etching in a HF bath a TFBG (10 degrees tilt angle), which allows changing the profile of the cladding modes. While the Bragg mode is substantially unaltered, the thinner fiber causes the wavelength difference between the cladding modes to expand, and to become more sensitive (at similar wavelength values) to the surrounding RI, therefore enhancing the sensitivity for biosensing applications. The e-TFBG has been then functionalized by means of a thrombin-binding aptamer to thrombin detection.

The rationale of e-TFBG biosensing is shown in Fig. 3.15, which reports the transmission-reflection spectrum of this type of grating, and the calibration to RI changes, at different values of etching times in a 48% HF solution. As etching progresses, we see no significant changes occurring on the Bragg wavelength; however, the leftmost part of the spectrum significantly changes, increasing the span between adjacent cladding modes and enhancing the sensitivity effect. The spectrum becomes broader and overall more sensitive to RI changes; however, this is challenging to handle for most interrogators due to the limitations of the bandwidth of the detectors, usually up to 100–140 nm for most interrogators. After 130 minutes of etching, the wavelength difference between adjacent modes has approximately tripled its original value. Subsequently, as evanescent waves become an increasing factor, the spectrum appears to deform significantly showing no clear peaks that can be tracked, albeit the sensitivity reaches its largest values. Fig. 3.15B shows the sensitivity to RI, measuring the peak at the leftmost wavelength value appearing on the interrogator (Luna OBR4600): as etching is deeper, the sensitivity appears to grow significantly, from the initial 1.25 nm/RIU to over 10 nm/RIU after 175 minutes of etching, and reaches values >20 nm/RIU when the grating is almost fully etched.

Overall, the e-TFBG structure has the drawback of increasing the fabrication complexity with one more step (wet-etching) and reducing the surface of the fiber available for interaction, but it can gather a significantly higher sensitivity without the need of plasmonic devices, and maintaining an interrogation based on wavelength shift. The work reported in Sypabekova et al. (2019) achieves a thrombin detection in the range of 2.5–40 nM with estimated LoD of 0.097 nM.

3.5.2 Tilted long-period grating

Tang et al. (Tang, Fu, Bai, Liao, & Wang, 2018) reported in 2018 an optical structure suitable for RI sensing and biosensing based on a tilted long-period grating (TLPG). The structure has been fabricated through a femtosecond laser, inscribing onto a tilted fiber prepared on a translation stage (with tilt angle around 3 degrees with respect to the fiber axis). The TLPG spectrum resembles the LPG spectra shown in Fig. 3.14, exhibiting multiple cladding modes that appear as spectral dips into the transmission spectrum. The tilt process appears to change the position of the spectral dips: increasing the tilt angle causes a shift of the cladding mode toward the shorter wavelength values. Overall, the sensitivity values measured in this work (−602.9 nm/RIU) is similar to the sensitivity recorded for standard LPG devices; however, the tilt angle allows shuffling the spectral position of the peaks, and therefore it is possible to position the mode corresponding to the highest sensitivity within the spectral window of the interrogator by acting on the tilt angle.

3.5.3 Partially etched chirped FBG

In 2018, Korganbayev et al. (Korganbayev et al., 2018) reported a partially etched chirped FBG (pECFBG), which has been fabricated by etching a linearly chirped FBG in a HF bath. A chirped FBG is a broadband FBG that has a nonuniform pitch Λ, which varies in each section of the grating. In this work, the authors etched the tip of a 1.2 cm chirped FBG in a HF bath, exposing only one region of the spectrum (around 80% of the total grating) to the outer RI. Thus the pECFBG performs a dual sensing function: it can detect the RI, by measuring the wavelength shift of the exposed region, with sensitivity up to 1.49 nm/RIU; and, simultaneously, it can detect the temperature changes across the grating region, using an algorithm that processes the spectral information across the whole grating. Although preliminary, a pECFBG probe is a promising structure, as it can detect the temperature and RI parameters across the whole grating length with a narrow spatial resolution.

3.6 Fabrication of gratings

3.6.1 Photosensitivity

In the majority of recent biosensors, the FBGs used for RI sensing are fabricated either using the phase mask technique, or by using direct inscription into the fiber with a femtosecond (fs) laser. The underlying principle behind FBGs is the *photosensitivity*, which is defined as the permanent change of the (effective) refractive index of an optical fiber when exposed to intense UV light (Hill et al., 1993). The exposure to UV light induces local damages to the crystal, at atomic level, causing a slight change or the RI (usually in the order of $\sim 10^{-6}$ for a silica fiber).

The photosensitive effect can be efficiently increased in order to have a short grating, capable of generating a substantial reflectivity in a short length. A common method is to use photosensitive fibers, characterized by a high Germanium concentration. Ge-doped fibers, designed in order to match the refractive index of a standard SMF fiber (e.g., Thorlabs GF1 and GF3 fiber classes, operating at 1500–1600 nm), yield a larger variation of effective refractive index (in the order of 10^{-5}–10^{-4}). In alternative, hydrogenation, or hydrogen-loading, can be used to artificially increase the photosensitivity of a standard fiber (Lemaire et al., 1993). Hydrogen-loading is achieved by placing the fiber in a hydrogen gas H_2-chamber at high pressure (around 150 atm), at a temperature around 20°C–75°C for several hours, and then inscribing the FBG immediately after the fiber is taken out of the chamber. As a result, the fiber has an excess of hydrogen, which facilitates the damages to the crystal structure under UV light, which yields a higher photosensitive effect. Hydrogen-loading is typically used to inscribe strong gratings onto standard or specialty fibers.

3.6.2 Phase mask method

The phase mask method is very popular in the fabrication of FBGs, which are subsequently etched and functionalized, and for the fabrication of TFBGs. The inscription method allows modulating the photosensitivity of the fiber along the fiber length, with a periodic modulation: in this case, we can create regions with lower refractive index and regions with higher refractive index, which form the periodic pattern described in Section 3.1 which has index contrast δn_{eff}.

The inscription based on this method makes use of a diffractive optical element, called *phase mask*, which is fabricated with electron-beam lithography or with holographic methods. When exposed to UV light, the phase mask is designed to cancel the 0th order diffraction, while maximizing the $+1$ and -1 orders of diffraction, creating an interference pattern within the fiber core. In the out-of-phase regions, the effect of the phase mask is minimal, while in the in-phase regions the exposure to UV light is maximized, hence having the maximum contrast in refractive index. With a phase mask having pitch (periodicity) Λ_{pm}, it is possible to inscribe a grating having Bragg wavelength $\Lambda_{pm} \cdot n_{eff}$, and for this reason FBGs operating in the third optical window with fibers having refractive index 1.464 have phase mask pitch of 1.02–1.09 μm. A typical setup based on the phase mask has been described in Tosi and Perrone (2017). The phase mask is the element that encodes the whole spectral response of the FBG, including the Bragg wavelength, the apodization pattern, and the type of spectral response. Optical setups are based on a UV or KrF free-space laser source, first expanded through an air path and then collimated onto the phase mask. The phase mask is mounted on top of the fiber, such that the refractive index modulation is impressed onto the fiber core. Then, the fiber and phase masks are mounted on a two-dimensional translation stage such that the UV light can scan the whole grating length, inscribing the FBG across the entire length. By acting on the translation stages, through a motion controller, it is possible to align the UV light onto the fiber core and to scan the grating at different speeds, varying the grating strength coefficient and the length of the FBG accordingly. By mounting the phase mask on a tilted surface, it is possible to inscribe TFBGs (Caucheteur et al., 2018), usually varying the tilt angle between 5 and 20 degrees.

Commercially, the phase mask technique is the most popular method to inscribe individual, as it allows fabricated large number of gratings all identical to each other, since each phase mask can generate one specimen of FBGs. The repeatability of the phase mask technique is also very accurate. However it does require multiple phase masks, as each different grating requires a different phase masks, limiting the flexibility of this method when fabricating custom gratings. Recently, the NORIA FBG inscription device (Northlab Photonics, Nacka, Sweden) has been industrialized: this device encapsulates the whole system for FBG fabrication, including a set of phase masks, which can be interchanged during fabrication, making the fabrication of large volume of FBGs and FBG arrays easier.

3.6.3 Direct inscription

While the phase mask shifts the complexity of generating the interfering pattern of the grating into a diffractive element, direct inscription (such as the point-by-point technique, PbP) uses the capability of modern fs lasers to create localized and permanent damages to the fiber structure to create periodical structures, such as the FBG.

Direct inscription of FBGs achieves a periodic modulation of the refractive index by means of a fs laser focused onto the fiber core. Martinez et al. (Martinez, Dubov, Khrushchev, & Bennion, 2004) reported a pivotal work on PbP inscription of an FBG into a silica fiber, a method that has been subsequently used in the fabrication of FBG and FBG arrays. With this method, a fs laser is used as a light source to induce localized photosensitivity; in Martinez's work, the laser was a 150-fs pulsed laser with 1 kHz repetition rate, 300–1000 nJ pulse energy, and 800 nm emission wavelength. The fiber (SMF) hosting the grating has been placed on a two-dimensional translation stage, which allows scanning the grating length, as it occurs for phase mask method as well. Each laser pulse produces one pitch of the grating, thus the translation stage is used to modulate the period of the Bragg grating. Given that f_{RR} is the repetition rate frequency of the laser, with the PbP method the speed v_z of the translation stage along the z direction, that is, the fiber length, is set as $v_z = \Lambda \cdot f_{RR}$, and therefore the

resulting Bragg wavelength is equal to $\lambda_B = 2n_{eff}\ v_z/f_{RR}$. Direct inscription method using pulses having length of few hundreds femtoseconds operate with typical repetition rate of 1–10 kHz, thus 1550-nm gratings are inscribed with axial speed of $v_z \approx 0.5-5$ mm/s. Poeggel et al. later in 2016 (Poeggel et al., 2016) showed the possibility of inscribing FBGs using PbP method, as well
as sawtooth-shaped scanning figures, into Fabry-Perot interferometers, opening the possibility for dual FBG-interferometer sensing, which can ensure temperature compensation in RI sensors.

Direct method inscription provides much more flexibility than phase mask method, since the scanning speed and the waveform applied on the two-dimensional translation stage encodes the whole properties of the grating, making it easier to fabricate gratings of any type as well as arrays of gratings. However, PbP-inscribed gratings have, in general, a nonideal shape and a lower repeatability, since much of the grating spectral characteristics depend on the focusing of the fs laser into the FBG core, which is hard to control and can deteriorate over time.

3.6.4 LPG fabrication

Since LPG have a much longer periodicity than FBGs, direct inscription methods are typically used while phase masks are not effective in inscribing such devices. A method that has been perfected by Parthenope University (Italy), and subsequently reported for LPG sensors on different types of fibers due to its simplicity and the fact that it does not require a UV/KrF light source, is based on arc-induced LPGs (Esposito et al., 2018).

The electric arc discharge (EAD) method is a PbP method that fabricates a series of defects into the fiber, which result in a periodical modulation of the refractive index having spatial periodicity equal to the distance between each perturbation. Each defect is fabricated by means of an EAD, a process that is very often used in fiber optics for standard splicing operations, and can be implemented on several fiber splicing machines. The formation of the LPG is due to the stress relaxation of the silica, and to the geometrical defects introduced in the core shape of the fiber exposed to the discharge process. The EAD method requires the electrodes of an electrical arc splicer, and a precision translation stage on which one side of the splicer is mounted. The peculiarity of this method is that it is widely compatible with most electrical splicers, which allow manual operation, while it is not suited for laser-based splicers based on CO_2.

During the EAD-induced fabrication of the grating, one end of the fiber is blocked by the translation stage controlled via software, while the other hand is held at constant tension. When the splicer is then set to perform a single-shot splice, it generates an electrical arc from the electrodes that cross the fiber section, with current of several mA and duration of few hundred milliseconds. The splice operation produces a slight deformation of the fiber, thus the arc is repeated several times in order to create a reasonable variation of the refractive index in the portion of the fiber exposed to the electrodes. In order to perform such operation, it is necessary to have manual control of the splicer, or to program the splicer in order to avoid the fiber alignments and postsplice routines, and directly perform the splice operation repeated times. The selection of the arc intensity, arc duration, and alignment of the electrodes to the fiber results in different type of geometrical defects, and therefore different amplitudes of the refractive index modulation steps. The modulation of the LPG is instead induced by the translation stage, which pulls the fiber backward by a predefined amount (which corresponds to the pitch of the grating). This way, multiple sections of the fiber are exposed to the repeated splices, all interleaved by the pitch of the grating Λ.

The EAD method has been applied to different types of fiber, and results in LPG having periodicity of 300–700 μm with good and repeatable spectral characteristics. The dual control of the splicer and the micropositioner (e.g., exploiting LabVIEW's GPIB interfaces) allows an automated fabrication of the LPG.

References

Allsop, T., Floreani, F., Jedrzejewski, K. P., Marques, P. V., Romero, R., & Webb, D. J. (2006). Bennion I. Spectral characteristics of tapered LPG device as a sensing element for refractive index and temperature. *Journal of lightwave technology, 24*(2), 870–878.

Ayupova, T., Sypabekova, M., Molardi, C., Bekmurzayeva, A., Shaimerdenova, M., Dukenbayev, K., & Tosi, D. (2019). Wavelet-based demodulation of multimode etched fiber Bragg grating refractive index sensor. *Sensors, 19*(1), 39.

Bekmurzayeva, A., Dukenbayev, K., Shaimerdenova, M., Bekniyazov, I., Ayupova, T., Sypabekova, M., ... Tosi, D. (2018). Etched fiber Bragg grating biosensor functionalized with aptamers for detection of thrombin. *Sensors, 18*(12), 4298.

Caucheteur, C., Loyez, M., González-Vila, Á., & Wattiez, R. (2018). Evaluation of gold layer configuration for plasmonic fiber grating biosensors. *Optics Express, 26*(18), 24154–24163.

Chryssis, A. N., Lee, S. M., Lee, S. B., Saini, S. S., & Dagenais, M. (2005). High sensitivity evanescent field fiber Bragg grating sensor. *IEEE Photonics Technology Letters, 17*(6), 1253–1255.

Cięszczyk, S., Kisała, P., & Mroczka, J. (2019). New parameters extracted from tilted fiber Bragg grating spectra for the determination of the refractive index and cut-off wavelength. *Sensors, 19*(9), 1964.

Dong, X., Zhang, H., Liu, B., & Miao, Y. (2011). Tilted fiber Bragg gratings: principle and sensing applications. *Photonic Sensors, 1*(1), 6–30.

Erdogan, T. (1997). Fiber grating spectra. *Journal of Lightwave Technology, 15*(8), 1277–1294.

Esposito, F., Ranjan, R., Campopiano, S., & Iadicicco, A. (2018). Arc-induced long period gratings from standard to polarization-maintaining and photonic crystal fibers. *Sensors, 18*(3), 918.

Guo, T., Liu, F., Guan, B. O., & Albert, J. (2016). Tilted fiber grating mechanical and biochemical sensors. *Optics & Laser Technology, 78*, 19–33.

Hill, K. O., et al. (1993). Bragg gratings fabricated in monomode photosensitive optical fiber by UV exposure through a phase mask. *Applied Physics Letters, 62*, 1035–1037.

Iadicicco, A., & Campopiano, S. (2015). Sensing features of long period gratings in hollow core fibers. *Sensors, 15*(4), 8009–8019.

Iadicicco, A., Cusano, A., Campopiano, S., Cutolo, A., & Giordano, M. (2005). Thinned fiber Bragg gratings as refractive index sensors. *IEEE Sensors Journal, 5*(6), 1288–1295.

Iadicicco, A., Cusano, A., Cutolo, A., Bernini, R., & Giordano, M. (2004). Thinned fiber Bragg gratings as high sensitivity refractive index sensor. *IEEE Photonics Technology Letters, 16*(4), 1149–1151.

Kersey, A. D., Davis, M. A., Patrick, H. J., LeBlanc, M., Koo, K. P., Askins, C. G., ... Friebele, E. J. (1997). Fiber grating sensors. *Journal of lightwave technology, 15*(8), 1442–1463.

Korganbayev, S., Ayupova, T., Sypabekova, M., Bekmurzayeva, A., Shaimerdenova, M., Dukenbayev, K., ... Tosi, D. (2018). Partially etched chirped fiber Bragg grating (pECFBG) for joint temperature, thermal profile, and refractive index detection. *Optics Express, 26* (14), 18708–18720.

Lemaire, P. J., et al. (1993). High-pressure H_2 loading as a technique for achieving ultrahigh UV photosensitivity and thermal sensitivity in GeO_2 doped optical fibres,". *Electronics Letters, 29*, 1191–1193.

Liang, W., Huang, Y., Xu, Y., Lee, R. K., & Yariv, A. (2005). Highly sensitive fiber Bragg grating refractive index sensors. *Applied Physics Letters, 86*(15), 151122.

Martinez, A., Dubov, M., Khrushchev, I., & Bennion, I. (2004). Direct writing of fibre Bragg gratings by femtosecond laser. *Electronics Letters, 40*(19), 1170–1172.

Meltz, G., Morey, W. W., & Glenn, W. H. (1989). Formation of Bragg gratings in optical fibers by a transverse holographic method. *Optics Letters, 14*, 823–825.

Othonos, A., & Kalli, K. (1999). *Fiber Bragg gratings: fundamentals and applications in telecommunications and sensing*. Boston, MA: Artech house.

Poeggel, S., Duraibabu, D., Lacraz, A., Kalli, K., Tosi, D., Leen, G., & Lewis, E. (2016). Femtosecond-laser based inscription technique for post Fibre-Bragg grating inscription in an extrinsic Fabry-Perot interferometer Pressure Sensor. *IEEE Sensors Journal, 16*(10), 3396–3402.

Shaimerdenova, M., Bekmurzayeva, A., Sypabekova, M., & Tosi, D. (2017). Interrogation of coarsely sampled Tilted Fiber Bragg Grating (TFBG) sensors with KLT. *Optics Express, 25* (26), 33487–33496.

Shen, F., Zhou, K., Gordon, N., Zhang, L., & Shu, X. (2017). Compact eccentric long period grating with improved sensitivity in low refractive index region. *Optics Express, 25*(14), 15729–15736.

Śmietana, M., Koba, M., Mikulic, P., & Bock, W. J. (2016). Towards refractive index sensitivity of long-period gratings at level of tens of μm per refractive index unit: Fiber cladding etching and nano-coating deposition. *Optics Express, 24*(11), 11897–11904.

Socorro-Leranoz, A. B., Santano, D., Del Villar, I., & Matias, I. R. (2019). Trends in the design of wavelength-based optical fibre biosensors (2008–2018). *Biosensors and Bioelectronics: X*, 100015.

Sypabekova, M., Korganbayev, S., González-Vila, Á., Caucheteur, C., Shaimerdenova, M., Ayupova, T., ... Tosi, D. (2019). Functionalized etched tilted fiber Bragg grating aptasensor for label-free protein detection. *Biosensors and Bioelectronics*, 111765.

Tang, J., Fu, C., Bai, Z., Liao, C., & Wang, Y. (2018). Sensing characteristics of tilted long period fiber gratings inscribed by infrared femtosecond laser. *Sensors, 18*(9), 3003.

Tosi, D., & Perrone, G. (2017). *Optical fiber sensors for biomedical applications*. Artech House, ISBN: 978-1630811525.

Viveiros, D., de Almeida, J. M., Coelho, L., Vasconcelos, H., Amorim, V. A., Maia, J. M., & Jorge, P. A. (2019). Spectral tuning of long period fiber gratings fabricated by femtosecond laser micromachining through thermal annealing. *Proceedings 2019, 15*(1), 4.

Yu, J., Wu, Z., Yang, X., Han, X., & Zhao, M. (2018). Tilted fiber Bragg grating sensor using chemical plating of a palladium membrane for the detection of hydrogen leakage. *Sensors, 18*(12), 4478.

4

Tapered and photonic crystal fibers

4.1 Tapered fiber

4.1.1 Introduction to tapered fibers

Conventionally, an optical fiber is defined as dielectric waveguide presenting cylindrical symmetry. The light propagation in such a structure is possible because an internal cylindrical structure, known as core, presents a refractive index higher than the surrounding structure. The characteristic of the light confinement and the number of modes that can propagate in the fiber are directly dependent on the radius of the core and the refractive index contrast between the core and the cladding (Saleh & Teich, 2019). A typical material for optical fibers is silica glass that can be doped in different way with other components to increase or decrease the optical index. Other materials, belong to plastic families, such as poly(methyl methacrylate), polystyrene, and polycarbonates, can be used for optical fibers. Because of the simple geometry of optical fibers and because of the versatility of the optical materials usually used for optical fibers, microfabrication and microstructuration of optical fibers can offer profound advantage for the use as fiber sensor. Microfabrication techniques include etching, tapering, side-polishing, and other more advanced micromachining techniques that make use of femtosecond lasers.

The process of fiber tapering is exploited for a large number of devices in photonics including power couplers, add-drop multiplexers, microresonators, sensors, and biosensors (Korposh, James, Lee, & Tatam, 2019; Love et al., 1991). Regarding fiber optics sensing, the use of tapered fibers has greatly increased in the last decades (Xu, Lu, Chen, & Bao, 2017), mainly because of the relative simplicity in fabrication, boosted by advanced equipment that permits a decent level of reproducibility. An example can be identified in the Fujikura LZM-100, a CO_2 laser splicer, which includes an automated routine for tapers (LaserFocusWorld, 2019). The sensing principles of tapered fibers can rely on two physical principles, one is the enhancement of the evanescent field and the second is the onset of an interferometric properties, both of them are related to the geometry of the tapered fiber.

Optical Fiber Biosensors.
DOI: https://doi.org/10.1016/B978-0-12-819467-6.00017-2

4.1.2 Geometry of tapered fibers

The process of tapering an optical fiber is generally achieved by heating a portion of the fiber while the fiber terminations undergo to a controlled traction. This operation results in the thinning of the heated portion of the fiber according to a profile depicted in Fig. 4.1. The tapered fiber, or fiber taper, or simply taper is divided into five regions. The external regions are represented by the unmodified optical fiber, characterized by a radius r_0, in this area the fiber does not present any evidence of stretching. The central area is represented by the thinned fiber or **taper waist region**, stretched by the combined action of the heat source and the applied tension. The waist region is uniformly thinned to a radius of r_w, for a length of l_w. The external and central regions are connected by two **transition regions**, presenting a length of z_0, called **down-taper** and **up-taper**. In these regions, the radius of the fiber is continuously modified from its maximum value of r_0 to its minimum value of r_w, according to a shape function $r(z)$ (Birks & Li, 1992). In Fig. 4.1, the two transition regions (up-taper and down-taper) are represented with mirror symmetry, which is the usual case for common tapers, so that also the left shape function presents mirror symmetry with the right shape function. When the shape function is approximately a straight line, which represents a sort of ideal case, the tapered fiber takes the name of **biconical-tapered fiber** (Latifi, Zibaii, & Hosseini, 2012). In this case, it is possible to identify a **taper angle** θ, such that $\theta = \tan^{-1}((r_0 - r_w)/z_0)$, that represents the slope which brings from the unstretched region to the waist region.

It is worth noting that the taper fabrication maintains, in principles, the ratio between the core and the cladding diameters of the optical fiber also in the waist region. As an example, we can consider an SMF-28 that presents a core with diameter of 10 μm and a cladding with diameter of 125 μm. If this fiber undergoes to a tapering process that scales the diameter of the fiber by a factor of 10, the final product will result in a tapered fiber that presents a waist region characterized by a cladding diameter of 12.5 μm and a core diameter of 1 μm. In this respect, the operation of tapering is structurally different from the operation of fiber etching, even if the geometrical result is comparable since both the

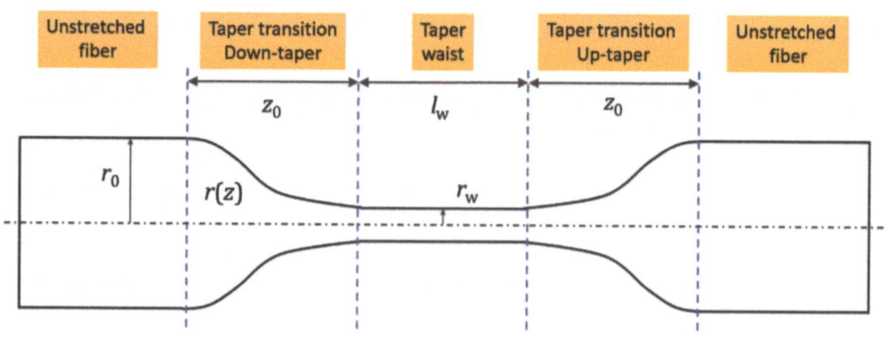

Figure 4.1 Schematic of the generic tapered fiber, with underlined the main geometrical parameters.

microfabrication methods arrive to create a thinned region in the fiber. However, the etching consists of the cladding removal to expose the fiber core while the fiber tapering consists of a scaling of the fiber which maintains the internal proportion. From the sensing principles point of view, the etched fiber works always as an evanescent field-based sensor, while the tapered fiber can be both an evanescent field sensor and an interferometric sensor. The discrimination is basically enclosed in the function that describes the transition region, or in the case of biconical tapers enclosed in the tapering angle θ.

4.1.3 Physical principles of tapered fibers

Despite the large number of different kinds of possible tapered fibers geometries, a tapered fiber can be classified into two different families following the physical nature of the light propagation: **adiabatic tapered fibers**, also known as **gradual taper**, and **nonadiabatic tapered fibers** or **abrupt taper**.

The difference between these two kinds of families is given by the behavior of light propagation. In an adiabatic taper, the core modes of interest that propagate in the fiber, typically LP_{01} and LP_{11} in a few modes fiber or simply LP_{01} in an SMF-28, experience negligible loses in the transition between the unstretched region and the waist region. Looking at the question from a different perspective, the mode confinement in the waist region remains of good level, and the energy transported by the mode is roughly preserved with respect to the energy of the mode in the unstretched fiber. For this reason, the taper is defined adiabatic. On the other hand, when the transition between the unstarched region and the waist region causes considerable losses of energy of the core modes in the cladding region of the waist (usually the LP_{01} mode of the unstretched fiber becomes coupled with HE_{11} and HE_{12} modes of the waist region), the taper is called nonadiabatic. The geometry of the taper is directly related to its adiabatic or nonadiabatic behavior. A transition region that connects the unstretched fiber to the waist with a gradual and smooth taper angle will foster the formation of an adiabatic taper, while a steep transition will result in the formation of a nonadiabatic taper. The difference between adiabatic and nonadiabatic tapered fibers is shown in Fig. 4.2 (Zibaii et al., 2010). From the

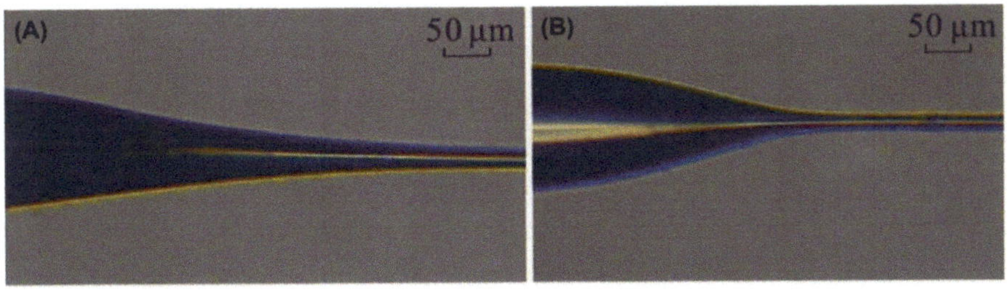

Figure 4.2 Microscope picture of an adiabatic taper (A) and of a nonadiabatic taper (B) (Zibaii et al., 2010) (Creative Commons CC).

microscope pictures depicted in Fig. 4.2A and B, it is easy to clearly identify the difference in the taper profile and the taper angle that results in a different taper behavior.

Nevertheless, a simple investigation of the taper angle is not enough to identify the adiabatic or the nonadiabatic properties of the fiber. A more specific **adiabatic criterion** can be used to verify the adiabatic properties. The criterion can be expressed using the following formula:

$$\Theta = \left|\frac{dr}{dz}\right| \leq \frac{r(\beta_1 - \beta_2)}{2\pi}, \tag{4.1}$$

where r represents the taper profile function $r(z)$, and β_1 and β_2 are, respectively, the local propagation constants, in the transition, of the mode of interest (LP_{01}) and the mode to which power is most likely to be lost becoming the first cladding mode of the taper region. The adiabatic criterion stated that the derivative of the profile function must be lower than radius divided by the beat length, so that no exchange of the core energy is allowed in the taper (Brambilla, 2010; Love et al., 1991).

Given the adiabatic criterion, strictly related to the onset of an exchange of energy between two modes mainly in the waist region, it is possible to identify the physical principles that make tapered fiber an adequate sensor and biosensor devices. Both adiabatic and nonadiabatic tapered fibers, presenting a thinned waist region that can come in contact with the analyte to measure, show an improvement of penetration of the evanescent wave field (EWF) in the waist region (Latifi et al., 2012; Leung, Shankar, & Mutharasan, 2007). Moar et al. investigated such an improvement of the EWF by using a near-field optical microscope (SNOM) and proposed a numerical analysis based on beam propagation method to estimate the intensity of the filed (Moar et al., 1999). The result of their measurement is shown in Fig. 4.3. The EWF presents an exponential increase by moving the SNOM probe near the surface of the taper waist region. The proposed numerical method is in close agreement with the experimental results.

The enhanced penetration depth is therefore the key to the sensing principle, as it permits a stronger interaction between the light propagating in the fiber taper and the external environment to test. In principles, there are two methods that can be used to measure the change associated with the interaction between the EWF and the external analyte:

- The detection of the light losses within the tapered region.
- The interferometric method which derives from the change of refractive indices of the modes propagating through the taper.

The second method is more suitable for the nonadiabatic tapers since the coupling between the mode LP_{01} to the cladding modes of the taper induces a periodic exchange of energy between core and cladding modes by producing an interference figure. The mechanism of the interference onset is shown in Fig. 4.4A (Korposh et al., 2019). The LP_{01} mode of the incoming unstretched fiber generally couples to the HE_{11} and HE_{12} modes of the tapered waist, which propagates with different effective indices along the taper waist and interferes when recombines to the outcoming unstretched end fiber. A typical interference pattern obtained from a tapered fiber with a waist diameter of 10 μm is shown in Fig. 4.4B (Jarzebinska et al., 2012).

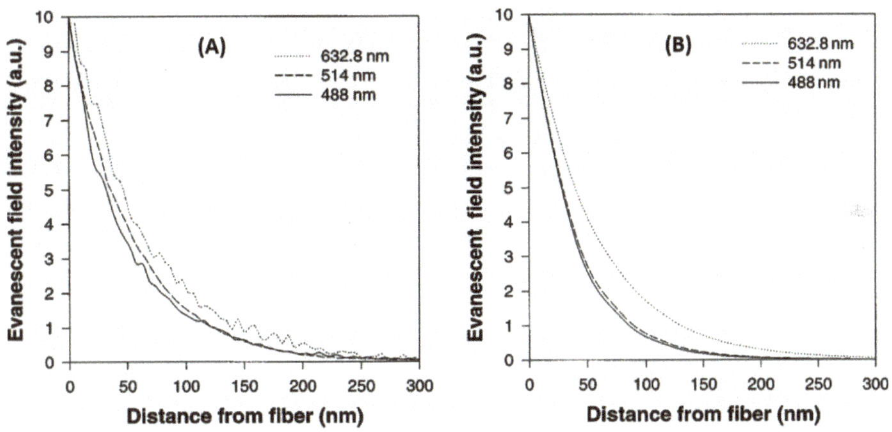

Figure 4.3 Measured evanescent field intensity versus the distance from the fiber surface located in the waist region (A); estimated field intensity by using a beam propagation algorithm (B) (Moar et al., 1999). Source: *Reproduced with the permission of AIP.*

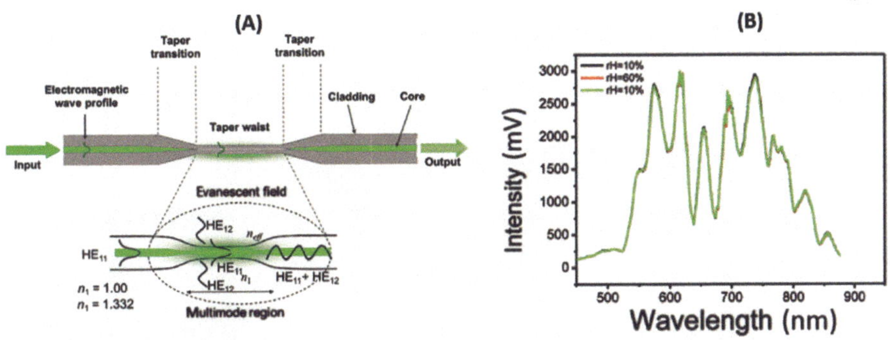

Figure 4.4 Schematic of the coupling of the LP_{01} mode to HE_{11} and HE_{12} modes in the tapered region. The interference patterns then channeled into the output fiber end (A) (Korposh et al., 2019) (Creative Commons CC). Typical transmission spectrum of a nonadiabatic taper of 10 μm of diameter (B) (Jarzebinska et al., 2012). Source: *Reproduced with the permission of T&F Online.*

Regarding adiabatic tapers, losses can be considered negligible, and the penetration depth of the EWF is more limited compared to the nonadiabatic tapers case, where the coupled waist modes can easily interact with the environment at the cladding interface. Reducing too much of the waist diameter can be detrimental since the adiabatic propagation of the LP_{01} mode is diffraction limited (Brambilla, 2010).

Said so, when such a tapered fiber is to be used as a sensor, it is convenient to coat the central part of waist region with an appropriate transducer (i.e., a thin metal layer or a functionalization layer). If the transducer is deposited uniformly around the taper waist, the fiber sensors become polarization independent. This strategy offers certain advantages in sensors on the basis of surface plasmon resonance (SPR) (Villatoro, Monzón-Hernández, & Mejía, 2003). Another method to enhance the interaction between the sensor and the external environment by using an adiabatic taper is to bend the fiber taper waist in an U-shape to improve the penetration depth of the EWF. This represents a good solution since the taper waist is not extremely thin, so that it maintains a certain robustness to permit the bending. In this case, the sensing principle can be identified in the fluctuation of output power at fixed wavelength (Villatoro et al., 2003).

4.1.4 Methods for tapered fiber fabrication

The main idea that brings to the fabrication of an optical fiber taper relies on the operation of **heating and stretching** the fiber. This fabrication method consists of simple operations. At the beginning, a short section, located in the middle of the fiber, is prepared by removing the external polymer coating by a mechanical stripper or by a proper chemical etching. Then the fiber tails are inserted in traction stages. Finally, a heat source is positioned under the section of the fiber where the coating has been removed as shown in Fig. 4.5. The heat sources can be different according to the quality of the taper that are expected. Typically, a heat source can be a flame given by a gas burner, or an arc discharge, or a CO_2 high power laser (Korposh et al., 2019).

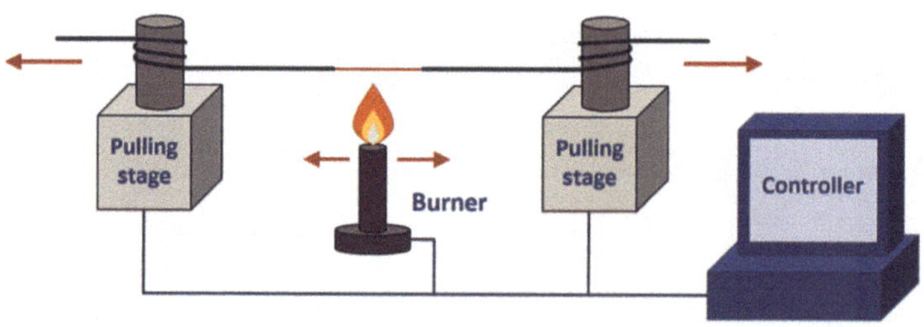

Figure 4.5 Schematic of heating and stretching technique to fabricate a tapered fiber. The fiber tails are connected to two pulling stages, while the uncoated fiber is placed over a heating source, in this case a gas burner. A controller stage is fundamental to achieve a good taper result.

The process of tapering maintains the ratio between the diameters of the core and the cladding of an untapered fiber. In case of adiabatic tapers used for sensing purposes, this results in a good coupling between the core modes of untapered fiber and core modes of tapered fibers, which consequently brings to a reduced exposure of the evanescent field to the external analyte. To facilitate the penetration of the evanescent field in the surrounding medium to sense, different fabrication techniques can be used. Some techniques involve adding a coating to the fiber taper and exploit the SPR. Other ones, that can be considered a sort of hybrid, involve in subsequent microfabrications, like polishing or chemical etching, whose target is to modify the ratio between the core and the cladding diameter in the taper region (Zhang, Dhawan, & Vo-Dinh, 2011).

By using the heating, a stretching tapers of different size and proportions can be fabricated. This is a very important aspect of the fabrication techniques because the characteristics of a tapered fiber, in particular when it is oriented for sensing applications, are determined by the final taper geometry. The taper diameter is fundamental to increase the penetration of the evanescent field in the surrounding material, while the taper transition, smooth or abrupt, determines the operation of the taper. A smooth and long transition region results in an adiabatic taper, whose sensing principles rely on the change of intensity of the evanescent field. An abrupt and short transition region brings the taper sensor to work as an interferometer, where the interference is between the core and the cladding modes excited by the imperfect coupling between the untapered core and the tapered region. In this context, the precise control of the fabrication process and of the choice of the heating source is fundamental to achieve the desired result, as well as the quality of the sensing performances.

The use of a gas burner flame, typically hydrogen, can bring to a tapered fiber with a very small diameter. Nevertheless, the control of the heating parameters is fundamental to achieve a consistent result, and the use of gas burners coupled to artisanal laboratory pulling setup not always can guarantee the required specifications. In fact, the tapers obtained by the use of gas flames are usually fragile and not uniform. To improve the result, more advanced fabrication techniques have been implemented. The most successful is the **flame-brushing technique**, where the gas flame is moved under an optical fiber that is stretched. A precise control of the pulling stage as well as of the flame stage can bring to remarkable results in terms of taper shape precision (Birks & Li, 1992; Brambilla, 2010). However, when taper geometry parameters are critical, or when long tapered region with particularly uniform waist is required, the use of equipment based on CO_2 laser, like the CO_2 laser splicers such as Fujikura LZM-100, brings to superior results. With Fujikura LZM-100, it is possible to fabricate long and uniform adiabatic tapers where taper diameter can be as small as 1/10 of the original fiber diameter, well-controlling the transition region. Moreover, the big advantage of using a CO_2 laser splicer, over other fabrication methods, is the consistency and the repeatability of the final result as well as the robustness of the obtained taper.

4.2 Biosensors based on tapered fiber

Tapered fibers represent an interesting platform for biosensing, since the thinned structure of the taper is well suitable to interact with an external biosample to detect. Among the two main principles of operation of a tapered fiber, the first one is based on the detection of the transmission fluctuation, typical of adiabatic tapers, and the second one is based on the onset of an interferometric pattern, occurring in nonadiabatic tapers, and can be successfully exploited for biosensing. Since both principles of operation rely on the enhancement of the evanescent field and its improved interaction with the external environment, the tapered region of the fiber represents a perfect place to develop the interaction with bio or the chemical samples. Typically, the interaction can be summarized in two kind of detections. The first one is when the biosample is in a liquid solution, so that the biosensor becomes a refractive index sensor for detecting the concentration of the sample in the solution. The second one is when the tapered region is functionalized by a proper chemical ligand which can capture and immobilized the biosample to detect. In this case, the detection relies on the change of propagation property given by the new external layer.

In principle, the interferometric sensors are preferred for the superior sensitivity. Moreover, in the case of transmission-based tapered sensors, the enhancement of the sensitivity is always accompanied to the extreme reduction of the taper waist, bringing to an enhancement of the fragility of the sensor (Latifi et al., 2012). Nevertheless, both the examples have been investigated and proposed in literature. In 2008, Leung et al. introduced the detection of bovine serum albumin (BSA), in a flow cell configuration, by using antibody-immobilized tapered fiber biosensor (Leung, Shankar, & Mutharasan, 2008). The taper has been fabricated with a waist diameter of roughly 5–10 μm, while the total lengths of the taper have been calculated in between 1000 and 1200 μm. The taper waist region has been housed in a close holder to permit the flow in the cell. The immobilization of the antibodies has been achieved after a process of silanization of the silica surface with APTES. Several detection experiments were performed by exposing the functionalized surface to flow of BSA solution varying from 1 pg/mL to 10 ng/mL and measuring the transmission at 1310 and 1550 nm. The results clearly show that the transmission of the tapered fiber is a function of the refractive index of the analyte solution surrounding the taper. The transmission is also dependent on the wavelength.

A different strategy has been followed by Zibaii et al. who fabricated a nonadiabatic fiber taper by the method of heat pulling and using a CO_2 laser as a heat source. Their sensor, therefore, exploits the interferometric effect of the taper. The experimental section has been organized to exploit the sensor to detect the variation in refractive index in solutions with low concentration of D-glucose and in solutions containing both amino acids and carbohydrates. The sensor has been demonstrated to be highly efficient because of the high sensitivity and the low cost of the fabrication. The limit of detection of refractive index measurement has been calculated to be 8.2×10^{-6} in a large range of indices going from 1.3330 to 1.3447. Moreover, the authors demonstrated the interaction between different amino acids with different carbohydrates solution in terms of variation of refractive index. With respect to the previous example, the interferometric effect permits a higher sensitivity of the measurement, but the functionalization, on the other hand, offers advantages in terms of selectivity of the analyte to be detected.

The detection method based on functionalization can be associated to the interferometric-based tapered fiber sensor. In 2019, Sun et al. proposed an aptamer biosensor for label-free thrombin detection (Sun, Sun, Guo, & Guan, 2019). The sensor has been fabricated from a commercial double cladding fiber with the flame-brushing technique, to obtain a nonadiabatic taper of 5 μm waist, which presents a clear interferometric pattern of transmission. The surface of the taper has been prepared by creating a functionalization of thrombin-binding aptamers. The results demonstrated a very high sensitivity of 1660 nm/RIU and a high level of accuracy, since the sensor has been able to detect the thrombin in solution containing concentration of 0.1 μm. Moreover, the sensor showed high specificity in various concentrations of pure and mixed thrombin solutions.

4.3 Photonic crystal fiber-based sensors

4.3.1 Introduction to photonic crystal fibers and microstructured fiber

To fully understand the scientific reason which have brought to the concept of **microstructured** fibers and, particularly to, p**hotonic crystal fibers** (PCFs), it is necessary to highlight one of the most important aspect of conventional step-index optical fibers, which is represented by the principle of guidance. In conventional fibers, the light is guided in the core because the presence of a cladding region around the core. Because core and cladding present different refractive indices, precisely the refractive index of the core is slightly higher with respect to the refractive of the cladding, the guidance is guaranteed by the total internal reflection (TIR) between core and cladding interface. Even if this is a simplified vision of step-index fiber guidance, whose complete understanding derives from the application of Maxwell equations, this guidance principle states two important concepts:

- The guidance can be achieved only in solid core fiber, with higher refractive index with respect to the surrounding material.
- The control of the guidance and modal properties is constrained by technological limitations of engineering the optical material of the fibers.

It is from the idea to overcome these two limitations that in 1996 a real breakthrough appeared in the optical fiber technology with the development of PCFs (Russell, 2003). A PCF, sometimes called microstructured fiber, is an optical waveguide that does not present a well-defined core as well a well-defined cladding. Instead, the PCFs present a cladding made of silica and a lattice of air holes, distributed in a periodic pattern, that go through all the length of the fiber along the propagation direction. PCFs are, therefore, a special kind of 2D photonic crystals that is built around the central area of the fiber which represents the core. Typical cross sections of PCFs and microstructured are depicted in the schematic of Fig. 4.6.

The advantages of PCFs are related to the fact that the fiber is made of a single material, usually pure silica, so there is no need for a complex optical material engineering to achieve the guidance. In fact, it is the geometry of the fiber, in particular the distance of the holes, called **pitch** Λ, and their **diameter** $\boldsymbol{d}$, to determine the guidance properties of the fiber, Fig. 4.6A. The presence of a microstructured holey cladding can be considered equivalent to a solid cladding where it is possible to finely tune the index contrast. Moreover, exploiting the physical properties derived by the photonic crystals, it is possible to confine the light in a hollow core, thus permitting the guidance in air as in Fig. 4.6B.

PCFs present interesting properties in terms of attenuation, in particular in the hollow core PCFs (HC-PCFs), and in terms of dispersion, which can be tuned by modifying the geometry of the holes. The advent of PCFs has not substituted the standard step index fibers, which remains a better and cheaper choice for telecom applications. Nevertheless, PCFs have gained an important role in

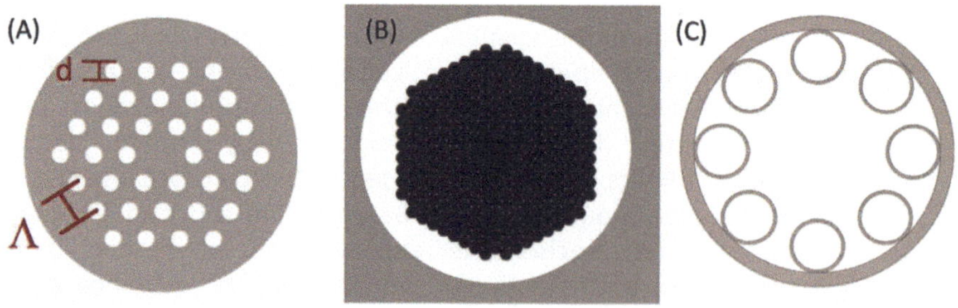

Figure 4.6 Schematic of a solid core photonic crystal fiber (PCF), the cladding is characterized by a regular pattern of holes, which present a distance hole-to-hole (pitch) Λ and diameter d (A). Schematic of a hollow core fibers: PCF with band-gap oriented design (B) and microstructured fiber presenting an antiresonant design (C).

optical fiber technology. There are, indeed, some fields of application that can be greatly benefitted from the PCFs properties. Among them, the request for very large mode area fibers in the last stage of amplification in high power fiber lasers has triggered the design of new and innovative PCFs, where it is possible to achieve extremely large cores while maintaining single mode operation (Coscelli, Molardi, Cucinotta, & Selleri, 2014; Jauregui, Limpert, & Tunnermann, 2013). Another interesting and growing field of application is the use of PCFs for sensing. Since PCFs present holes in their geometric structures, not only in the cladding but also the core in the case of HC-PCFs, they represent a perfect platform for sensing. The holes can be infiltrated with gas or with chemical solutions, and because the guidance properties can significantly change according to the refractive index of the solution, the capability of PCF sensors are huge (Cubillas et al., 2013). Moreover, the holes in the microstructured fiber can be functionalized with reagents for selectively capturing of biomolecules, so that to permit the creation of sensitive label-free sensors (Barozzi et al., 2017). In general, it is possible to address the PCF as a versatile structure for sensing applications, where the interaction of the evanescent field with the analyte to be detected can be enhanced by properly designing the geometry of the microstructure of the fiber.

4.3.2 Type, geometry, and guidance of photonic crystal fibers

Microstructured fibers can be divided into two big families, those presenting a solid core and those presenting a hollow core. Before to continue the explanation, it is better to clarify a point which is of fundamental importance for understanding the principles of guidance in microstructured fibers. There is a common practice to interchange indifferently the term "photonic crystal fiber" with "microstructured fibers," which derives by the observation that the principles of guidance can be assimilated under some macrocategories. In a more precise description, the term "microstructured fiber" refers to all the optical fibers that present a microstructuration of the cladding, while the term "photonic crystal fiber" refers to the fibers that present a microstructured cladding whose pattern is periodic and can be assimilated to a 2D photonic crystal, like the schematic of the fiber shown in Fig. 4.6A which demonstrates a pattern of hole arranged according to a triangular pattern. Therefore a PCF is a microstructured fiber, but a microstructured fiber is not, in strict sense, necessarily a PCF. An example can be retrieved in the work of Coscelli et al. where a microstructured solid core fiber with an aperiodic holey cladding has been studied to increase the mode area (Coscelli, Molardi, Masruri, Cucinotta, & Selleri, 2014). Similar consideration can be done in the domain of hollow core fiber. Fig. 4.6B and C depicts two schematics of hollow core fibers, the first one is a PCF, in the strict definition, the second one is an antiresonant microstructured fiber.

The tendency to use indifferently the terms PCF or microstructured fiber is extensively justified by the mechanisms of guidance of this kind of fibers presenting patterns of holes in the cladding regions, which can be, under certain hypothesis, considered similar. There are basically three mechanisms guidance, the **modified total internal reflection** (mTIR), the p**hotonic band gap** (PBG) guidance, and a**ntiresonant reflecting optical waveguide** (ARROW).

4.3.2.1 Modified total internal reflection

The guidance by mTIR is given by the presence of holes in the cladding while the core is represented by a solid silica region. The mTIR is, indeed, comparable to the standard TIR of step index fibers. The mechanism of TIR relies on the presence of two different glasses, one used for the core and another used for the cladding, whose refractive indices are slightly different. In particular, the refractive index of the core is larger than the one of the cladding. This permits to obtain, at the interface between core and cladding, a TIR. The propagation constant β of the modes guided in the step index fiber is limited by the properties of the core and cladding materials, according to the following formula:

$$n_{cl}k_0 \leq \beta \leq n_{co}k_0, \tag{4.2}$$

where n_{co} and n_{cl} are, respectively, the refractive index of the core and the cladding, and k_0 is the wavevector of the vacuum. In a PCF, because of the presence of air holes, the virtual refractive index of the cladding is, again, lower with respect to the refractive index of the central area made of silica, which represents the core. In this case, the difference is that the virtual refractive index of the cladding is a function of the wavelength of the light propagating inside the fiber.

$$n_{cl}(\lambda)k_0 \leq \beta \leq n_{co}k_0. \tag{4.3}$$

This fact presents a fundamental consequence in the guidance of the PCF, which is related to the distance between the holes Λ, and to the diameter of the holes d. It is well-known that in an optical fiber the number of propagating modes can be estimated by the use of the V-number. This is also valid in a PCF and the V-number assumes the following formula:

$$V = \frac{2\pi\Lambda}{\lambda}\sqrt{n_{co}^2 + n_{cl}^2(\lambda)}. \tag{4.4}$$

Since the virtual refractive index of the cladding is wavelength dependent, it is clear that the geometric parameters of the cladding hole pattern are fundamental for understanding the guidance properties of modes. In particular, a deep analysis of this kind of PCF brings to the conclusion that, for values of $d/\Lambda < 0.43$, the PCF supports the propagation of only one mode, the fundamental mode. Moreover, since the d/Λ does not depend on λ, the PCF remains single mode for virtually every wavelength. This peculiar property, typical of PCFs, is called **endlessly single-mode**. The mTIR is, therefore, similar but not identical to the standard TIR, and it permits to understand the guidance of the PCF and microstructured fibers.

4.3.2.2 Photonic band-gap guidance

An HC-PCF presents a cladding composed by a periodic lattice of glass capillaries. This creates a structure comparable to a photonic crystal that surrounds a region that is maintained empty, called hollow core. It is evident that in a hollow core fiber, the guidance cannot be explained by the principle of mTIR, since the refractive index in the core is lower than the average of the refractive index of the cladding. The effective index β/k_0 of the guided modes in the hollow core is less than the refractive index of the air which is equal to 1. To explain the guidance in the empty core in this condition, it is necessary to invoke the theory of PBG. Like band gap in electronic structures, where electrons can achieve only particular energies located in specific bands, PBG is defined as the wavelength range where the structure cannot absorb light or allow light propagation. In photonics structures, this particular behavior is obtained by the use periodic dielectric structures. The periodicity of the photonic crystal cladding defines the range of wavelengths that are not allowed to propagate in the fiber. The physical mechanism of light diffraction can be effectively used to explain the origin of the PBG. Because of the multiple diffraction imposed by periodic structure, which implies the formation of PBG, the light is reflected and confined inside the core. As a matter of principle, the band gap can be tailored by acting on the structure periodicity and on the refractive index of the thin glass structure used to create the photonic crystal. The bridges of silica are necessary to create a robust structure, nevertheless their excessive thickness can be detrimental for the onset of the band gap, so a significant filling fractions of holes over silica is necessary to permit the propagation in the core. The HC-PCFs usually present a large core, extremely low propagation losses and they are relatively insensitive to bending (Russell, 2003).

4.3.2.3 Antiresonant reflecting optical waveguide

There are microstructured hollow core fibers whose guidance cannot be justified with the presence of a PBG. An example is shown in Fig. 4.6C, which depicts a negative curvature hollow core fiber. The core of this fiber is not characterized by a photonic crystal-like structure. The numerical analysis shows that this family of fibers does not present a band gap. The confinement of the modes inside the hollow core is similar to the one obtained in the HC-PCFs, but the propagation presents higher losses, which justifies the absence of a band gap. To explain the guidance in this fiber, it is possible to use the ARROW model (Yu & Knight, 2016). Each higher refractive index layer, such as the ones of the silica bridges used to create the structure, can be assimilated as part of a Fabry–Perot resonator. The presence of multiple resonators can be used to explain the confinement in the air core. In particular, the wavelengths that cannot resonate with the silica bridges are rejected and confined in the hollow core of the fiber. These microstructured hollow core fibers, even not presenting a photonic crystal cladding and a PBG guidance, are compared to HC-PCF in terms of properties and applications. In the field of fiber sensing, in fact, hollow core fiber can be effectively used as sensors by filling the holes with the analyte to detect, by functionalizing the wall of the holes to selectively detect some molecules. The modification of the properties of the holes induces a change of guidance properties that can be detected and analyzed.

4.3.3 Photonic crystal fiber and microstructured fiber for sensing

PCFs and microstructured fibers are relatively new as a sensing device in the field of optical sensing technology. However, for many reasons including the variety of possible designs, the unique guidance characteristics, and the presence of holes that can be used to increase the evanescent field interaction with the external environment, PCFs and microstructured fibers have awakened the interest in the field of optical and photonics sensing technology.

The first major reason that makes PCFs so attractive, and superior to the standard optical fibers, is their cladding geometry that can be varied by changing the size, and the pattern of the holes. The manipulation of the cladding permits to tune several propagation properties of the fibers such as:

- the transmission spectrum,
- the number of modes,
- the attenuation,
- the nonlinear properties,
- the dispersion properties, and
- the birefringence.

In conventional step index fiber, such properties and parameters are far more difficult to be manipulated, and when it is possible the tunability is limited. The second main reason of PCFs attractiveness is the presence of air holes, which play multiple roles in the use of microstructured fiber for sensing applications. The holes give a large possibility to control the interaction between the light and the sample to be analyzed, and therefore, enhancing the penetration of the evanescent field in the analyte. Moreover, microstructured fibers can be hollow core and this fact gives the possibility to directly infiltrate the core with the analyte to be detected. Therefore it is possibly a direct interaction between the guided mode and the sample, difficult to obtain in a standard fiber without complex microfabrications.

Due to the fact that the PCFs and, in general, the microstructured fibers present a large variety of features, many sensing applications are achievable. These include physical and biochemical sensing applications (Pinto & Lopez-Amo, 2012).

4.3.3.1 Physical optic sensors

Physical optical sensors are usually designed to measure parameters like temperature and strain, but other derived properties can be detected as well. This includes physical parameters like displacement, bending, torsion, pressure, and vibration. A special discussion must be opened on the measurement of refractive index, which is a physical parameter that is mostly used to conceptualize and fabricate biological and biochemical optical sensors.

The measurement and monitoring of strain, and the derived properties like bending, displacement, and pressure, are of great interest for a large number of applications, ranging from long range application and structural engineering to precision applications in biomedical engineering. With fiber optics sensors network, it is possible to monitor, in multiple points, civil structures like building and bridges, or controlling the state of kilometers long pipelines, so that improving and simplifying the operation of maintenance. On the other hand, optical fibers strain sensors can be embedded in the medical tool for shape sensing and precision applications (Beisenova et al., 2019). PCFs can be effectively used to detect strain. Han proposed a PCF-based strain sensor that exploits the birefringence of the fiber (Han, 2009). The setup of this sensor is shown in Fig. 4.7. The strain measurement is achieved by configuring a birefringent interferometer based on a polarization maintaining PCF. The interferometric pattern is achieved by inserting the PCF between two linear polarizers. The proposed scheme shows a strain sensitivity of 1.3 pm/$\mu\varepsilon$ in a wide range of strain values ranging from 0 to 1600 $\mu\varepsilon$. This scheme also offers an additional, and interesting property, which is the insensitivity to the temperature variation, so that permitting to decouple the strain and the temperature measurement.

The measurement of temperature is also of great importance. Fiber optics sensor technology offers consistent advantages in terms of precision and accuracy of temperature measurement. The form factor of optical fiber, as well as its compactness, permits a fast measurement over a wide range of temperature. This can involve a large span of applications going from material processing in chemical industries to aerospace applications for monitoring the structure

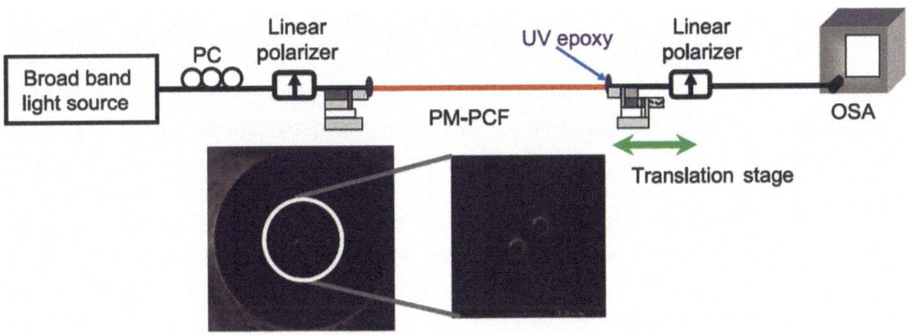

Figure 4.7 Experimental setup proposed by Han for temperature-insensitive strain measurement. The sensors use a birefringent interferometer fabricated using a polarization maintaining PCF (Han, 2009). Source: *Reproduced with the permission of Springer Nature.*

health. The use of PCF for temperature sensing aims to produce new sensors with improved stability and sensitivity. In 2011, Nalawade et al. proposed a high temperature sensor based on modal interferometric technique (Nalawade & Thakur, 2011). The sensor makes use of a strongly nonlinear PCF spliced with a multimode fiber from the broadband source side, and with a single mode fiber from the spectrum analyzer side. The sensor performances show a quite high temperature sensitivity of 73 pm/°C and a remarkable low strain sensitivity of 0.93 pm/$\mu\varepsilon$. Such a sensor permits to obtain a strong decoupling between the measurement of strain and the measurement of temperature, becoming useful in strain applications where an accurate temperature measurement is strictly required.

4.3.3.2 Biological and biochemical sensors

Fiber-based optical sensors represent a consistent platform for bio and chemical sensing. Among the advantages of fiber optics sensors, it is possible to mention the reduced size, the flexibility, the capability of remote sensing, the biocompatibility, and the immunity to electromagnetic interference. The last property is very useful in biomedical applications that involve the simultaneous use of electric and magnetic field, such as magnetic resonance imaging. The main approach for exploiting standard fiber sensors for bio and chemical sensing is to expose the core of the fiber for interacting with the analyte. Another approach involves the enhancement of the evanescent field to interact with the surrounding environment. To achieve such characteristics, standard optical fibers need further microfabrication such as chemical etching, polishing, or tapering. Once the core of the fiber is exposed and the evanescent field penetrates the analyte, the bio and chemical sensing rely mainly on a measurement of refractive index, in case of solutions containing a certain concentration of chemical elements to be detected. On the other hand, the sensor selectivity can be improved by using a coating or a functionalization to bind and enhance the measurement of the molecules or elements to be detected.

In this context, the use of standard optical fibers, with or without fiber Bragg grating (FBG) inscribed inside, represents a solution that presents advantages in terms of cost and reliability and disadvantages in terms of robustness, accuracy, and sensitivity. However, PCFs and microstructured optical fibers offer several unique advantages in chemical and biosensing applications. The presence of air holes along its entire length of the fiber gives the ability to receive samples that present themselves in liquid or gas form. The presence of holes naturally enhances the capability of penetration of the evanescent field, so that, in case of solid core PCF, the first ring of holes can be a perfect space to interact with the light guided in the core. Sometimes, microstructured fibers are purposely built to improve such an interaction. As an example, it is possible to mention suspended core fibers, where a small core is surrounded by oversized holes whose function is both to confine the light in the core and to host the analyte.

But the most interesting advantage of PCFs is the possibility to simultaneously guide light and interact with the analyte such as in the case of HC-PCF, where the core can be filled with the sample to be measured. In this case, the overlap between the light and the sample to measure is maximum, bringing to a very high sensitivity. Eventually, the small size of holes in microstructured fibers, and the strong interaction with the analyte, permit to measure very small quantity of samples, making the PCF sensing solution very attractive for bio applications, such as the detection of protein and DNA in solutions.

4.4 Biosensors using photonic crystal fiber and microstructured fibers

Several demonstrations have been proposed to show the capability of microstructured and PCF to enhance the detection of biomaterial, so that to demonstrate the superior capability of those fibers as selective biosensors. One of the main targets, to make microstructured fibers a consistent platform for biosensing, is to enhance the overlap between the sample to be detected and the guided light in the fiber. This involved the use and the chemical preparation of the hole of the fiber to accept the target samples. This treatment is called functionalization and is mainly required to allow the binding of biological species to the internal glass surface of the holes. Good fiber candidates for this kind of operation are PCFs and microstructured fiber that presents small solid core and large surrounding holes or hollow core fibers, where there is a direct interaction between the guided modes and the analyte.

4.4.1 Functionalized suspended core fiber for specific DNA detection

A particularly good microstructured fiber sensor platform for DNA detection is represented by the **suspended core fiber**, a microstructured fiber that presents a small triangular core, literally suspended in the center of the cross section by three small bridges of silica. The cross section is shown in Fig. 4.8A. The guidance in this small core is guaranteed by the presence of three large holes that characterize the cross section. The big holes represent a good opportunity to functionalize the internal part of the fiber to selectively detect biosamples.

In 2012, Nguyen et al. proposed the use of a suspended core fiber to detect a specific sample of DNA sequence (Nguyen et al., 2012). To achieve the result, the authors immobilized on the internal surface of the core, mainly in the proximity of the core, a molecular beacon (MB). The MB is a type of hairpin structured DNA probe. The immobilization to the external wall of the core is guaranteed by the presence of biotin–streptavidin–biotin attachment technique. The cross section of the fiber, as well as the schematic of immobilization chain is depicted in

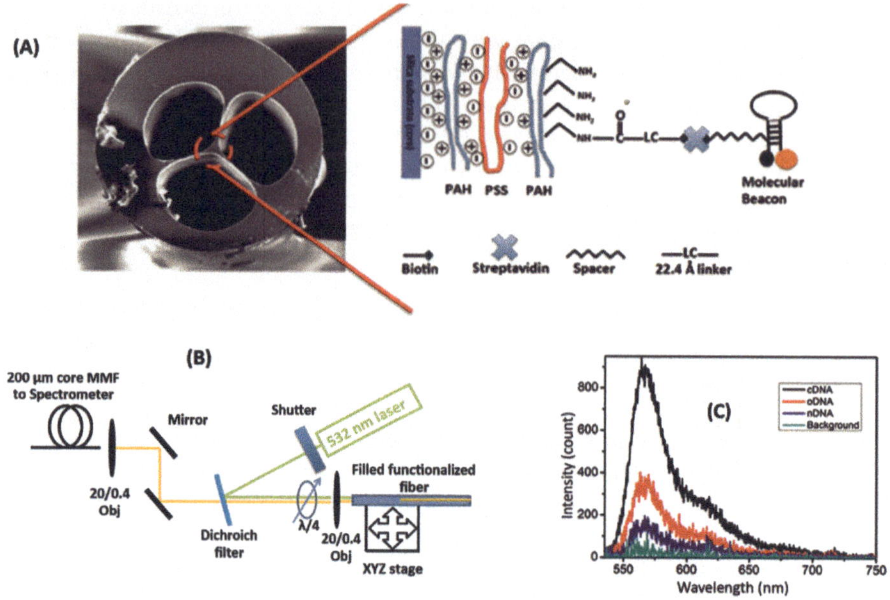

Figure 4.8 SEM cross section of the suspended core microstructured fiber (A), the schematic on the left represents the structure of the functionalization for attaching the molecular beacon. Setup to simulate the fluorescence and detect the backscattered signal to be analyzed (B). Intensity of the detected signal, it is possible to see that the matching DNA sample is prevalent with respect the nonmatching ones (Nguyen, Warren-Smith, Cooper, & Monro, 2012). Source: *Reprinted with permission from © The Optical Society. Nguyen, L., Warren-Smith, S., Cooper, A., & Monro, T. (2012). Molecular beacons immobilized within suspended core optical fiber for specific DNA detection. Optics Express, 20(28), 29378–29385.*

Fig. 4.8A. The MB probe is provided by a mechanism of fluorescence that is activated when the matching DNA is captured by the MB. Three samples of 4 cm functionalized fiber have been tested using three different solution of DNA sequences, a complementary DNA (cDNA), a DNA differing by only one nucleotide with respect the complementary DNA (oDNA), and a nonmatching DNA (nDNA). The setup for detecting the fluorescence derived by the hybridization of the DNA is shown in Fig. 4.8B. A green laser is collimated in the core of the fiber, while the backscattering of the fluorescence is collected and transported by a multimode fiber to the spectrum analyzer. The results of the measurement are depicted in Fig. 4.8C. It is possible to see the effectiveness of the microstructured fiber sensor to detect the matching cDNA, in fact the derived fluorescence is roughly 10 times larger than the one obtained with the detection of the nonmatching nDNA, and roughly 20 times larger with respect to the background fluorescence. A different consideration must be done regarding the oDNA that is detected with a ration 1:3 with respect to the complementary DNA. Nevertheless, the microstructured fiber shows a good degree of selectivity and the capability to capture prevalently the matching complementary DNA.

4.4.2 Label-free DNA biosensor by using a microstructured optical FBG

A weak point emerged by the previous microstructured fiber sensor device is that the propagation properties of the light guided in the fiber core are not exploited, since there is not a real interaction with the guided light and the anality. Instead, the core is used to collect the back-scattering light coming from the fluorescence emitted by the MBs. In this regard, the sensor is not label-free.

A possible solution for the above-mentioned issue has been developed by Candiani et al. (2013). In their work, the authors used a nonlinear microstructured fiber known as Penta fiber, Fig. 4.9A. The fiber presents the core surrounded by five big holes located like a flower shape. The core of the fiber has been provided with a 22 mm long Bragg grating, inscribed using a

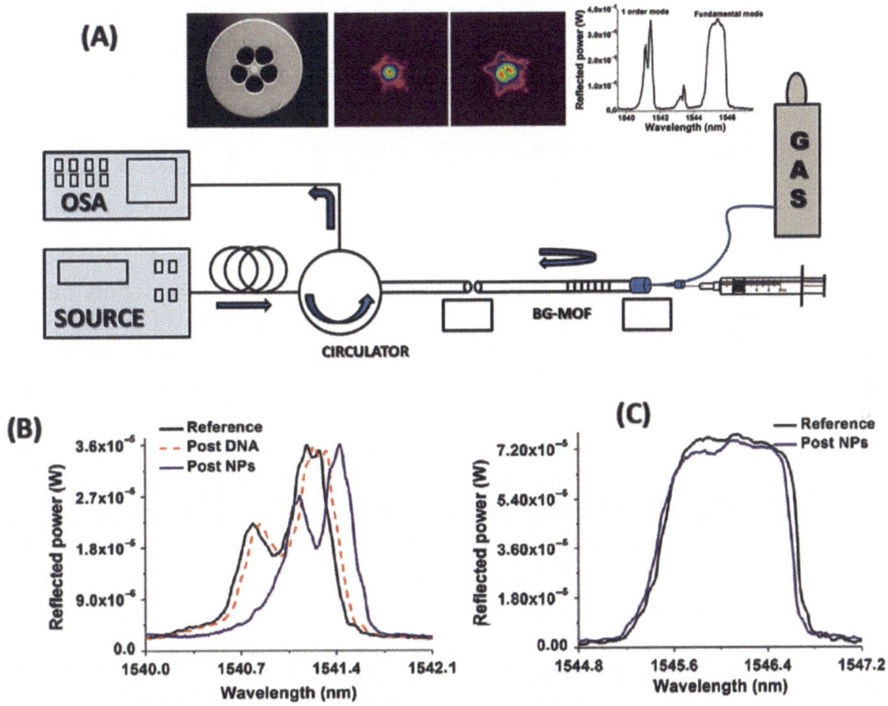

Figure 4.9 Setup of the experiment, the functionalized Penta fiber has been infiltrated with a solution of matching DNA and gold nanoparticles. The fiber has been excited with a large spectrum source around 1550 nm, and the signal reflected by the FBG is collected and redirected to a spectrum analyzer. The cross section of the Penta fiber is shown in the inset (A). Spectral shift of the first higher order modes (B) and spectral shift of the fundamental mode (C) (Candiani, Bertucci, Giannetti, & Label-free, 2013). Source: *Reproduced with the permission of SPIE.*

1067.73 nm phase mask and a 193 nm excimer laser. The period of the fiber Bragg grating, combined with the guidance property of the fiber is suitable for reflecting wavelengths around 1545 nm. The internal layers of the holes have been factionalized with a peptide nucleic acid, immobilized with a carboxylic acid functional group to the silica of the fiber. The fiber has been infiltrated, using a pressurized gas with a solution of 100 nM DNA biotinylated matched DNA and gold nanoparticles. Then the system has been connected to a high pressure microfiltered nitrogen line, to dry the fiber after infiltration. The fiber has been excited with a large spectrum source around 1550 nm, and the signal reflected by the FBG is collected and redirected to a spectrum analyzer. The setup is shown in Fig. 4.9A. The results show interesting achievements. The first one is that the fundamental mode, more confined in the core of the fiber, poorly interacts with the DNA layer formed in the holes, as shown in Fig. 4.9C. The second one is that the first higher order modes, less confined in the core, interact much better with the analyte showing a clear shift in the spectrum, as shown in Fig. 4.9B. The third one is that the presence of gold nanoparticles significantly improves the spectral shift. The experiments have been repeated by infiltrating a nonmatching DNA and the authors found any shift nor in the fundamental mode and in the first higher order mode. This result demonstrates the high selectivity of the microstructured fiber-based sensor and shows the possibility to achieve a label-free detection.

4.4.3 Biological optical sensing using hollow core microstructured fiber

In the previous example to achieve a consistent interaction between guided light and analyte, and to permit the detection, the fiber has been equipped with an FBG that has functioned as a transducer. It is well-known that microfabrication like the FBGs can increase the complexity of the sensors compromising the advantage to have a PCF structure. It is also well-known that the peak of interaction between the guided light and the sample to detect can be only achieved in the core, and this is possible only in the case of hollow core fibers. Starting from this consideration, Giovanardi at al. proposed a fiber sensor based on an antiresonant tube lattice fiber, similar to the one shown in Fig. 4.6C (Giovanardi et al., 2019). This fiber presents a structure composed by a minimal cladding made of eight tubes organized in a symmetric lattice. The idea has been to functionalize the internal part of core of the fiber (represented by the hollow space between the tubes). As a proof of concept of the feasibility of their work, the authors decided to detect streptavidin molecule. This can be achieved by functionalizing the internal layer of the fiber with biotin molecule. The reason of this choice is because the streptavidin–biotin system is a very well-known system, strongly used as a benchmark of biomolecular interactions. A cut of 25 cmcentimeter of fiber has been prepared by a silanization procedure, then the hollow core has been infiltrated with a solution of biotin. After

2 hours, the fiber has been washed and a new solution of streptavidin has been infiltrated. The fiber has been washed again, dried and inserted in an optical setup, as shown in Fig. 4.10A.

The simple setup consists of supercontinuum broadband laser source and an optical spectrum analyzer to detect the transmitted signal. It is possible to see, from the results depicted in Fig. 4.10B that the presence of the target molecule (streptavidin) captured by the functionalization layer (biotin), drastically change the transmission spectrum. In particular, the high attenuation window of the fiber is red shifted with respect to the case where no target molecule has been infiltrated. The results demonstrated the effectiveness of the label-free system based on a hollow core fiber to be effectively used as a biosensor.

4.5 Discussion

Tapered fiber sensors and biosensors represent a reliable and easy-to-fabricate solution to enhance the interaction between the light propagating in the fiber and the analyte to measure. It has been discussed that taper operation can be divided into two different behavior according to the geometry of the taper. When the taper is abrupt and nonadiabatic, the taper operation is mainly related to the formation of an interferometric pattern, whose spectrum shift can be successfully used for precise measurement of the external sample. On the other hand, when the taper is smooth and adiabatic, the taper remains in single mode operation so that no interferometric pattern is visible. In this case, the detection is related to the variation of the optical intensity transmitted by the taper, after the interaction with the analyte. This kind of detection is intrinsically less sensitive with respect to the previous one. Both the described taper operations present some disadvantages. The first one is related to the

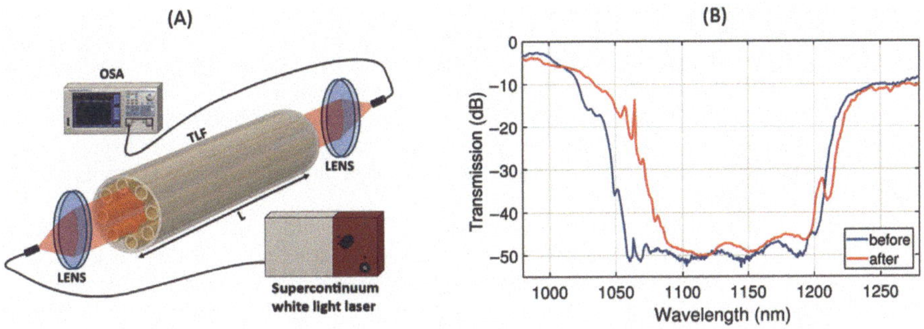

Figure 4.10 Setup of the experiment. A cut of 25 cm of hollow core ant resonant fiber, functionalized with biotin and infiltrated with streptavidin is coupled with a broadband light source coming from a supercontinuum laser. The output is collected and sent to a spectrum analyze (A). Transmission of the fiber before and after the infiltration of streptavidin (B) (Giovanardi et al., 2019). Source: *Reproduced with the permission of IEEE.*

enhancement of sensitivity that comes with a strong reduction of the taper waist, making the taper less robust and usable. The second one is related to the use of tapers for selective biosensors. In this case, the selectivity is given by a functionalization of the sensor that, in the case of a fiber taper, offers a small area to be functionalized, so a limitation of the detectable limit is expected.

Microstructured fibers, such as PCFs, show a great potential in the field of fiber sensing and biosensing. The geometry of their cross section, characterized by a pattern of holes in the cladding, can be engineered to finely tailor every single property of the fiber including guidance, attenuation, dispersion, birefringence, and nonlinearity. The presence of holes inside the fiber increases the appeal for the sensing and biosensing operation. In fact, some fibers are designed to have very large holes that can be infiltrated with the analyte to be detected. The same holes can also be functionalized for selective biosensing. The holes, as well as the tunability of microstructured fiber design, represent a big advantage in terms of sensing capability, by offering an unmatched surface to functionalize and a consistent interaction with the guided light. Moreover, some microstructured fibers present guidance inside a hollow core, so that the analyte can come in direct contact with the guided light. Microstructured fiber and PCF-based sensors can be considered a sort of microlab inside the fiber itself. Nevertheless, this fiber family presents disadvantages, related to their high cost of production, and to their non–user-friendly deployment. In fact, it is complicated to infiltrate the holes, and it is also complicated to couple and collect the light from the fiber. This operation involves precise setup and expensive optical components.

References

Barozzi, M., Manicardi, A., Vannucci, A., Candiani, A., Sozzi, M., Konstantaki, M., ... Cucinotta, A. (2017). Optical fiber sensors for label-free DNA detection. *Journal of Lightwave Technology, 35*(16), 3461–3472.

Beisenova, A., Issatayeva, A., Iordachita, I., Blanc, W., Molardi, C., & Tosi, D. (2019). Distributed fiber optics 3D shape sensing by means of high scattering NP-doped fibers simultaneous spatial multiplexing. *Optics Express, 27*(16), 22074–22087.

Birks, T. A., & Li, Y. W. (1992). The shape of fiber tapers. *Journal of Lightwave Technology, 10*(4), 432–438. Available from https://doi.org/10.1109/50.134196.

Brambilla, G. (2010). Optical fibre nanowires and microwires: A review. *Journal of Optics (Online), 12*(4), 19.

Candiani, A., Bertucci, A., Giannetti, S., Konstantaki, M., Manicardi, A., Pissadakis, S., ... Selleri, S. (2013). Label-free DNA biosensor based on a peptide nucleic acid-functionalized microstructured optical fiber-Bragg grating. *Journal of Biomedical Optics, 18*(5), 057004.

Coscelli, E., Molardi, C., Cucinotta, A., & Selleri, S. (2014). Symmetry-free Tm-doped photonic crystal fiber with enhanced mode area. *IEEE Journal of Selected Topics in Quantum Electronics, 20*(5), 544–550.

Coscelli, E., Molardi, C., Masruri, M., Cucinotta, A., & Selleri, S. (2014). Thermally resilient Tm-doped large mode area photonic crystal fiber with symmetry-free cladding. *Optics Express, 22*(8), 9707–9714.

Cubillas, A. M., Unterkofler, S., Euser, T. G., Etzold, B. J. M., Jones, A. C., Sadler, P. J., ... Russell, P. S. J. (2013). Photonic crystal fibres for chemical sensing and photochemistry. *Chemical Society Reviews, 42*(22), 8629–8648.

Giovanardi, F., Cucinotta, A., Rozzi, A., Corradini, R., Benabid, F., Rosa, L., & Vincetti, L. (2019). Hollow core inhibited coupling fibers for biological optical sensing. *Journal of Lightwave Technology., 37*(11), 2598–2604.

Han, Y.-G. (2009). Temperature-insensitive strain measurement using a birefringent interferometer based on a polarization-maintaining photonic crystal fiber. *Applied Physics B: Lasers and Optics, 95*(2), 383–387.

Jarzebinska, R., Korposh, S., James, S., Batty, W., Tatam, R., & Lee, S.-W. (2012). Optical gas sensor fabrication based on porphyrin-anchored electrostatic self-assembly onto tapered optical fibres. *Analytical Letters, 45*(10), 1297–1309.

Jauregui, C., Limpert, J., & Tunnermann, A. (2013). High-power fibre lasers. *Nature Photonics, 7*(11), 861–867.

Korposh, S., James, S. W., Lee, S.-W., & Tatam, R. P. (2019). Tapered optical fibre sensors: Current trends and future perspectives. *Sensors., 19*(10), 2294.

LaserFocusWorld. (2019). *Fiber optics: CO_2 laser technology increases the flexibility of fiber end cap splicing and fiber array assembly.* https://www.laserfocusworld.com/fiber-optics/article/14071886/co2-laser-technology-increases-the-flexibility-of-fiber-end-cap-splicing-and-fiber-array-assembly

Latifi, H., Zibaii, M. I., Hosseini, S. M., & Jorge, P. A. S. (2012). Nonadiabatic tapered optical fiber for biosensor applications. *Photonic Sensors, 2*, 340–356. Available from https://doi.org/10.1007/s13320-012-0086-z.

Leung, A., Shankar, P. M., & Mutharasan, R. (2007). A review of fiber-optic biosensors. *Sensors and Actuators, B: Chemical, 125*(2), 688–703.

Leung, A., Shankar, P. M., & Mutharasan, R. (2008). Model protein detection using antibody-immobilized tapered fiber optic biosensors (TFOBS) in a flow cell at 1310 nm and 1550 nm. *Sensors and Actuators B: Chemical, 129*(2), 716–725.

Love, J., Henry, W., Stewart, W., Black, R., Lacroix, S., & Gonthier, F. (1991). Tapered single-mode fibres and devices. I. Adiabaticity criteria. *IEE Proceedings Journal., 138*, 343–354.

Moar, P. N., Huntington, S. T., Katsifolis, J., Cahill, L. W., Roberts, A., & Nugent, K. A. (1999). Fabrication, modeling, and direct evanescent field measurement of tapered optical fiber sensors. *Journal of Applied Physics, 85*(7), 3395–3398. Available from https://doi.org/10.1063/1.369695.

Nalawade, S. M., & Thakur, H. V. (2011). Photonic crystal fiber strain-independent temperature sensing based on modal interferometer. *IEEE Photonics Technology Letters, 23*(21), 1600–1602.

Nguyen, L., Warren-Smith, S., Cooper, A., & Monro, T. (2012). Molecular beacons immobilized within suspended core optical fiber for specific DNA detection. *Optics Express, 20*(28), 29378–29385.

Pinto, A. M. R., & Lopez-Amo, M. (2012). Photonic, crystal fibers for sensing applications. *Journal of Sensors, 2012*, art. no. 598178.

Russell, P. St. J. (2003). Photonic crystal fibers. *Science (New York, N.Y.), 299*, 358–362.

Saleh, B. E., & Teich, M. C. (2019). *Fundamentals of photonics.* John Wiley & Sons.

Sun, D., Sun, L., Guo, T., & Guan, B. (2019). Label-free thrombin detection using a tapered fiber-optic interferometric aptasensor. *Journal of Lightwave Technology, 37*(11), 2756–2761.

Villatoro, J., Monzón-Hernández, D., & Mejía, E. (2003). Fabrication and modeling of uniform-waist single-mode tapered optical fiber sensors. *Applied Optics, 42*(13), 2278–2283.

Xu, Y., Lu, P., Chen, L., & Bao, X. (2017). Recent developments in micro-structured fiber optic sensors. *Fibers, 5*(1), 3.

Yu, F., & Knight, J. C. (2016). Negative curvature hollow-core optical fiber. *IEEE Journal of Selected Topics in Quantum Electronics, 22*(2), 146–155, Art no. 4400610.

Zhang, Y., Dhawan, A., & Vo-Dinh, T. (2011). Design and fabrication of fiber-optic nanoprobes for optical sensing. *Nanoscale Research Letters, 6*(1), 18.

Zibaii, M. I., Latifi, H., Karami, H., Gholami, M., Hosseini, S. M., & Ghezelayagh, M. H. (2010). Non-adiabatic tapered optical fiber sensor for measuring the interaction between α-amino acids in aqueous carbohydrate solution. *Measurement Science and Technology, 21*(10), Art no. 105801.

5

Surface plasmon resonances

5.1 Surface plasmon resonance in fiber optics

5.1.1 Introduction

In the context of modern technological applications, ranging from telecommunication to laser industrial applications, and from medical imaging to optical sensing, the great versatility of optical fibers technology is well known (Udd & Spillman, 2011). Optical fibers present interesting and unusual advantages with respect to other technologies such as reduced size, robustness, immunity to external electromagnetic interference, and biocompatibility. Typically, optical fibers can be efficiently used to detect physical properties like temperature and strain, but with some modifications of the configuration in the detecting medium, it is also possible to detect other properties like pressure, lateral forces, and refractive index of external analytes. For these reasons, Fiber Optics Sensing (FOS) technology is becoming more and more appetible for biological and medical applications. According to their structural configuration, optical fiber sensors can be divided in the following categories: interferometric sensors, grating-based sensors, microstructure sensors, and scattering-based sensors (Bao & Chen, 2012; Lee, Roh, & Park, 2009; Lee et al., 2012). All of these families of fiber sensors present advantages and disadvantages. For instance, fiber Bragg grating (FBG) sensors are cheap, robust, scalable, easy to use. They are perfect for detecting single and multipoint variation of temperature and strain. However, to detect the refractive index of an external analyte, they require subsequent microfabrication that can compromise their robustness and their reliability. On the other hand, microstructured fiber sensors, like photonic crystal fiber (PCF) sensors, permit a strong interaction between the evanescent field and the analyte to detect, so that they present good capability for refractive index sensing. However, PCF sensors are expensive and not practical to insert in optical setups.

In this context, characterized by a large multiplicity of fiber sensing solutions, several considerations must be taken into account to determine which fiber sensor represents the optimum for the required application. Applications in

Optical Fiber Biosensors.
DOI: https://doi.org/10.1016/B978-0-12-819467-6.00005-6

biological and medical fields usually require the precise detection of the refractive index of a solution or the detection of molecules such as proteins or DNA fragments. These requirements, moreover, must be evaluated with respect to the goals that the sensor aims to achieve. The first, and most important, goal of a fiber biosensor is the achievement of lowest limit of detection, which implies the capability to detect very low concentration of a particular molecule interacting with the sensor. The second goal is related to the environment of application, which can be summarized to identify where the sensor is designed to work. It is possible to identify two main environments of application: laboratory-based applications and field-based application. The difference between these two is significant. Since laboratory represents a controlled environment for sensing, the sensor can be designed to have elevated sensitivity characteristics, ignoring other peculiar characteristics that can be useful for field applications, such as portability and easiness of use. A good fiber biosensor aims to be inexpensive, portable, and versatile, so to adapt for field-based applications. The last goal is related to the simplicity of the detection method. Biosensors, in particular those designed for selective detection of biomaterial, can be separated in two classes: sensors that use a labeled detection method and sensors that use a label-free detection method (Caucheteur, Guo, & Albert, 2015). Labeled detection implies the use of a sort of tag, such as a fluorescent protein, added to the analyte in order to enable its detection. Label-free detection, instead, is direct and does not require any modification of the analyte. In this regard, label-free detection is in line with the basic characteristics of fiber biosensing. Therefore the requirements for the optimum fiber sensor for bioapplications can be summarized into the following characteristics:

1. low cost and simple design,
2. versatility and use in field-based application,
3. easiness of application and label-free detection, and
4. lowest possible limit of detection.

It is worth noting that the above-mentioned requirements are difficult to be matched all together by the same fiber sensors. Some fiber sensor technologies are more focused on the improvement of the limit of detection, and some others on the versatility and simplicity of the use.

In the last few years, in the landscape of fiber sensor technology, a new category of fiber sensors has emerged. This category, which can be called plasmonic-based fiber sensor, is based on the nanoscale interaction between the light (photons), propagating in the fiber, and the superficial electrons of a thin metal film in contact with the fiber. The interaction is known as surface plasmon resonance (SPR). This class of fiber sensors represents a good compromise to fit the above-mentioned characteristics, by offering impressive limit of detection, while maintaining versatility, easiness of application, and simple design (Esfahani Monfared, 2020).

5.1.2 Physical principles of surface plasmon resonance

The term *plasmonics* refers to the science that describes the interaction, at nanoscale level, between photons and surface electrons. In a broader meaning, it is the description of an unconventional interaction between light and matter. This phenomenon usually appears when a dielectric and a thin metal surface or metal nanostructure came in contact under certain conditions. In this case, the incoming light of the source can push the surface electrons to create a collective oscillation, which is called *surface plasmon* (SP) (Stockman, 2011). Since this interaction is better described by using quantum mechanics, the plasmon is usually described as the quantum particle of the surface wave. This kind of interaction between light and matter, that specifically involves the excitation of a plasmon, is referred as SPR.

There are two distinct physical phenomena that can be associated to the family of SPR, and for this reason both are usually referred as SPR. The first one involves the excitation of SPs on a thin metal film that is in contact with a dielectric material. The excited plasmon wave propagates at the interface between metal and dielectric. This phenomenon, presenting such a configuration, is known as *surface plasmon polariton* (SPP), shown in Fig. 5.1A. The second kind of plasmon resonance is, instead, generated in nanostructures, such as nanoparticles or nanorods, which involve strong localization of the oscillation. This kind of resonance is called *localized surface plasmon resonance* (LSPR), depicted in Fig. 5.1B. Even if the physical mechanisms of LSPR and SPP are slightly different in the practical applications, both these resonances can cause energy transfer between light and matter in form of absorption or scattering. This energy transfer is one of the main reasons of the SPR success in the field of optical sensors.

Surface plasmon polariton: In order to explain the SPR in the case of an interface between thin film metal and dielectric, precisely in the case of SPP, it is useful to illustrate the Kretschmann–Raether configuration, one of the first example

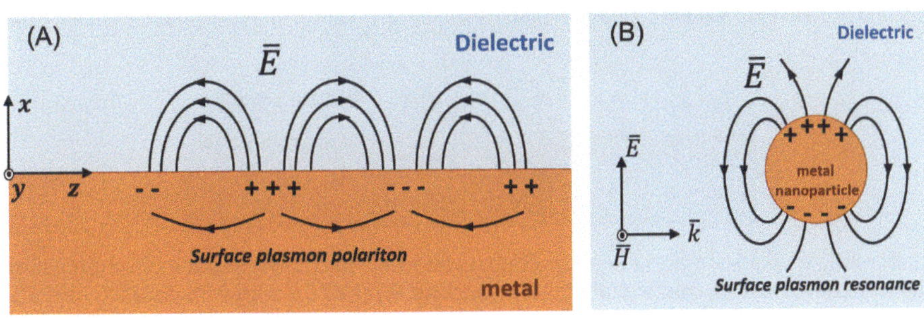

Figure 5.1 Schematic of the formation and propagation of a Surface Plasmon Polariton along the interface between the dielectric and the metal film (A). Diagram of the interaction between an external optical field and a metal nanoparticle, with the onset of a localized surface plasmon resonance (B).

of effective excitation of a SP (Kretschmann & Raether, 1968). Moreover, Kretschmann–Raether schematic presents the advantage to be extended to the model of SPR-based optical fiber sensors, without drastic changes of the mathematical model. As shown in Fig. 5.2, this method of excitation makes use of a dielectric prism.

There are other methods of SPR excitation, including waveguide coupling, optical fiber coupling, and diffraction-grating coupling, but under some consistent hypothesis, these methods can all refer to the coupling through prism. In Kretschmann–Raether configuration, a prism of dielectric material, typically a glass, is coated in one of its surfaces by a film of metal. The film shall be very thin, in the order of hundreds of nanometers or less. Metals that can be used for SPR are aluminum, copper, silver, and gold. Gold and silver are usually preferred because of their unique characteristics and because the SPR is achieved in the visible spectrum. Silver presents a very sharp peak of resonance, while gold is easier to be applied as coating and presents an excellent stability. The second surface of the thin film is in contact with a second dielectric, that can be, in the case of optical sensors, a solution whose refractive index can vary according to the concentration of a particular molecule to be detected. It is possible to consider the following parameter referred to the materials involved in Kretschmann–Raether configuration:

$$n_p = \sqrt{\varepsilon_p}, \quad \text{refractive index of the prism} \tag{5.1a}$$

$$n_s = \sqrt{\varepsilon_s}, \quad \text{refractive index of the solution} \tag{5.1b}$$

$$\varepsilon_m, \quad \text{electric permittivity of the metal} \tag{5.1c}$$

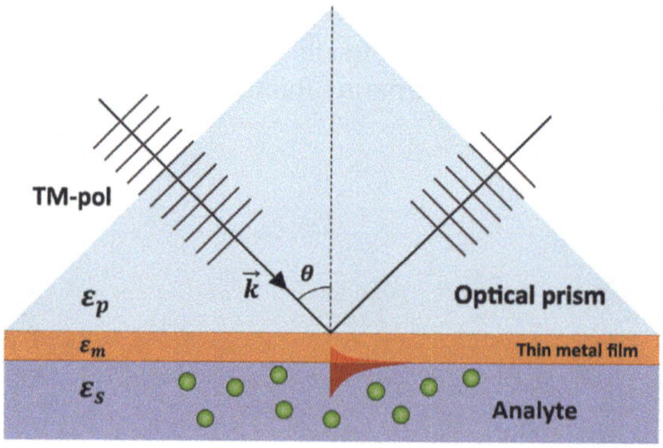

Figure 5.2 Schematic of Kretschmann–Raether configuration for exciting a surface plasmon using an optical prism. The prism is coated with a thin metal film. The second layer of the film is in contact with a solution whose refractive index must be determined. The incoming light must be TM-polarized and totally internally reflected by the prism-metal interface. When the matching condition between the evanescent wave of the prism-metal interface and the plasmonic wave of the metal-solution interface is satisfied, then a SPP on the external metal surface can be excited.

The basic idea of prism coupling is to arrive to the prism-metal interface with an angle that is larger with respect to the critical angle of total internal reflection. To obtain this condition, it is necessary to analyze the structure. The prism-metal interface is composed of a dielectric with refractive index n_p and a metal characterized by a permittivity ε_r, presenting a complex value according to Drude model at optical frequencies (Saleh & Teich, 2019). Since the metal layer is supposed to be thin in the order of nanometers, the light is transmitted through the metal, reaching the second interface between metal and solution, characterized by a reflective index n_p. This implies that the light is reflected back in the prims by the second dielectric (the solution). The condition of total internal reflection is, therefore given by the refractive indices n_p and n_s, and necessarily $n_p > n_s$. At the condition of total internal reflection, an evanescent field, tangential to the prism-metal interface, is formed. The evanescent field can penetrate the thin metal layer and excite a SP wave on the other boundary between metal and solution. To permit the excitation of a SPP, it is necessary to fulfill two conditions. The first one is related to matching condition between the evanescent wave propagation constant and the propagation constant of the SP. The second one is related to the polarization of the incoming light, which must be inevitably TM-polarized in order to satisfy the tangential conditions of the evanescent wave.

The propagation constant of the SP, propagating along the metal-solution boundary, is described by the following equation:

$$k_{sp} = \Re\mathrm{e}\left(\frac{2\pi}{\lambda}\sqrt{\frac{\varepsilon_p\varepsilon_m}{\varepsilon_p + \varepsilon_m}}\right), \tag{5.2}$$

where ε_p and ε_m are the permittivity of the prism dielectric and the permittivity of the metal, respectively. While λ is the wavelength of the incident light. This propagation constant must match the propagation constant of the evanescent wave, occurring at prism-metal interface, in order to excite the SPP and transferring energy to the plasmonic wave. The propagation constant of the evanescent wave is described by the following equation:

$$k_{ev} = \frac{2\pi}{\lambda} n_p \sin\theta, \tag{5.3}$$

where θ is the angle of incidence of the TM-polarized light to the prism-metal interface. Regarding Eq. (5.3), it is important to underline that one of the ways to match the condition of SPR, in the case of prism coupling, is to vary the angle of light incidence.

The evanescent wave, penetrating through the metal layer, can induce, at the correct matching condition, an SPP at the metal-solution boundary. The SPP can radiate back part of the light into the thin metal layer. This kind of reflected radiation can interfere, in a destructive way, with the reflected component of the incident light. The effect is to reduce the light that is transmitted outside the prism, so that at the matching condition for the onset of the SPR, the output spectrum of the system presents a dip. Going to the limit of this reasoning, in the ideal case of extremely thin metal layer, all the energy of the incident light is transferred to the SPR, so that the output becomes null.

Kretschmann–Raether prism-based configuration is, under certain circumstances, the most convenient in term of capability of SP excitation and sensing efficiency. However, it presents disadvantages because it is bulky and not somewhat expensive. Moreover, it is not adapted for remote and multiple sensing. A way to reach a better compactness is with the use of fiber optics technology, since optical fibers present small size and versatility for short- and long-range use. Optical fiber SPR sensors can be directly derived from the prism configuration. It is necessary to substitute the prism with the core of the fiber and operating a microfabrication in order to remove or modify the cladding to expose the core. Typically, etching or tapering is suitable for this purpose, but many other fabrication methods have been explored by the scientific community. Fig. 5.3 is shown a schematic of microfabrication for SPP excitation in optical fiber. In this case, a small portion of the optical fiber has been etched in order to expose the core, then the etched section has been coated with a thin layer of metal. Outside the metal layer, it is possible to put the analyte, which can be a solution whose refractive index is to be detected.

The principle of operation of the SPR optical fiber sensor remains consistent with the one of Kretschmann–Raether design, and the SPR is achieved at the matching condition of the modes propagating in the fiber, according to the following formula:

$$\frac{2\pi}{\lambda} n_{eff} \sin\theta = \Re e\left(\frac{2\pi}{\lambda}\sqrt{\frac{\varepsilon_p \varepsilon_m}{\varepsilon_p + \varepsilon_m}}\right), \tag{5.4}$$

In an optical fiber, the propagating modes are confined in the structure because of a mechanism of total internal reflection. Exposing the core, and

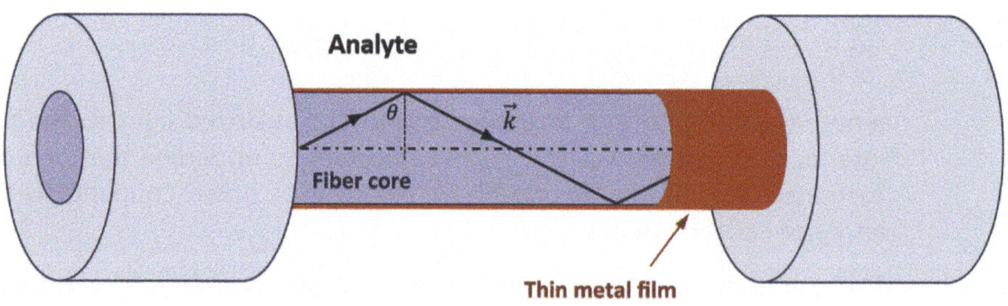

Figure 5.3 Example of microfabrication of an optical fiber for the use as SPP-based sensors. A small portion of the optical fiber has been exposed by a procedure of etching. Then, the exposed core is coated by a metal layer. The SPP excitation in given by the interaction between the propagating modes and the interface core-metal.

creating a core-metal interface, it is possible to recreate the same condition, for the SPP excitation, existing in the prism configuration. One of big difference between SPR fiber sensors and prism-based SPR sensors is the detection method. Usually, in a prism-based sensor, the angle of the incident of a monochromatic light is varied to match the SPR condition. This permits to obtain a very precise and sharp dip in the transmission spectrum. In an optical fiber, it is not possible to control the angle of incidence of the modes, so the result is a broader resonance curve in the transmission spectrum. To counteract this drawback, so that improving the characteristics of the sensor, it is suggested the use of a single mode fiber. In this case, it is also necessary to inject in the fiber a large spectrum source, like a white light or a supercontinuum source, in order to monitor the shift of the resonant wavelength given by the refractive index change of the analyte (Jorgenson & Yee, 1993; Sharma, Jha, & Gupta, 2007).

Localized surface plasmon resonance: LSPR is a phenomenon appearing when light is trapped inside a conductive nanostructure like nanoparticles or nanorods. This creates a significant difference with respect to SPP, where evanescent waves propagate along a thin and continuous metal interface. LSPR is the result of a strict interaction between the incident light and the free electron on the surface of the nanostructure. Necessarily the wavelength of the light must be longer than the size of the nanostructure (Willets &Van Duyne, 2007). The presence of resonant nanostructures, interacting with the incident light, can create a coherent plasmon group oscillation. In this case, the resonance condition is strongly dependent on several parameters, including:

1. the geometry of the system,
2. the composition of the nanostructures,
3. the size of the nanostructures,
4. the concentration and the separation of the nanostructure, and
5. the characteristics of the external environment.

Commonly, for sensing purpose, the chosen nanostructure is represented by gold or silver nanoparticles, which exhibit the SPR in the visible spectrum. Similarly to SPP, the detection consists in the measurement of the absorption spectrum of a broadband light source. To achieve the detection, the nanoparticle can be deposited on a solid substrate, interacting with the analyte, or dispersed directly in the solution to measure. The use of LSPR and nanoparticles is, in general, more complicated and less versatile than the SPP counterpart, but it offers the advantage of a larger surface in contact with the analyte, thus improving the limit of detection.

5.1.3 Basic sensing principles of surface plasmon resonance-based fiber sensors

A SPR-based fiber sensor consists of an optical fiber, properly modified through microfabrication or microstructuration, that is used to excite a SP exploiting the interaction between the light propagating in the fiber and a metallic nanostructure properly arrange on the fiber. The most common configuration is related to the excitation of SPP over a thin metal layer deposited on the fiber. Under this point of view, the optical fiber is a perfect platform for SPR, since the light, which propagates in the core of the fiber, is confined by total internal reflection, thus permitting a dielectric-metal interaction similar to the one proposed by Kretschmann–Raether with a prism-metal configuration. The main question here is related to the modality of fabrication and location of the metal interface. The subject is interesting, and it has pushed the scientific community to suggest several different designs, which can be divided into three main categories:

1. Designs that involve a partial or total removal of the cladding, in order to create a dielectric-metal interface in proximity of the core.
2. Designs with microfabrication that induces the core mode to leak in the cladding, so that the dielectric-metal interface can be fabricated on the cladding.
3. Designs that involve microstructuration, like PCF, where the dielectric-metal interface can be built in the microstructured channels of the fiber.

The above-mentioned classification is not so strict, and hybrid designs, which involve characteristics of different categories, have been explored.

The SPP resonance is extremely convenient for optical fiber sensors and biosensors, since it permits to have a significantly large metal surface that can be exploited to detect the analyte. Typically, the SPP fiber sensors are designed to measure a refractive index of a solution. This fact can be exploited to build biosensors able to detect the concentration of a particular molecule inside a solution. On the other hand, in optical biosensors, the metal layer can be factionalized to selectively capture biomaterial like proteins or DNA. In this case, the physical properties of the SPR are modified by the label-free interaction between the analyte captured by the functionalization and the metal layer. In both of these sensing configurations, the sensing principles are similar, the modification of the external analyte induces a shift or a modification of the SPR wavelength, like in the plot shown in Fig. 5.4.

In this regard, most of the SPR-based fiber sensors work in transmission. It is convenient to inject a broadband light, such as a white light or a supercontinuum source, in the fiber and detect the light that is transmitted after the SPP sensing section. At the matching condition, the input light is coupled with the SPP so that part of the energy is transferred to the SP. The matching condition, therefore corresponds to a minimum in the transmission spectrum (Fig. 5.4). By changing the characteristics of the analyte environment, for instance by changing the concentration of the analyte inside a solution, the resonance wavelength shifts. The shift can be detected and correlated with the change in the analyte, as shown in the inset of Fig. 5.4. Under this consideration, the sensitivity can be expressed as:

$$S = \frac{\Delta\lambda_{SPR}}{\Delta n}(\mathrm{nm/RIU}), \tag{5.5}$$

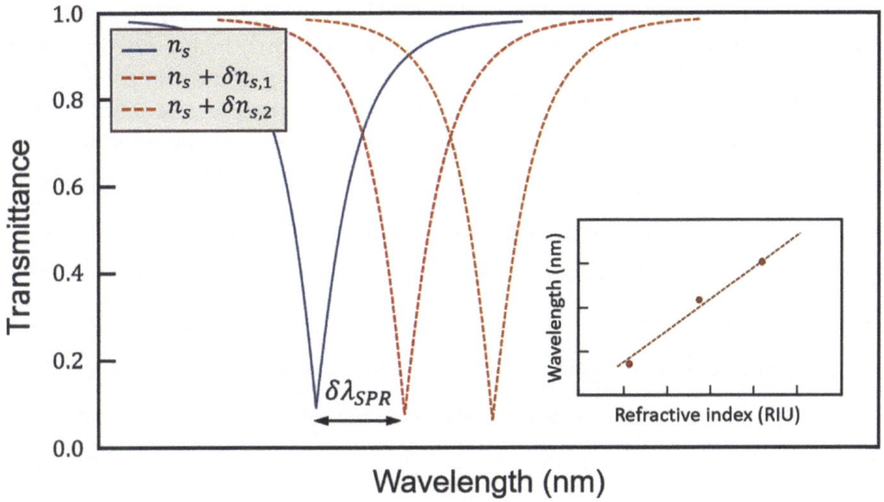

Figure 5.4 Typical transmission spectrum of the light interacting with a surface plasma polariton, obtained by coating the transmitting medium with a thin metal layer. The spectrum presents a dip corresponding to the SPP resonance, where part of the incoming light energy is transferred to the plasmon. By changing the refractive index and/or the environment of the external analyte, it is possible to detect a shift of the resonant wavelength. In case of measurement of the refractive index of the external analyte, the refractive index is given in term of wavelength shift, while the sensitivity is $\Delta\lambda_{SPR}/\Delta n$ (nm/RIU).

in case of detection of the refractive index. Clearly, other properties of the analyte, such as its concentration, can be retrieved as well, and the sensitivity expression can be modified in this regard.

One of the key features of the SPR-based fiber sensor is the excellent sensitivity, strictly correlated to the limit of detection. Clearly, there is not a unique output in terms of sensitivity, since there are a large number of possible configurations and implementations of this family of sensors. However, SPR technology permits to reach in sensitivity of hundreds or sometimes thousands of nanometers over refractive index unit. These extreme values of sensitivity permit the SPR technology, applied to fiber sensing, to detect very small changes of refractive index, or equivalently, very small changes in the concentration of a particular molecule inside a solution. For this specific reason, the SPR-based fiber sensors have grown a large interest in the scientific community, permitting to improve the limit of detection and maintaining the versatility of typical optical fibers.

5.2 Geometry of fiber sensors based on surface plasmon resonance

The large number of SPR-based fiber sensor design as well as its configurations makes the classification of this kind of sensors a hard task. The main reason is that the SPR technology, both SPP and LSPR, is flexible and versatile and can be applied to a large number of fiber designs, including those provided with inscribed grating, those with microfabrication, and those presenting microstructured features. So, it is not uncommon to read in scientific literature different descriptions of SPR-based fiber sensors, based on fiber geometry, the sensor behavior, or the SPR principles of applications. It is worth noting that the operation of classification does not separate the SPR-based fiber sensors in a separated set. In fact, some sensors present characteristics common to more than one identifying family. In this section, it has been decided to mainly analyze the SPP designs and to present the different SPR-based fiber sensors following the approach of identifying the position of dielectric-metal interface. In this regard, it is possible to divide the SPR sensors into following categories:

1. Sensors that present dielectric-metal interface in proximity of the fiber core.
2. Sensors where dielectric-metal interface is on the cladding.
3. Sensors based on microstructured fiber, where the dielectric-metal interface is in the microstructured channels.

5.2.1 Dielectric-metal interface in proximity of the fiber core

In this family of SPR-based optical fiber sensors, the basic idea is to exploit the total internal reflection of the guided fiber modes in order to excite the SPP occurring on a thin metal layer when the matching condition between the evanescent wave of the modes and the SPP is satisfied. Clearly, this modality of SPP excitation can be fulfilled when the thin metal layer is in contact of in proximity to the core, so that it can be influenced by the evanescent field of the guided modes, considering the limited capability of the evanescent field to penetrate the cladding. The idea is, therefore to exploit the evanescent field when it presents maximum intensity in order to obtain a robust SPR.

The most used configurations, to achieve the correct contact with the core, consist of removing the cladding entirely or in part. The cladding can be completely removed with a mechanical operation of stripping or by using a chemical etching process. Then the exposed core can be entirely coated by a proper metal layer, a similar configuration is shown in Fig. 5.5A. On the other hand, the process of stripping or etching the fiber can weaken the structure, in particular in single mode fibers where the core has a diameter of around 10 μm. A second configuration consists to partially remove the core by polishing one side of the fiber creating a D-shape structure. This process is precise and safe, and it permits to decide the depth of the cladding removal, so that it is possible to engineer the exposure of the core. This mechanical process results in a robust structure that has a relatively large planar surface that can be easily coated with a metal layer, like the one shown in Fig. 5.5B. Another possible configuration, that offers advantages in terms of technological and manufacturing repeatability, involves the use of adiabatic tapered fibers. In this case the

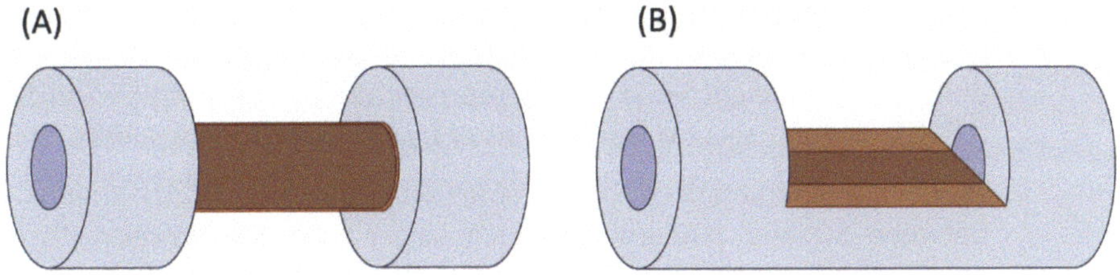

Figure 5.5 Examples of surface plasmon resonance-based fiber sensors where the thin metal layer is in proximity to the core. In the left figure the cladding is stripped or etched in order to expose the core and the metal layer is deposited all around the core (A). The right figure shows a fiber with a D-shape microfabrication (B). The fiber is side-polished to reach the core and a flat metal layer is deposited on the fiber.

core is not exposed, but at the taper waist the penetration of the evanescent field is improved, so that the metal film can be deposed on the tapered area in proximity of the thinned core (Jha, Verma, & Gupta, 2008).

D-shape and exposed core sensors are mostly used in the region of operation of visible light and near infrared, ranging from 500 to 800 nm. Both single mode and multimode fibers can be used for this purpose. Multimode fibers having a larger core permit to obtain firmer structure, but the SPR spectrum has the tendency to become broader and less defined, since many modes propagate with different angles. On the other hand, single mode fiber can achieve a sharper spectrum, but the structure becomes weaker to mechanical solicitations. In this kind of SPR-based fiber sensors, the resonances in the transmitted spectrum lie in a span of 100 nm. The sensitivity, in terms of refractive index measurement, can be very high, reaching thousands of nm/RIU.

5.2.2 Dielectric-metal interface on the cladding

A different solution to excite the SPP on the metal surface of a thin layer, which preserves the integrity of the fiber structure, is to force the core modes to spread inside the cladding. This configuration offers the advantages to permit an easier deposition of the metal layer over the cladding, covering a larger area. The target of having the dielectric-metal interface over the cladding can be reached by several configurations. Two of them have shown a better reliability and, therefore they catch the interest of the researchers' community.

The first one, which is very conservative and easy to implement, consists of the photoinscription of special grating, in the core of the fiber. The grating is able to couple the core light to the cladding modes. The mechanical resistance of the fiber, with such a solution, is basically preserved. The use of inscribed grating offers further advantage to select particular guided wavelengths, thus selectively improving the capability of the modes to excite the SPP. Short-period gratings, like FBGs, are not suitable for this operation, since the light remains confined in the core, acting as a notch filter, transmitting all the light except of a very narrow band that is reflected back by the grating. Fortunately, there are two grating structures that are suitable to couple the core light into the cladding, in an efficient way: one is represented by the long-period fiber grating (LPFG), and the second is represented by TFBG (Erdogan, 1997).

LPFGs are characterized by a refractive index periodicity that is roughly in between 50 and 500 μm, so much larger than the wavelength of the light propagating in the core. The effect of this inscribed structure is to couple the forward core modes into forward cladding modes. The transmitted spectrum results to present multiple resonances, usually with relatively large band. By coating the cladding in the correspondence of the LPFG, it is possible to stimulate the SPP by the mediation of the cladding modes, coupled in the cladding from the core by the effect of the LPFG (Li et al., 2016). The schematic is illustrated in Fig. 5.6A. The second and most used grating for this purpose is the TFBG, which is made by a periodic alternation tilted fringes with high and low refractive index. The tilt angle is very small with respect to the propagation direction. The effect of the tilted grating is to generate modes that are backward coupling in the core and modes that are backward coupling in the cladding. The number of modes, coupled in the cladding, are quite large, in the order of hundreds. Their spectrum results in a sort of large comb, occupying a band of roughly 100 nm. Similarly to SPR-based fiber sensors that make use of LPFG, also in the TFBGs configuration, shown in Fig. 5.6B, it is possible to coat the cladding with a thin metal layer in order to create an interaction between cladding modes and SPP of the layer. Thanks to the large spectrum of cladding modes, it is possible to observe that only a small fraction of those modes can couple to the metal structure by exciting the SPP. This results in a clear absorption in the transmission spectrum, like the one shown in Fig. 5.7 (Caucheteur et al., 2015). The sensitivity offered by this configuration is in the order of hundreds of nm/RIU, in terms of refractive index measurement.

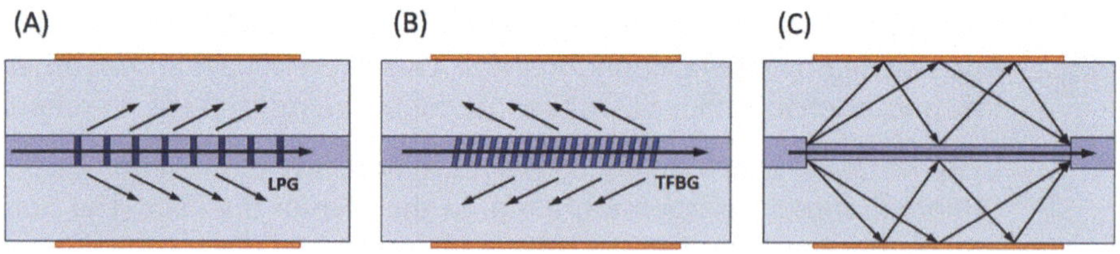

Figure 5.6 Surface plasmon resonance-based fiber sensors where the thin metal layer is deposited on the cladding. To enable this behavior, it is necessary to have a core feature that permits to couple the core light to the cladding modes. This effect can be achieved by the use of inscribed gratings, like long-period fiber gratings (A), or like tilted fiber Bragg gratings (B). Another possibility is to create a hetero structure, where a piece of fiber with smaller core is spliced into two pieces of fiber with larger core. This mismatch permits to couple core modes in the cladding (C).

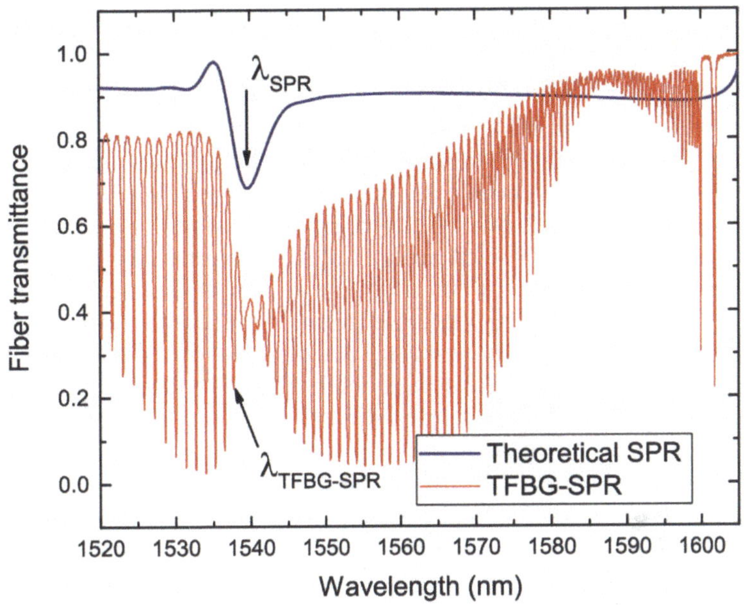

Figure 5.7 Example of surface plasmon resonance achieved by coupling the cladding mode of a Tilted Fiber Bragg Gratings and a thin metal layer. The transmission spectrum presents a decrease of intensity in correspondence of the resonance (Caucheteur et al., 2015). Source: *Image reproduced with the permission of Springer Nature.*

Fiber gratings are not the only way to couple the core modes into the cladding in order to excite the SPP on a dielectric-metal interface located on the cladding. It is also possible to exploit microfabricated heterostructures composed by one piece of single mode fiber and two pieces of multimode fibers, as shown in Fig. 5.6C. The piece of single mode fiber is, clearly, the trigger of the cladding coupling. The principle of operation of such a structure derives by the fact that, moving form a larger core to a smaller core, part of the light is leaked in the cladding. This fact permits to excite a large number of cladding modes that can, subsequently, interact with the thin metal layer coated on the cladding. The refractometric sensitivity of this hybrid structure can be quite high reaching values of more than 1000 nm/RIU (Iga, Seki, & Watanabe, 2004).

5.2.3 Dielectric-metal interface in the microstructured fiber features

PCF, or more generally microstructured fibers, presents unique characteristics that can be coupled in a very efficient way with the SPR technology. Microstructured fibers are characterized by microstructured cladding, which presents a pattern of holes that go along the length of the fiber. If the pattern of the cladding holes follows a 2D periodicity, the cladding assumes the characteristics of a photonic crystal. The light is guided in the central region of the fiber, that it is identified as a core. The principles of guidance in microstructured fibers differ according to the geometry of the fiber. For a solid core microstructured fiber, the guidance is guaranteed by the modified Total Internal

Reflection (mTIR). In case of a hollow core fiber, the principles of guidance rely on Photonic Band Gap (PBG) guidance, or on guidance for Antiresonant Reflecting Optical Waveguide (Arrow) (Russell, 2003).

Because of their microstructured nature, microstructured fibers present a unique versatility for tuning their guidance characteristics and their properties. It is, in fact, possible to modify parameters like the number of propagating mode, the attenuation, the dispersion, and the birefringence by simply operating on the geometric parameters of the microstructured cladding. Moreover, the presence of holes can be effectively used to enhance the sensing properties of the fiber, by triggering a more effective interaction between the propagating light and the analyte to measure. For the above-mentioned reasons, microstructured fibers are a good platform to work in combination with the SPR technology. Because of their advantage of flexibility in the design, SPR microstructured fiber geometry can be tuned and optimized to reach the optimum evanescent field. The holes in microstructured fiber can be considered a good location for growing the dielectric-metal interface. The distance between the holes and their diameter can be varied to tailor the propagation characteristics of the leaky modes, thus optimizing the interaction between the core modes and the holes interface, improving both the sensitivity and the limit of detection (Rifat et al., 2017).

Regarding the SPR microstructured fiber design, the natural choice is to exploit the internal holes to become the metal-dielectric interface. Nevertheless, the operation of coating the internal holes, with a thin metal film, can be of difficult realization, since holes usually present small diameter. For this kind of operation, microstructured fibers that present oversized holes have selected as a preferential choice. An example is the use of suspended core fiber, which presents three large holes, separated by small glass bridges, that confine the light in a small triangular core (Hautakorpi, Mattinen, & Ludvigsen, 2012). However, microstructured fibers can be designed to optimize the geometry for the deployment of the metal layer, thus creating mixed design where both the guidance properties of the fiber and the localization of the metal layer can be tailored to achieve a better performance in terms of sensing. Typical designs, which go in this direction, are shown in Fig. 5.8. In these designs the main

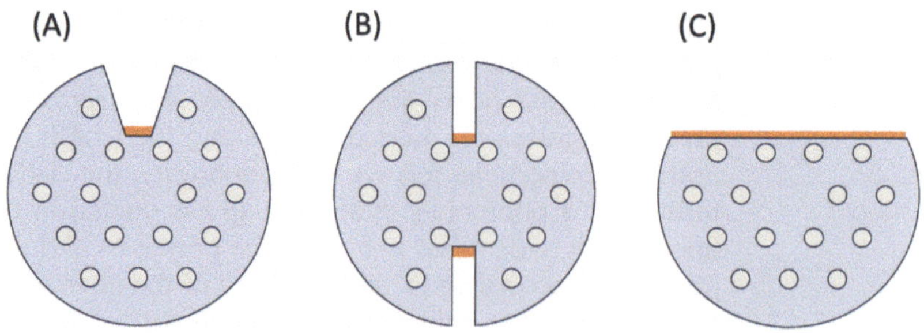

Figure 5.8 Typical designs of surface plasmon resonance microstructured fiber sensors. Channel design (A), H-shape design (B), and D-shape design (C).

properties of the guided modes, in particular the attenuation and the polarization, can be tuned by acting on the cladding holes, while the fiber can be subsequently microfabricated to arrange a convenient location for the dielectric-metal interface. It is worth noting that the D-shape design on a microstructured fiber permits a better interaction between the light and the SPP.

Currently, a conspicuous amount of effort is spent by the scientific community to numerically demonstrate the most suitable design that incorporates SPR principles by operating on microstructured fibers (Esfahani Monfared, 2020).

5.3 Application of surface plasmon resonance-based fiber sensors and biosensors

SPR-based fiber sensors are mainly used for detecting refractive indices of external solutions. This is possible because of the principles of SPP resonance applied to the optical fiber medium coated by a thin metal layer. SPR-based fiber sensors present very good characteristics in terms of sensitivity and limit of detection. Moreover, this family of sensors maintains the versatility typical of optical fibers. For this reason, SPR-based fiber sensors received a strong technological and scientific interest, pushing the research to find new and more efficient designs. The efficiency, in terms of refractive index measurement, makes SPR-based fiber sensors good and versatile chemical sensors. In fact, the sensitivity of the SPR-based fiber sensors, that can be identified as a shift of the resonance dip over the refractive index of the external analyte, presents usually values of the order of 1000 nm/RIU or more. This means that SPR-based fiber sensors can detect minimal variation of the concentration of a particular molecule inside a chemical solution. For similar reasons, SPR-based fiber sensors can be an excellent and effective platform for biosensing. The external surface of the metal film, in fact, can be functionalized to selectively detect biocomponents like proteins and DNA. Moreover, the reduced size of SPR-based fiber sensors represents an advantage in term of quantity of analyte to be detected, guaranteeing a fast and reliable detection.

5.3.1 Refractive index sensors using a surface plasmon resonance-based single mode etched fiber

The simplest, however, effective, SPR-based optical fiber sensor is based on the use of microfabricated optical fibers, where the cladding is removed to expose the core in order to create a thin metal coating and directly excite the SPP by using the interaction with the core modes. One of the most efficient and technically reliable technique of cladding removal is represented by the chemical etching. By using this technique, Coelho et al. have designed, fabricated, and demonstrated an efficient refractive index sensor suitable for chemical and biological sensing, working in near-infrared region at the typical wavelength used for telecommunication (Coelho et al., 2015).

The schematic of the sensors in shown in Fig. 5.9A. The sensor is designed to work in transmission, but the reflection operation is also possible by cutting one of the fiber ends and fabricating a mirror on the tip. For this sensor, 10 mm of a standard telecom SMF28 fiber has been etched by using a solution of 48% of HF. The thickness of the final etched region is 13 μm. The etched region has been coated with 2 nm layer of chromium (Cr). Then, a gold film with thickness of 16-nm has been deposited around the fiber. The gold layer has been covered with a dielectric layer of 120 nm of TiO_2. With this configuration the resonance dips are expected to appear at a wavelength around 1500 nm, when the refractive index of the external solution to measure is around 1.3.

The experimental session, to demonstrate the sensor, has been performed by using water solutions with addition of ethylene glycol. The refractive index of the solution to detect has been varied from 1.335 to 1.374. The progression of the dips, in the transmitted spectra, is shown in Fig. 5.9B. To such a large spectral shift of 200 nm, it corresponds a very high sensitivity of 5100 nm/RIU, as shown in

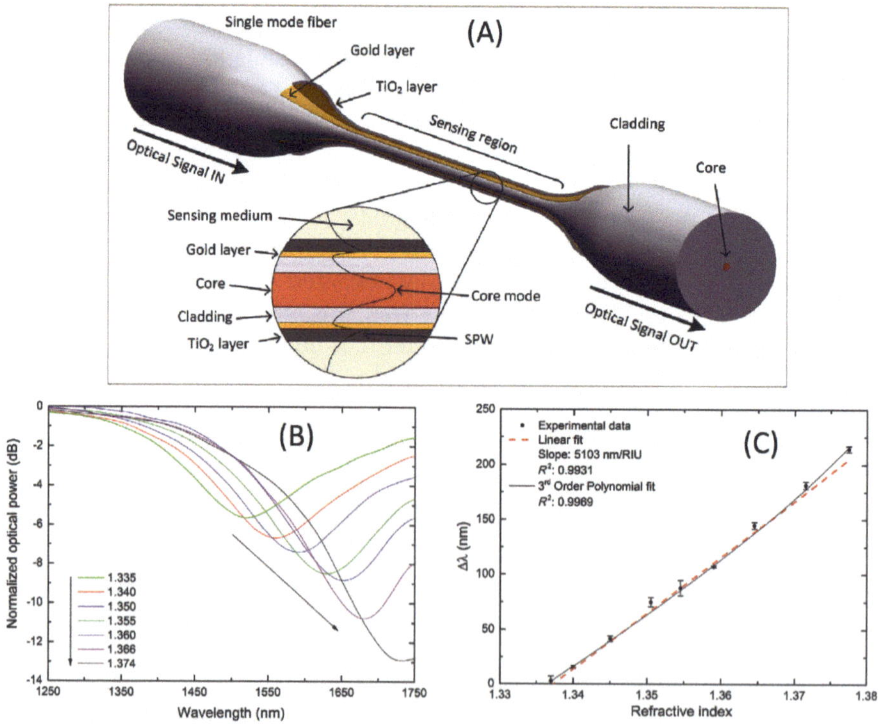

Figure 5.9 Surface plasmon resonance-based fiber sensor realized by etching a single mode optical fiber. Schematic of the sensor working in transmission mode (A). Normalized transmission spectra obtained by varying the refractive index of the analyte (B). Sensitivity of the sensor (C) (Coelho et al., 2015). Source: *Image reproduced with the permission of Springer Nature.*

Fig. 5.9C. The proposed SPR-based fiber sensor shows an excellent performance in terms of sensitivity, and it presents two fundamental advantages. The first one is related to the use of a standard telecom SMF28, which is the one cheaper and reliable fiber on the market. The second, instead, is related to the process of fabrication, which is simple and repeatable.

5.3.2 Label-free monitoring of cellular behavior by using a surface plasmon resonance-based fiber sensor

The most relevant application domain for SPR-based fiber sensors is by far biosensing. The reason for this success must be found in the number of significant advantages that SPR-based fiber sensors offer compared to other biosensing methods. The main one is the label-free aspect, but also the possibility of sensing small volume of analyte, the possibility of in situ measurement, and the capability of real-time measurement. To enable a proper SPR response in a biosensor, the thin metal layer surface must be functionalized with a bioreceptor, designed to selectively interact with a specific analyte. The result is a measurable change in terms of refractive index of the measurand. Bioreceptors of interest for biomedical applications include aptamers, proteins, DNA, enzymes, and antibodies. Often, fiber-based biosensors need to interact with the analyte a prolonged amount of time to get a relevant measurement. In this case, the sensor must present a large surface of interaction and be able to resist to external mechanical and chemical stresses. A good choice for biosensing applications is represented by SPR-based fiber sensors where the dielectric-metal interface is located on the cladding. This family of sensors shows an intrinsic robustness and a large surface to functionalize.

In 2014 Shevchenko et al. proposed an interesting application of an optical fiber biosensor for real-time analysis of cellular behavior. The authors used SPR-TFBG sensor for monitoring of cellular responses to chemical stimuli. The proposed sensor is designed to be used into conventional cell culture dishes and to be used for label-free sensing. The sensor is obtained by inscribing a TFBG in a standard telecommunication fiber. The period of the grating is set to work in the spectral region around 1500 nm. Then, the region of the cladding in proximity of the TFBG has been coated by a thin metal layer of 50 nm. The TFBG induces a coupling between the core modes and the backward cladding modes, thus redirecting the light to the dielectric-metal interface located over the cladding. At the matching condition, a SPP can be excited into the external surface of the metal film. The schematic of the sensors is shown in Fig. 5.10A. The gold surface has been treated with fibronectin to favor cell attachment, then the sensor has been inserted in a cell culture of fibroblast cells.

The rationale of the work is real-time monitoring, by measuring the change in the sensor transmission spectrum, the interaction between the fibroblast cells, captured by the surface of the sensor, and other chemicals that induce stimuli

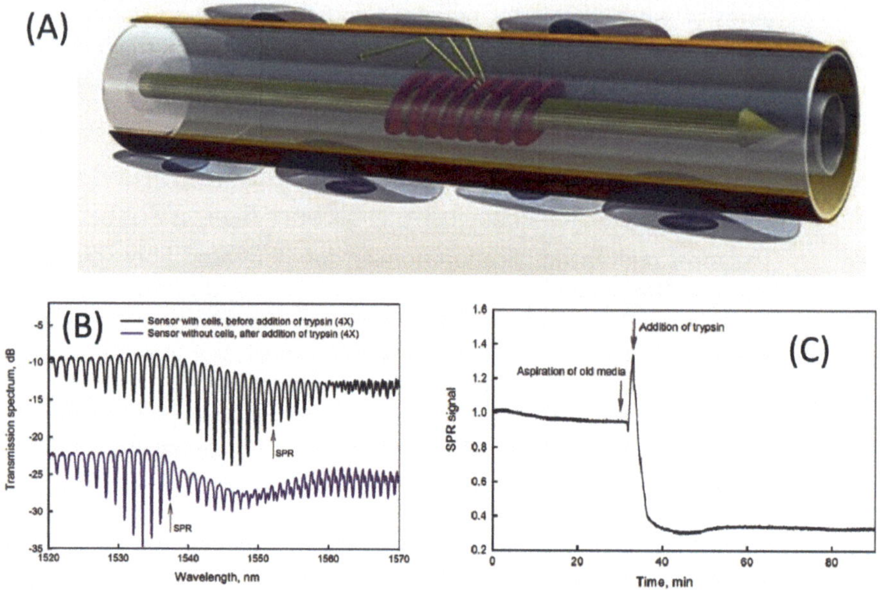

Figure 5.10 Label-free surface plasmon resonance-Tilted Fiber Bragg Gratings sensor (SPR-TFBG) for real-time monitoring of cellular responses to external chemical stimuli. Schematic of the sensors (A). Typical SPR-TFBG transmission spectra when the analyte is attached or not to the sensor (B). Real-time response of the sensor after the chemical interaction with the analyte (C) (Shevchenko et al., 2014). Source: *Image reproduced with the permission of Elsevier.*

on the cells. In between the various tests performed by the authors, the use of trypsin has been shown to detach the cells from the surface and the sensor. This behavior has been properly recorded by the sensor. In Fig. 5.10B, it is possible to see the clear resonant spectral shift given by the detachment of the cells from the surface of the sensors, while in Fig. 5.10C, it is possible to see the time evolution of the cell detachment. The LPG-TFBG sensor has been demonstrated to be a good solution, cheap and practical, for biosensing real-time applications.

5.3.3 Hybrid surface plasmon resonance-based photonic crystal fiber biosensor

Sometimes it is not a straightforward work to classify a particular configuration of an optical fiber sensor, particularly in the classification of SPR-based fiber sensors, which present a large number of designs and configurations. In many cases SPR-based fiber sensors show characteristics that embrace multiple technologies. It is the case of the sensor proposed by Wong et al. (2013), which presents a hybrid configuration where the central cut of the sensor is obtained by a piece of PCF.

In their work the authors fabricated a SPR-based fiber biosensor for selectively detecting anti-IgG antibodies. The sensor is composed by a small cut (5–20 mm) of large mode area PCF whose terminations have been collapsed. The PCF cut is then spliced on both sides to a multimode graded index optical fiber. Multimode fibers and PCF present the same cladding diameter. The goal of the central cut of the sensor, composed by the PCF, is to create a hybrid structure to direct the guided mode to the cladding interface. The PCF is then coated with a thin layer of gold of 50 nm. The schematic of the structure is shown in Fig. 5.11A. Before the functionalization of the external surface of the gold layer, the sensor has been calibrated using a solution with refractive index varying from 1.330 to 1.377. The absorbance spectra of calibration are shown in Fig. 5.11B. The shift of the SPR peak spans over 100 nm. This corresponds to an average sensitivity of roughly 2300 nm/RIU, as shown in Fig. 5.11C. It has also demonstrated that the sensitivity is poorly influenced by the thickness of the gold layer, under a certain range.

Later the thin metal surface has been functionalized by using bovine serum albumin, protein G, and immunoglobulin G (IgG). Several experiments have been conducted to test the selectivity of the sensor. The sensor has been put in contact with solutions containing concentration anti-IgG varying from 1 to 20 mg/L. The device demonstrated a good performance, showing a limit of detection of 0.267 mg/L.

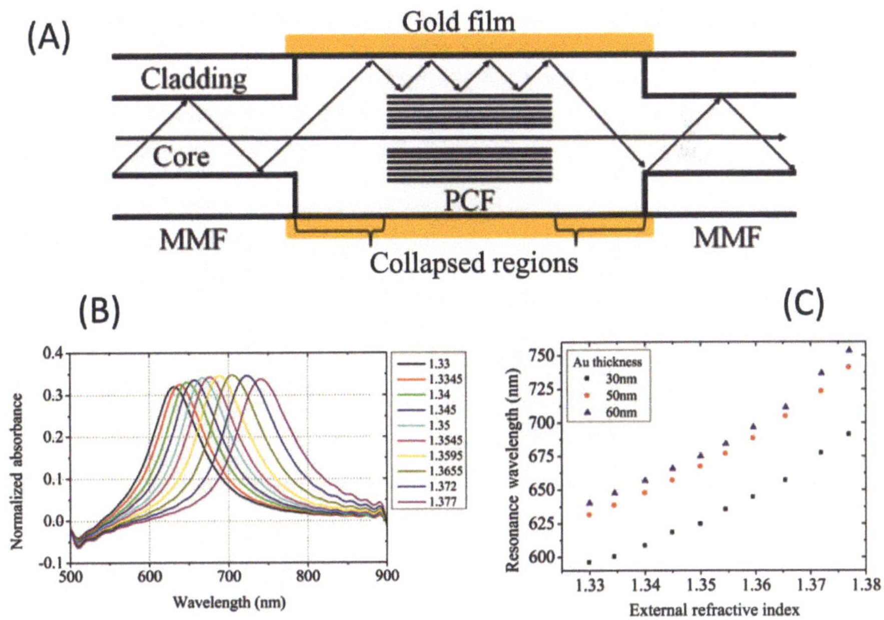

Figure 5.11 Hybrid configuration of surface plasmon resonance-based photonic crystal fiber sensor. Schematic of the sensor configuration (A). Absorbance spectra used for calibration (B). Sensitivity of the sensor (C) (Wong et al., 2013). Source: *Image reproduced with the permission of IEEE.*

5.4 Discussion

SPR-based optical fiber sensors currently represent one of the most investigated technology in the field of fiber optics, particularly in the field of fiber sensors and biosensors. The big advantage arising from the use of SPR applied to optical fiber sensor technology is represented by the extreme sensitivity of the plasmon resonance with respect to the external analyte to detect. In this regard SPR-based fiber sensors give their best in the detection of external refractive indices. These facts represent the major reason of the success of SPR-based fiber sensors in the field of biosensing. The detection of biomaterial, such as proteins, DNA fragments, or bacteria, usually requires a high sensitivity and a very low limit of detection. Moreover, most of the biosensing applications, such as the detection of molecules in a solution, or the selective capturing of a biomarker on a functionalized surface, come down to a measurement of refractive index. Other advantages of SPR-based fiber sensors are intrinsically related to the nature of optical fibers that represent an elite platform in term of versatility.

The scientific community has recently incremented the research on SPR-based fiber sensors proposing a large number of different fiber designs, in order to find the optimum sensor, which combines high sensitivity, mechanical and chemical durability, easiness of interrogation, and low cost of production. From the point of view of sensor design, indeed, the SPR technology can be coupled with basically all the other kinds of fiber sensors. It is possible to combine SPR with etched and tapered fibers to obtain highly sensitive sensors that, however, present reduced mechanical properties. It is possible to improve the SPR-based fiber sensors by exploiting the cladding modes without the necessity of microfabrication of the fiber. This fact increases the sensor robustness at the expense of the sensitivity. It is also possible to think to combine SPR technology with the versatility of microstructured fibers. This is, theoretically, a good solution to preserve both the sensitivity and the resilience of the sensor. However, the use of microstructured fibers comes with the drawback of high cost of production, and difficulties related to the interrogation of the fiber. In general, the optimum fiber biosensor does not exist. However, according to the particular application of interest, it is possible to choose the best design. In this regard, SPR-based fiber sensors offer a large fan of high-quality options.

References

Bao, X., & Chen, L. (2012). Recent progress in distributed fiber optic sensor. *Sensors, 12*(7), 8601–8639.

Caucheteur, C., Guo, T., & Albert, J. (2015). Review of plasmonic fiber optic biochemical sensors: Improving the limit of detection. *Analytical and Bioanalytical Chemistry, 407*(14), 3883–3897.

Coelho, L., de Almeida, J. M., Santos, J. L., Ferreira, R. A., André, P. S., & Viegas, D. (2015). Sensing structure based on surface plasmon resonance in chemically etched single mode optical fibres. *Plasmonics, 10*, 319–327. Available from https://doi.org/10.1007/s11468-014-9811-3.

Erdogan, T. (1997). Fiber grating spectra. *Journal of Lightwave Technology, 15*(8), 1277–1294. Available from https://doi.org/10.1109/50.618322.

Esfahani Monfared, Y. (2020). Overview of recent advances in the design of plasmonic fiber-optic biosensors. *Biosensors, 10*(7), 77.

Hautakorpi, M., Mattinen, M., & Ludvigsen, H. (2012). Surface-plasmon-resonance sensor based on three-hole microstructured optical fiber. *Optics Express, 16*(12), 8427–8432. (2008).

Iga, M.; Seki, A.; Watanabe, K. (2004). Hetero-core structured fiber optic surface plasmon resonance sensor with silver film. Sensors and Actuators B: Chemical, 101, 368–372.

Jha, R., Verma, R. K., & Gupta, B. D. (2008). Surface plasmon resonance-based tapered fiber optic sensor: Sensitivity enhancement by introducing a teflon layer between core and metal layer. *Plasmonics, 3*(151).

Jorgenson, R. C., & Yee, S. S. (1993). A fiber-optic chemical sensor based on surface plasmon resonance. *Sensors and Actuators B: Chemical, 12*(3), 213–220.

Kretschmann, E., & Raether, H. (1968). Notizen: Radiative decay of non radiative surface plasmons excited by light. *Zeitschrift für Naturforschung A, 23*(12), 2135–2136. Available from https://doi.org/10.1515/zna-1968-1247.

Lee, B., Roh, S., & Park, J. (2009). Current status of micro- and nano-structured optical fiber sensors. *Optical Fiber Technology, 15*(3), 209–221.

Lee, B. H., Kim, Y. H., Park, K. S., Eom, J. B., Kim, M. J., Rho, B. S., & Choi, H. Y. (2012). Interferometric fiber optic sensors. *Sensors, 12*(3), 2467–2486.

Li, Z., Chen, T., Zhang, Z., Zhou, Y., Li, D., & Xie, Z. (2016). Highly sensitive surface plasmon resonance sensor utilizing a long period grating with photosensitive cladding. *Applied Optics, 55*(6), 1470–1480.

Rifat A.A., Ahmed R., Yetisen A.K., Butt H., Sabouri A., Amouzad Mahdiraji G., ... Mahamd Adikan F.R., (2017). Photonic crystal fiber based plasmonic sensors, *Sensors and Actuators B: Chemical*, 243, pp. 311–325.

Russell, P. S. J. (2003). Photonic crystal fibers. *Science (New York, N.Y.), 299*, 358–362.

Saleh, B. E., & Teich, M. C. (2019). *Fundamentals of photonics*. John Wiley & Sons, Feb 27.

Sharma, A. K., Jha, R., & Gupta, B. D. (2007). Fiber-optic sensors based on surface plasmon resonance: A comprehensive review. *IEEE Sensors Journal, 7*(8), 1118–1129.

Shevchenko Y., Camci-Unal G., Cuttica D.F., Dokmeci M.R., Albert J., Khademhosseini A. (2014). Surface plasmon resonance fiber sensor for real-time and label-free monitoring of cellular behavior, *Biosensors and Bioelectronics*, 56, pp. 359–367.

Stockman, M. I. (2011). Nanoplasmonics: Past, present, and glimpse into future. *Optics Express, 19*(22), 22029–22106.

Udd, E., & Spillman, W. B., Jr (2011). editors *Fiber optic sensors: An introduction for engineers and scientists*. John Wiley & Sons.

Willets, K. A., & Van Duyne, R. P. (2007). Localized surface plasmon resonance spectroscopy and sensing. *Annual Review of Physical Chemistry, 58*, 267–297.

Wong, W. C., Chan, C. C., Boo, J. L., Teo, Z. Y., Tou, Z. Q., Yang, H. B., ... Leong, K. C. (2013). Photonic crystal fiber surface plasmon resonance biosensor based on protein G immobilization. *IEEE Journal on Selected Topics in Quantum Electronics, 19*(3), art. no. 6425403.

6 Interferometers

6.1 Introduction to interferometry

Interferometry is an important branch of photonics, with a wide range of applications that ranges from the very small, such as subpicometer displacement measurement, to the very large, such as the measurement of high energy levels (Udd, 1995; Udd & Spillman, 2011); for example, even the recent observation of gravitational waves has been performed through the LIGO (Laser Interferometer Gravitational-Wave Observer) interferometer structure. In the interferometric system, we measure the interference of two or more waves, which are coherently overlapping in the sensing structure, each wave traveling through a different optical path.

In fiber-optic biosensing, interferometry plays the role of an essential technology thanks to its direct encoding of the effective refractive index (RI) and the wavelength into the phase of the interfering waves. Considering a simple propagation of a lightwave in a lossless medium with effective RI n_{eff} and length L. If we consider the input electric field E_{in}, the output electric field E_{out} will be perturbed by a phase shift φ, as $E_{out} = E_{in} \times \exp(-j\varphi)$ (Ulaby, Michielssen, & Ravaioli, 2010). The phase shift contains both the wavelength λ and n_{eff}: $\varphi = 2\pi n_{eff} L/\lambda$. In an interferometer, we observe the interference due to the overlap of at least two waves traveling through different optical paths; since each wave has a different phase pattern, itself function of λ and n_{eff}, when we combine waves having different phase terms, we observe a difference in spectrum (due to the λ term) that changes with the effective RI. Interferometry is a powerful biosensing tool, since a small change of n_{eff} gives rise to a relevant spectral change. Different sensing methods will result in different ways to combine the multiple waves giving rise to the interferent pattern within an optical fiber device, and the techniques to engineer the external (surrounding) RI change into a change of the n_{eff} term. Modern fiber-optic biosensors use interferometric schemes, usually exploiting low-finesse low-reflectivity mirrors built by creating small gaps or cavity within the fibers, compacting the interferometer structure into a miniature-sensing probe.

Optical Fiber Biosensors.
DOI: https://doi.org/10.1016/B978-0-12-819467-6.00006-8

6.2 Principles and theory of interferometry

6.2.1 Principles of interferometry

In order to introduce the practical concepts of interferometry, we first discuss the simplest implementation of interferometric schemes in a generic waveguide, which are visually described in Fig. 6.1 reporting the main classical schemes of interferometry.

The first scheme is the Mach–Zehnder interferometer (MZI), which is a transmission interferometer. The input is connected to an 1×2 splitter, forming two separate branches of different lengths (L_1 and L_2), which are collected with a 2×1 combiner, symmetrical to the input splitter. The interference beams are collected on the output side, hence the device is working in transmission mode. We can observe the interference pattern at the 2×1 output, where the two beams intersect. The Michaelson interferometer has a similar architecture, and substantially adapts the MZI to work in reflection. It is formed by a 2×2 device (or a 2×1 followed by an 1×2), allowing to collect the output from the same side of the input. Two mirrors, on both arms, form the optical path by reflecting the light back toward the input side; the intersection point is located at the center of the 2×2 splitter. We can notice that the Mach–Zehnder and Michaelson are similar interferometric structures, in optical terms: if we use the image plane method and we "rotate" the left side of the interferometer around the mirrors, we obtain the MZI structure. The theory of the two devices is very similar, taking into account that the interference path is run across once in the MZI, and twice (forward and backward) in the

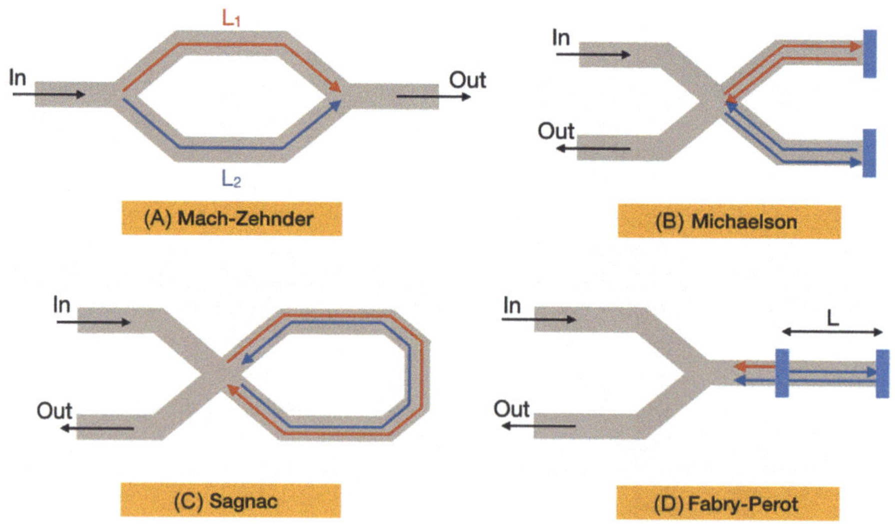

Figure 6.1 Schematic of the main fiber-optic interferometer architectures. The chart shows the fiber setup and two main optical paths, indicated with red and blue colors. (A) Mach–Zehnder interferometer; (B) Michaelson interferometer; (C) Sagnac or loop interferometer; (D) Fabry–Perot interferometer.

Michaelson architecture. Also, the optical paths of the two interferometers are spatially separated, since they run through two different fibers or waveguides.

The Sagnac interferometer, often referred as ring, loop, or gyro, is formed with a 2×2 splitter closed on a loop. The left sides lead to the input and the output, which can be collected in reflection. The right side forms a loop, closed between the input and the output. The two optical paths are not spatially separated, but run across the same loop: the first path runs from the upper toward the lower side, and the second path in the opposite direction but within the same fiber.

Finally, the other common structure is the Fabry–Perot interferometer (FPI), formed by a cavity, that is, the cascade of two (or more) mirrors having distance L. The figure sketches a reflection interferometer, but we can simply collect the light after right mirror to work in transmission. Unlike previous interferometers, the FPI is a multipath interferometer: at the intersection point (on the left mirror, in the figure) we see the overlap of (1) light being reflected by the first mirror, (2) light being transmitted through the first mirror, reflected by the second mirror, and transmitted through the first, (3) light being transmitted through the first mirror, reflected three times, and transmitted through, etc. Hence, we overlap light running 0, 2, 4, 6,... times through the inner cavity of length L. The optical paths run through the same cavity, and the mirror reflectivities weight the order of each interference; if mirrors have low reflectivity, we only "see" two optical paths as higher orders would be significantly attenuated, but if mirrors have high reflectivity we "see" the contribution of many orders of the transmission-reflection process.

6.2.2 Mach–Zehnder interferometer

To better understand the effect of interferometry, we now study the working principle of the MZI (Martinez, Griol, Sanchis, & Marti, 2003; Udd & Spillman, 2011). Consider an ideal lossless MZI, having 50/50 splitter and 50/50 combiner; the length of the upper side is L_1 and the effective RI of the upper waveguide is n_1; similarly, length and effective RI of the lower side are L_2 and n_2. The input field carries a power P_{in}, and an electric field E_{in}; we know that the optical power, which is the parameter that we measure, is proportional to the square of the electric field intensity.

We now consider the two electric fields, interfering at the intersection point. At the point of output intersection, the two fields $E_{out,1}$ and $E_{out,2}$ are:

$$E_{out,1} = \frac{1}{\sqrt{2}} E_{in} e^{-j2\pi\frac{L_1 n_1}{\lambda}} \tag{6.1}$$

$$E_{out,2} = \frac{1}{\sqrt{2}} E_{in} e^{-j2\pi\frac{L_2 n_2}{\lambda}}$$

where we observe the phase shift due to the propagation through the interferometer arms, and the splitting ratio of each channel. The output field E_{out}, measured at the outer side of the interferometer, is based on the linear combination of the fields $E_{out,1}$ and $E_{out,2}$ weighted by the combiner:

$$E_{out} = \frac{1}{\sqrt{2}}\left(E_{out,1} + E_{out,2}\right) \tag{6.2}$$
$$= \frac{1}{2}E_{in}\left(e^{-j2\pi\frac{L_1 n_1}{\lambda}} + e^{-j2\pi\frac{L_2 n_2}{\lambda}}\right)$$
$$= \frac{1}{2}E_{in}e^{-j2\pi\frac{L_1 n_1}{\lambda}}\left(1 + e^{-j\frac{2\pi}{\lambda}(L_2 n_2 - L_1 n_1)}\right)$$

where we highlight the term $\Delta\varphi = 2\pi/\lambda\ (L_2 n_2 - L_1 n_1)$ as the *optical path difference*, which is the phase differential between the waves traveling the two arm of the interferometer. Since the output power P_{out} is proportional to $|E_{out}|^2$ we can now calculate the output power as:

$$P_{out} = \frac{1}{4}P_{in}\left|1 + e^{-j\Delta\varphi}\right|^2 \tag{6.3}$$

and, unfolding the right term using Euler's formula, we obtain a sine-wave expression for the output term:

$$P_{out} = \frac{1}{2}P_{in}(1 + cos\Delta\varphi) \tag{6.4}$$

Therefore we can see the effect of the interferometer in action: a change in the optical path difference, either a length stretch of L_1 or L_2, or a RI change of n_1 or n_2, results in a change of $\Delta\varphi$, which in turns result in a change of the output power. The P_{out} term, which is the parameter measured in the interferometer, has a periodic pattern, characterized by peaks and valley. The maxima of P_{out} occur when $\Delta\varphi = 0,\ \pm 2\pi,\ \pm 4\pi,\ \ldots$, while minima occur for $\Delta\varphi = \pm\pi,\ \pm 3\pi,\ \pm 5\pi, \ldots$. If we consider the power maximum values, they occur for $(L_2 n_2 - L_1 n_1) = \pm m\lambda$, where m is an integer, which means that the difference in optical path is a multiple of the wavelength.

In the MZI-based measurement devices, one arm of the interferometer usually serves as reference, while the second arm contains the sensing point. If we consider the first arm as the reference, having L_1 and n_1 fixed, then the second arm can act as a sensor; in RI sensors, we fix L_2 and consider a variation of n_2 as $n_2 = n_{2,ref} + \Delta n$, where Δn is the small RI variation that we want to measure. So we can rewrite the term "OPD" as $\Delta\varphi = \Delta\varphi_{ref} + \delta\varphi$, where $\Delta\varphi_{ref} = 2\pi/\lambda\ (L_2 n_{2,ref} - L_1 n_1)$ and $\delta\varphi = 2\pi\ L_2\Delta n/\lambda$.

The derivative of P_{out} with respect to Δn shows how sensitive is the power variation with respect to small Δn variations:

$$\frac{\partial P_{out}}{\partial(\Delta n)} = -\frac{\pi P_{in} L_2}{\lambda} sin(\Delta\varphi_{ref} + \delta\varphi) \tag{6.5}$$

which is maximum when the argument of the sine function is equal to odd multiples of π. However, in most modern interferometers the full spectrum is measured, hence the detection method aims at measuring spectral shifts rather than intensity changes. The periodicity of the $\Delta\varphi$ term is such that any two adjacent maxima are always spaced by a phase change of 2π, that is, when $(L_2n_2 - L_1n_1) = \lambda$.

In an MZI, the properties of the interferometers are therefore tuned by the choice of L_1 and L_2, as well as on the choice of the splitting ratio. By reducing the asymmetry of the splitter (e.g., choosing a 80/20, 90/10, or 95/5), the power modulation reduces its amplitude with respect to the mean value; the periodicity is instead encoded in the choice of L_1 and L_2.

The MZI theory can apply also to the Michaelson interferometer, by replacing L_1 and L_2 with $2L_1$ and $2L_2$, since the light runs twice the optical path, and adjusting each field by the reflection coefficient of the mirror.

6.2.3 Fabry–Perot interferometer

The FPI is a multipath structure formed by a cavity of length L and refractive index n, closed by two mirrors having reflectivity R_1 and R_2. As such, we cannot limit our analysis to two interfering beams, but we need to account the whole amount of reflections occurring between the cavity mirrors. The number of reflections that we can see in practice depends on the coherency of the source used in the interrogation system; laser sources have a deep coherency length and can detect several orders of reflections, while white light sources have a shallow coherency length and therefore limit the analysis to few reflections.

In order to account for a generalized FPI model for a single cavity, which, however, can be easily extended to multiple cavities, we can consider the FPI as the cascade of the first mirror, a propagation term, and the second mirror. We can consider each item as a two-port device, and write the transmission matrix of each element (Tosi, 2016). The transmission matrix is a generalized method to express the input/output relations of a multiport device; it is generated from the scattering (or S) matrix, but allows resolving cascade of devices in a simpler way (Fricke, 2010).

Considering Γ_1 and Γ_2 as the reflection coefficients of the mirrors, and τ_1 and τ_2 as the transmission coefficients of the mirrors, and assuming lossless conditions, that is, $|\Gamma_1|^2 + |\tau_1|^2 = |\Gamma_2|^2 + |\tau_2|^2 = 1$; we can write the transmission matrices of the mirrors as:

$$T_{M1} = -\frac{j}{\tau_1}\begin{bmatrix} -1 & \Gamma_1 \\ -\Gamma_1 & 1 \end{bmatrix} \tag{6.6}$$

$$T_{M2} = -\frac{j}{\tau_2}\begin{bmatrix} -1 & \Gamma_2 \\ -\Gamma_2 & 1 \end{bmatrix}$$

The transmission matrix of the propagation within the cavity can be simply written as

$$T_P = \begin{bmatrix} e^{j2\pi Ln/\lambda} & 0 \\ 0 & e^{-j2\pi Ln/\lambda} \end{bmatrix} \tag{6.7}$$

The transmission matrix of the whole FPI can be calculated by multiplying each element of the cascade:

$$T_{FPI} = T_{M1} \times T_P \times T_{M2} \tag{6.8}$$

$$= -\frac{1}{\tau_1 \tau_2} \begin{bmatrix} e^{j2\pi Ln/\lambda} - \Gamma_1\Gamma_2 e^{-j2\pi Ln/\lambda} & \Gamma_1 e^{-j2\pi Ln/\lambda} - \Gamma_2 e^{j2\pi Ln/\lambda} \\ \Gamma_1 e^{j2\pi Ln/\lambda} - \Gamma_2 e^{-j2\pi Ln/\lambda} & e^{-j2\pi Ln/\lambda} - \Gamma_1\Gamma_2 e^{j2\pi Ln/\lambda} \end{bmatrix}$$

The reflection coefficient of the FPI can be calculate from the transmission matrix:

$$\Gamma_{FPI} = \frac{T_{FPI}(1,2)}{T_{FPI}(2,2)} = \frac{\Gamma_1 - \Gamma_2 e^{j4\pi Ln/\lambda}}{1 - \Gamma_1\Gamma_2 e^{j4\pi Ln/\lambda}} \tag{6.9}$$

The phase term $\exp(j4\pi Ln/\lambda)$ is the optical path difference between each order of reflection, and corresponds to a two-way (forth and back) run across the interferometer. In the noteworthy case of the two mirrors having the same reflectivity, that is, $|\Gamma_1|^2 = |\Gamma_2|^2 = R$, then we can obtain the spectrum of the FPI as a closed-form expression:

$$R_{FPI} = \frac{4R\sin^2(2\pi Ln/\lambda)}{(1-R)^2 + 4R\sin^2(2\pi Ln/\lambda)} \tag{6.10}$$

and the transmission spectrum is equal to $(1 - R_{FPI})$. Multiple-cavity FPI interferometry can be resolved by applying the transmission matrix method to each element of the cascade.

The spectra of FPI, simulated with the transmission matrix method, are shown in Fig. 6.2. We observe that the spectra have a periodicity, with period growing proportionally to the wavelength due to the phase change. The envelope of the spectrum is similar to a sine wave, for small reflectivity values: in this condition, the interferometer spectrum tends to the shape of a sine wave since second and higher orders of reflection are substantially attenuated. This is also explainable from Eq. (6.10): for small values of R, the denominator of the R_{FPI} term tends to 1, hence $R_{FPI} \approx 4R\ \sin^2(2\pi Ln/\lambda) = 2R\ (1 - \cos(4\pi Ln/\lambda))$ and we obtain the same expression of Eq. (6.4) of an MZI. For high values of reflectivity, instead, the reflection spectrum appears to have a more pronounced lobe, with a narrow transmission dip. When the mirror reflectivity grows over 90%, the FPI becomes a transmission filter with a narrow bandwidth, increasing the contrast of the modulation of the amplitude.

The second chart shows the spectrum of an FPI in operative condition, when either the cavity length L varies, or the cavity RI n is changed; for simplicity, we

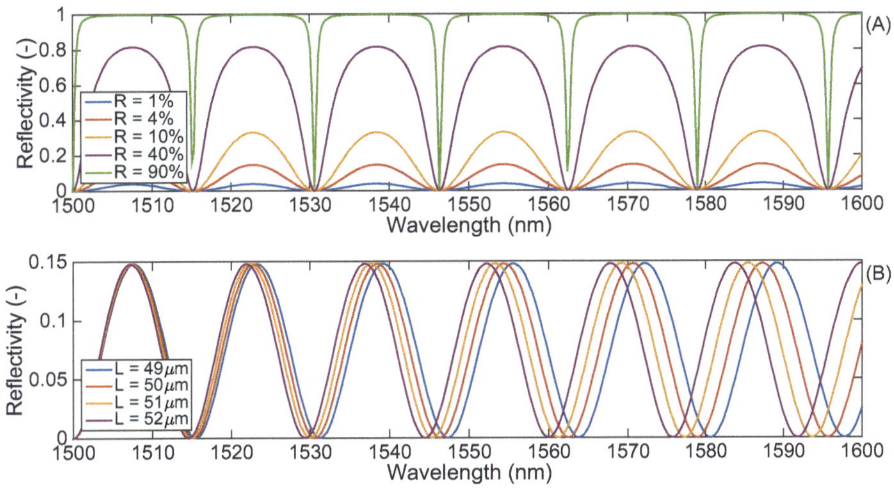

Figure 6.2 Reflection spectrum of a simulated FPI, reporting the reflectivity as a function of the wavelength over 1500–1600 nm range. (A) FPI having $L = 50$ μm and $n = 1.5$, for different values of mirror reflectivity ranging from 1% to 90%. (B) FPI having $n = 1.5$ and $R = 4\%$, for L ranging from 49 to 52 μm. *FPI*, Fabry–Perot interferometer.

report the case of cavity length variation, but a similar effect would be observed with the variations of n. We observe that the change of the optical path results in a change of the periodicity of the interferometer: the spectra appear to spread in wavelength, and each peak or valley shifts toward longer wavelengths. While the whole envelope of the interferometer appears to change, interferometer-based biosensors in general operate under small-signal analysis, that is, small variations of the optical cavity length.

6.2.4 Definitions and characterization of an interferometer

The definitions of interferometers used in optical fiber sensors are similar to their counterparts used in spectrometry or displacement measurements, and can be applied for any practical implementation of the device. In general, interferometers having a low reflectivity, and therefore a low finesse, are used in sensing, due to the presence of air/glass (4% reflectivity) or glass/water (0.4% reflectivity) interfaces; however, the following definitions can apply to any interferometric device. They are also used to define the main quality parameter of the interferometer, and are evaluated from the reflection or transmission spectrum as shown in Fig. 6.3.

Free spectral range (FSR): It is the difference, in wavelength or frequency, between two adjacent peaks or valleys of the reflection or transmission spectrum of the interferometer. As in Fig. 6.3, the FSR is calculated from the two valleys of the second envelope. The FSR is popular definition in high-reflectivity

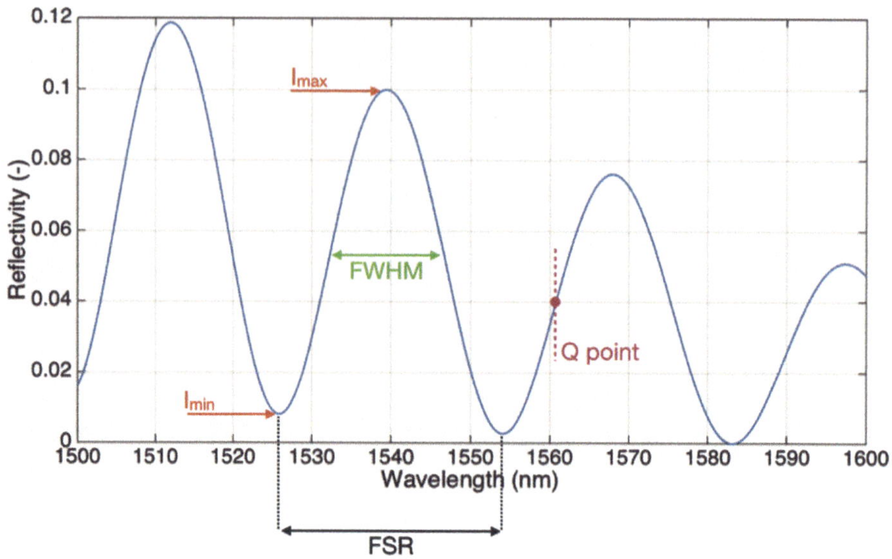

Figure 6.3 Visualization and definition of the main parameters of a generic interferometer, based on the reflection spectrum.

FPI devices used for absorption spectrometers, but since all interferometers have a periodical shape it can be extended to any device by simply computing the periodicity. It is important to underline that since the optical path difference terms of interferometers are proportional to $1/\lambda$, and the periodicity is for multiples of 2π for the MZI (and for all transmission interferometers that run once through the optical path) or π for the FPI or Michaelson (and for all interferometers that forward and backward through an optical path), the FSR is proportional to λ. This means that when working with broadband analyzers, the interferometer has more fringes at short wavelengths, which become coarser as the wavelength increases.

Fringe visibility: The fringe visibility defines the *contrast* of the interferometer, that is, the difference between the maximum and minimum intensity values of the interferometer. Here, for intensity we define either the reflectivity or transmittivity, or the power, or the return loss depending on which device is used for interrogation. The fringe visibility υ, shown in Fig. 6.3 for the second fringe, is equal to:

$$\upsilon = \frac{I_{max} - I_{min}}{I_{max} + I_{min}} \tag{6.11}$$

where I_{max} and I_{min} are, respectively, the maximum and minimum value of the intensity of the fringe. The fringe visibility is a normalized figure of merit of the interferometer, because it affects the quality of detection: interferometer with a clear fringe as in Fig. 6.3, where the fringe visibility is equal to 0.42, can easily detect the spectrum even in presence of noise or interference, while interferometer with a shallow fringe ($\upsilon < 0.05$) cannot be easily detected as the fringe is almost invisible.

Full-width half maximum (FWHM): The FWHM of the interferometer refers to the extension of the interferometer at half of the peak power (normalized by the lowest power). The FWHM measures the bandwidth of the spectral fringes: interferometers with a weak reflectivity have a large FWHM, but the bandwidth of the spectral peaks significantly restricts for high-reflectivity interferometers.

Finesse: The finesse F of the interferometer is a quality parameter, that relates the FSR and FWHM:

$$F = \frac{FSR}{FWHM} \tag{6.12}$$

For a Fabry–Perot structure with identical mirror, F is equal to

$$F = \frac{\pi\sqrt{R}}{1 - R} \tag{6.13}$$

Selective interferometers, having a high reflectivity, have a low finesse value, usually in the order of 0.2–1; however, the finesse can significantly rise over 10 when $R > 75\%$.

Quadrature (Q) point: The Q point is located the spectral points of the interferometer spectrum at which the rate of change of the spectrum can be located; they correspond to the maxima and minima of $\partial P_{out}/\partial\lambda$, that is, to the zeros of the second-order derivative $\partial^2 P_{out}/\partial\lambda^2 = 0$. The Q point is usually the spectral location monitored for monochromatic interrogation of interferometer, since we observe the maximum intensity change for a given change of RI.

Wavelength shift: The most popular approach for interferometer detection is to detect the wavelength shift of an interferometer spectral peak, or valley, upon measuring the whole reflection spectrum. Although, as from the previous theory, a change of RI and therefore of the optical path results in a change of periodicity of the whole spectrum, when the RI change Δn is small it results in a spectral shift $\Delta\lambda$. This allows calculating the sensitivity as $\Delta\lambda/\Delta n$, as for many of the other sensors.

6.3 Fiber-optic interferometric biosensors

Mach–Zehnder, Michaelson, Sagnac, and FPIs represent the key principle of optical interferometry that can be used for RI sensors and biosensors; in all of them, the change of the RI affects the length of the optical path, causing a shift of the interferometer fringes. In order to fabricate probes that have high sensitivity, compact form factor, and do not rely on circuits with multiple fibers, we can design interferometers that modify the design or the implementation of the classical interferometers, improving the performance. In this section, we review the most effective design methods for fiber-optic biosensors based on interferometry.

6.3.1 All-glass extrinsic Fabry–Perot interferometer

The most elegant design of an FPI cavity on an optical fiber has been reported by Poeggel et al. as an extrinsic Fabry-Perot interferometer (EFPI) (Poeggel et al., 2014); the term extrinsic refers to the fact that the cavity makes use of an external element to close the structure.

The EFPI structure is shown in Fig. 6.4, reporting the schematic and the simulated reflection spectra. The structure is formed as an all-glass probe with three distinct mirrors and two cavities. The inner cavity is formed between the tip of an single mode fiber (SMF) fiber, and the facet of a second fiber serving as a tip diaphragm: both mirrors have a ~4% reflectivity and form an air-gap with length L that constitutes the main cavity. The second cavity is the diaphragm, having length d, and closed by the third mirror, which is the Fresnel reflection between the diaphragm and the external RI; as the external RI changes by a quantity Δn, we observe a change of reflectivity of the third mirror, which alters the spectral pattern (by reducing or increasing the visibility of the second cavity). The whole structure is encapsulated by a glass capillary, which seals the inner air-gap.

The structure proposed by Poeggel et al. is compact and all-glass, making it a biocompatible sensor easy to fabricate. In this implementation, the lead-in fiber is a standard SMF (10/125 μm core/cladding diameter), and the diaphragm is a multimode fiber (MMF) (62.5/200 μm core/cladding diameter), with the capillary matching the diaphragm outer size and allowing sliding the SMF inside of it (130/200 μm inner/outer diameter). The whole structure is fabricated by splicing and polishing; the fiber surfaces are first prepolished, and a manual splicer is used to splice the diaphragm to capillary, as well as to fuse the SMF to the capillary far from the air-gap. When the diaphragm is short, the EFPI has a high pressure sensitivity, but long diaphragm lengths (>5 μm) ensure that the sensor is RI-sensitive only.

Fig. 6.4B shows a simulated EFPI spectrum, for a sensor having cavity length 30 μm, diaphragm length 7 μm, and immersed in water with external RI changes between 0 and 0.08 RIU. We observe that the fringes of the interferometer change in intensity in a quite significant way, particularly on the second fringe due to the different visibility of the second cavity, resulting also in a wavelength shift of the peak wavelength. The inset on the inner part of the fringe shows that the peak wavelength shifts from 1556.89 to 1558.14 nm for a 0.08 RIU change, hence with a sensitivity of 15.7 nm/RIU.

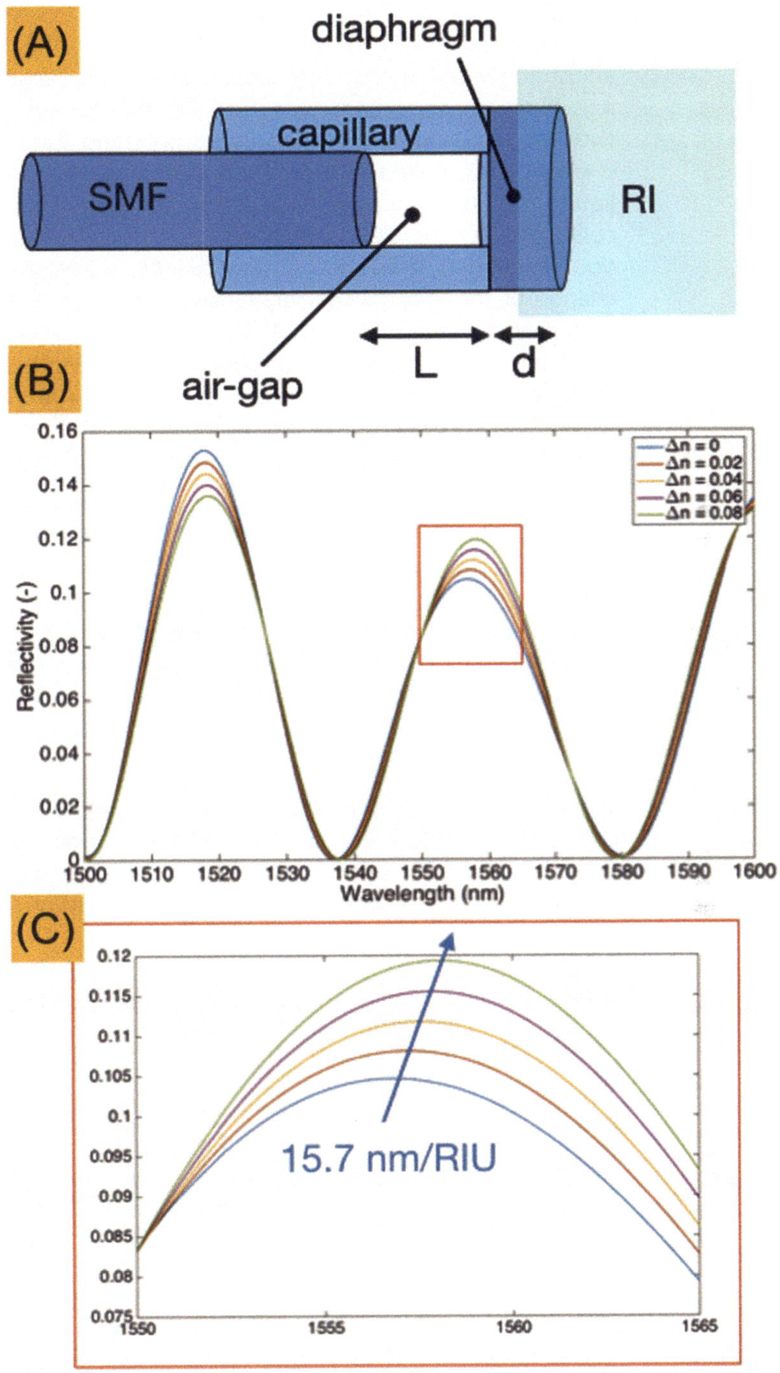

Figure 6.4
Design and analysis of an EFPI all-glass sensor. (A) Schematic of the structure; (B) simulated EFPI reflection spectrum for different values of RI change Δn; (C) zoom on the reflection peak wavelength shift with sensitivity estimation.

The EFPI structure achieves RI sensing with a good sensitivity, and it is possible to vary the number of spectral fringe within the interrogation window by adjusting the value of *L*. This can be done on a standard telecom fiber. Overall, it is a simple and cheap structure to fabricate and interrogate in reflection, with modern splicers and automated polishing stations; the choice of capillary is essential to make the sensor robust and seal the inner air-gap from external liquids. The main disadvantage is that the sensor is a two-step fabrication process (splicing + polishing), hence cannot be automated in a single-step fabrication. The other drawback is that the RI change is encoded in a reflectivity change of the external mirror, rather than in an in-line change of the optical path length; that means that the intensity change of the spectral fringes is more effective than the corresponding wavelength shift, as can be observed from Fig. 6.4B, limiting the sensitivity in terms of nm/RIU.

6.3.2 Spherical resonator

A spherical resonator is a multipath interferometer formed by fabricating a sphere at the tip of an optical fiber. The sphere having diameter a few times larger than the fiber itself acts by triggering multiple resonant modes in the tip, which act as a cavity and interfere. In this type of interferometer, the generation of modes is governed by the shape of the sphere and its ellipticity, as well as by the coating around the fiber, which affects the reflectivity of each path. As the light rebounds multiple times inside a spherical resonator, the types and number of excited modes are not well controllable, but rather similar to a "random" resonator.

The simplest fabrication method was proposed by Nazarbayev University and is shown in Fig. 6.5. The resonator has been fabricated with a CO_2 laser splicer (Fujikura LZM-100) using a splicing mode designed for spherical lenses, used in laser-based microscopy methods (LaserFocusWorld, 2019). This recipe is an

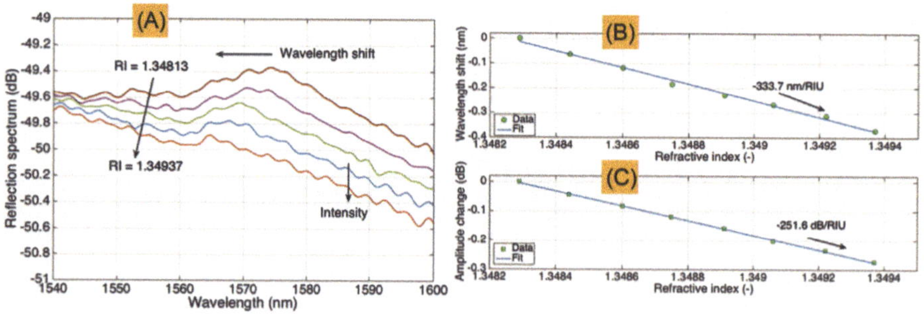

Figure 6.5 Characteristic and performance of a spherical resonator, fabricated at Nazarbayev University with a CO_2 laser splicer. (A) Reflection spectrum, for different RI values from 1.34813 to 1.34937; (B) wavelength shift as a function of the RI, estimating the sensitivity to −333.7 nm/RIU; (C) intensity change as a function of the RI, estimating the sensitivity to −251.6 dB/RIU. *RI*, refractive index.

one-step fabrication, as two-standard SMF fibers are fused together to form a resonator with 0.4%–4% reflectivity (water–air) at each wall. The figure shows the spectrum of a resonator with diameter 547 μm fabricated on an 125 μm fiber, and interrogated with an optical backscatter reflectometer. Rather than observing a clear spectrum as in traditional FPI structures, we see shallow fluctuation of the reflection spectrum, which, however, appear to have a clear shift in wavelength and amplitude. In Fig. 6.5A, we observe a peak at 1562–1572 nm when operating in water, which shifts toward the lower wavelengths as the RI increases. The peak has a very shallow visibility, with $v = 0.002$, but it is possible to track its wavelength shift; the result in Fig. 6.5B shows a very linear pattern with sensitivity of −333.7 nm/RIU, which is a high result as the interrogator can detect around 2 pm shifts. Besides the wavelength shift, as the increase of RI reduces the wall reflectivity of the sphere/liquid interface, resulting in a change of the reflected intensity that can be measured at the Q point, around 1586 nm. The interrogation of the amplitude change leads to a sensitivity of −251.6 dB/RIU, visualized in Fig. 6.5C.

The spherical resonator, fabricated with a CO_2 laser splicer, has the advantage of a very straightforward and cheap fabrication (30 seconds to 20 minutes per probe, depending on the target ellipticity of the sphere), and achieves sensitivities well in the order of several hundreds of nm/RIU. From the point of view of probe fabrication, spherical resonators have excellent properties: they work in reflection, which is the easiest mode to fabricate a probe, and since spheres have shape in the order of half millimeter, they are both mechanically robust when used and small enough to be package in minimally invasive devices. The main drawback is the lack of well-detectable modes with a high fringe visibility, which forces the interrogation to either detect shallow spectral shifts or track an intensity change, therefore leading to a less robust method for detection; in addition, while FPI spectra are repeatable and usually well defined, each resonator has a different spectral pattern, which comes as a result of the random reflection occurring in the sphere. The other key drawback is the low reflectivity of the structure; since light rebounds more than once on each interface, the amount of reflected light is small and below the limit of detection of common FBG interrogators. Users need to resort to a different method of interrogation, based on either a spectrometer with a large integration time (which, however, reduces the reliability of amplitude detection and introduces more noise), an optical spectrum analyzer operating on a wide bandwidth (which limits the resolution bandwidth), or an optical backscatter analyzer that can detect very low power levels.

6.3.3 Microstructured Mach–Zehnder interferometers

The MZI structure is based on the interference of two light beams traveling in transmission, along two arms. In order to avoid using two separate fibers for reference and sensing, which would be unpractical in several applications and would reduce the robustness of the sensing method, current research addresses the fabrication of in-fiber MZI structures, in which we still have two separate light beams interfering but within the same fiber. By combining the high figures of merit of the MZI, and the fact that the FSR can be easily designed by selecting the cavity length, with an all-in-one-fiber form factor we can obtain a highly sensitive compact probe with a straightforward principle of operation.

The work reported by Song, Zhang, Liu, Lin, and Wu (2016) reports an MZI sensor, functionalized for DNA sensing, which uses a microfiber cavity. The sensor scheme and performance are shown in Fig. 6.6. The sensor, shown photographically in Fig. 6.6A, is formed by two SMF fibers, with an inner cavity made by a microfiber of 51.4 μm diameter, obtained by tapering a SMF fiber. The fabrication process is entirely splicer-based, with a fusion splicer (Fujikura FSM-60). At first, a SMF fiber is tapered, forming a microfiber of thickness about 2/5 of the initial SMF. The tapered microfiber is then spliced to an SMF, forming the left part of the sensor; the right side of the sensor is formed in a similar way. Finally, the two sides are spliced together with a slight misalignment, which can be seen from the microscopic view of the sensor. The authors fabricated three sensors of different cavity lengths (176.88, 272.81, and 434.72 μm).

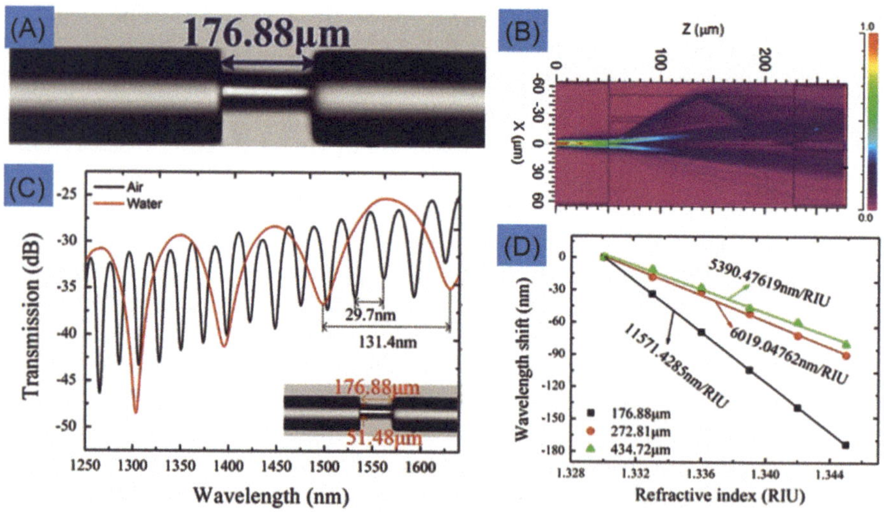

Figure 6.6 Characteristics of an MZI based on a fiber microcavity. (A) View of the microfiber cavity MZI sensor, with cavity length 176.88 μm; (B) simulation of the electrical field propagation within the cavity along direction of propagation *z*; (C) transmission spectra of the MZI sensor, in air and water; (D) RI sensitivity of the MZI, for cavities having different lengths (176.88, 272.81, and 434.72 μm). *MZI*, Mach–Zehnder interferometer; *RI*, refractive index. Source: *Image reproduced with permission. Proposed by Song, B., Zhang, H., Liu, B., Lin, W., & Wu, J. (2016). Label-free in-situ real-time DNA hybridization kinetics detection employing microfiber-assisted Mach-Zehnder interferometer.* Biosensors and Bioelectronics, 81, *151–158.*

The sensor having microfiber cavity within two SMFs behaves as an MZI, as shown in Fig. 6.6B, which simulates the propagating field within the structure. Entering into the microfiber from the SMF, the light is split into three beams; the lower beam is not coupled into the second SMF, while the upper beam and the light rebounding from the cladding of the microfiber form the two arms of the interferometer. This phenomenon is well visible on the upper side of the chart, where the light reflected at the upper bound interferes with the beam propagating from the SMF to the microfiber and to the second SMF. As a result, the structure behaves as an MZI, and its transmission spectrum shown in Fig. 6.6C has a periodic pattern with clear fringes; the FSR of the resonator is 29.7 nm and the interferometer contrast is about 10 dB and $\upsilon \approx 0.8$ (in water). The RI calibration in water shows sensitivity values ranging from -5390 to 11,571 nm/RIU, the latter value recorded for the shortest cavity length.

Another approach has been proposed by Li et al. (2017) and shown in Fig. 6.7. In this work, a microstructured MZI has been proposed, having an inner cavity of length 98 μm fabricated with an fs laser. The method proposed in this work combines the MZI with an optofluidic device, where four channels drilled by the laser are connected directly to the cavity formed in the fiber core. The cavity, as shown in the schematic, has four channels formed by an 800-nm laser with energy 65 nJ, which allows drilling at 5 μm/s speed into the core. After the channel is formed, hydrofluoric acid is injected in the channels, to form the inner cavity and obtain a change of inner RI in proximity of the fiber core.

When a liquid solution is introduced into the inner cavity, around the core of the fiber, through the channel, the device works as an MZI; the two optical paths here are represented by the light propagating across the cavity through the fiber, and the light propagating in the liquid within the cavity. As a result, at the end of the cavity the field interference is observed, and the transmission show the RI dependence. The transmission fringes, shown in Fig. 6.7B, have

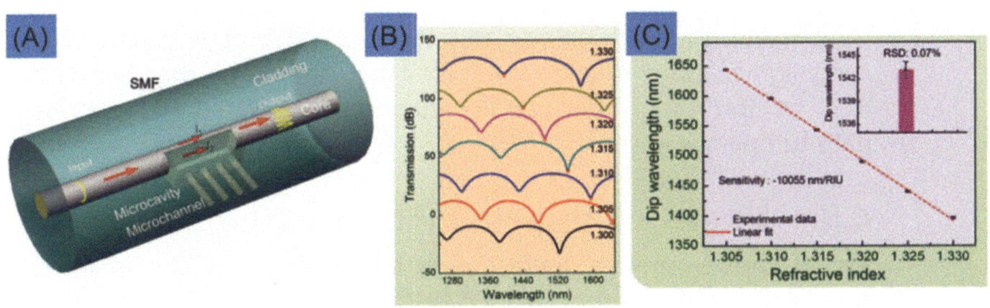

Figure 6.7 Characteristics of a microstructured MZI fabricated with an fs laser. (A) Schematic of the sensor; (B) transmission spectra of the interferometer at different values of RI (1.30–1.33); (C) estimation of the RI sensitivity. *MZI*, Mach–Zehnder interferometer; *RI*, refractive index. Source: *Image reproduced with permission. Proposed by Li, Z., Liao, C., Chen, D., Song, J., Jin, W., Peng, G. D., ... Wang, Y. (2017). Label-free detection of bovine serum albumin based on an in-fiber Mach-Zehnder interferometric biosensor.* Optics Express, *25(15), 17105–17113.*

fringes in the order of 15–25 dB, and the sensitivity can be estimated by tracking the deeper spectral valley. Due to the large variation of RI between the fiber core and the liquid, the FSR of the interferometer is large, about 130 nm at 1500 nm, which requires a broadband interrogator in order to achieve a detection. The sensitivity of the device, shown in Fig. 6.7C, is 10,055 nm/RIU.

A common point of the microstructured MZI is that $FSR = \lambda^2/(L\Delta n_{eff})$ where L is the cavity length and Δn_{eff} is the difference in effective RI between the two elements composing the optical path. In Song et al. (2016) the difference in the effective RI can be visible by the large difference between the light steered toward the end-side of the cavity, and the angle of incidence of the light into the microfiber; in Li et al. (2017) Δn_{eff} is approximately equal to 0.13 (the difference between 1.464 of glass and 1.333 of water). Hence, in order to have a spectrum with multiple fringes and shorten the FSR to tens of nanometers, longer cavities should be fabricated.

Microstructured MZI devices achieve a high sensitivity, in the order of several thousands of nm/RIU, and therefore are suitable for biosensors with low limit of detection. The spectra of MZI devices are well clear, with fringes in order of >10 dB and an easily interpretable shape, which simplifies the detection. Another advantage is that they can be fabricated with a relatively simple setup: Song et al. (2016) propose an all-splicer fabrication, with the cavity, tapers, and interfaces all manufactured with an advanced arc-fusion splicer, while Li et al. (2017) implement an fs-laser fabrication method, which is relatively fast. The main disadvantage is that MZI interferometers work in transmission, rather than in reflection; hence, they are not well suitable to design a sensing probe but rather to work as a benchtop device, where the analyte is injected into the cavity from an external device. Another drawback is that, although the setup for fabrication can be found in many laboratories, the process of fabrication is relatively slow and not scalable, since it requires the handling of many splices or precision micromachining with a laser. Finally, while other interferometers such as spherical resonators have a mechanically robust structure, microstructured MZIs have require thinning the fiber sizes or removing part of the solid fiber core, significantly reducing the forces that can act on the fiber without breaking it, or compromising the shape of the cavity; hence, they are a less good candidate to operate in situ.

6.3.4 Single-multisingle-mode interferometers

Modal interferometers operate with a working principle similar to microstructured MZI, with a short cavity fabricated in a fiber. The interferometer, however, is not formed with a fluid-filled cavity or a microstructured fiber, but rather by splicing an MMF between two spans of SMF fiber. The key principle of this interferometer is that, in a short stretch of few millimeters, the fundamental mode launched by the SMF is forced to propagate in a multimode

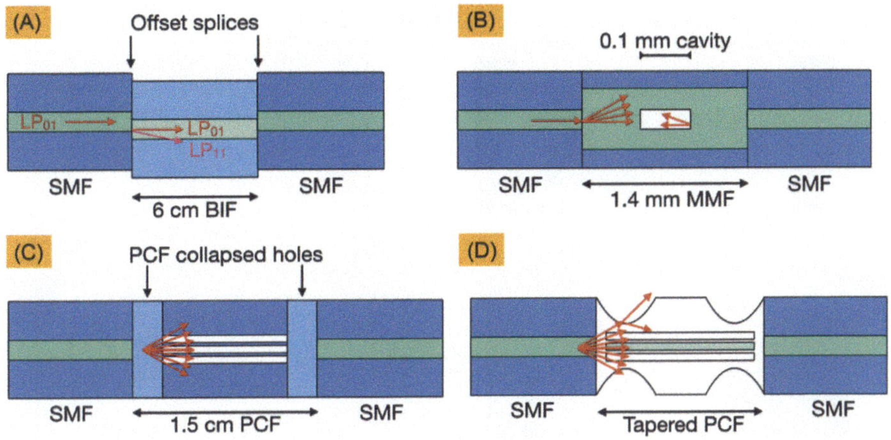

Figure 6.8 Schematics of the main SMS architectures for interferometric biosensors. (A) Two-mode SMS structure, withBIF; (B) SMS with cavity within the multimode fiber; (C) SMS implemented with a PCF collapsed within two SMF fibers; (D) SMS with tapered PCF. *BIF*, bend-insensitive fiber; *PCF*, photonic crystal fiber.

structure, which excites several modes having different n_{eff}, and therefore different OPD. When light is recoupled back into an SMF, the modes interfere, resulting in an interference pattern similar to a classical interferometer. The behavior of the structure depends on the cavity length, and on the geometrical properties of the fiber used to excite the multimodality in the cavity. A generic nomenclature for this sensing principle is single-multisingle-mode (SMS), referring to a stretch of MMFs fused to two SMF fibers. The main architectures for SMS sensors are shown in Fig. 6.8, reproducing in schematic form the interferometers proposed in Hu et al. (2019); Liu, Wu, Gao, and Qu (2017); Olivero, Vallan, Orta, and Perrone (2017); and Wang et al. (2016).

The simplest interferometer form has been proposed by Olivero et al. (2017) and is a two-mode interferometer, hence behaving as an MZI. The cavity is formed by a 6 cm bend-insensitive fiber (BIF), with an offset splice on both sides. As the light travels from the SMF to the offset splice, both the fundamental mode LP_{01} and the second-order mode LP_{11} are excited. The BIF behaves as a two-mode fiber, hosting both of the excited modes along its length. Hence, the structure behaves as an MZI, having $\mathrm{FSR} = \lambda^2/(L\Delta n_{01-11})$, where Δn_{01-11} is the difference in effective RI of the LP_{01} and LP_{11}.

The interferometer proposed by Liu et al. (2017) instead uses a short 1.4 mm MMF spliced within two SMF fibers, and a cavity of 100 μm length drilled with an fs laser. The role of the cavity is to enhance the sensitivity, combining the SMS effect to the inner cavity. The resulting spectra, recorded around 1300 nm, have a 35 dB contrast and FWHM around 3 nm, resulting in an interferometer with a very high contrast and easily detectable spectrum. The RI

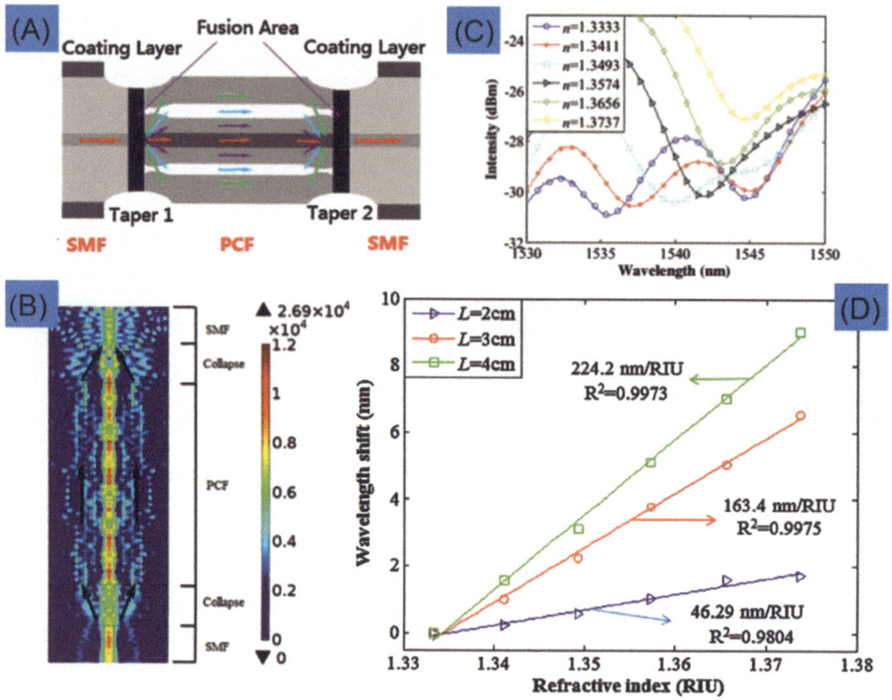

Figure 6.9 SMS sensor implemented with an SMF—tapered PCF—SMS architecture. (A) Schematic of the sensor; (B) electric field distribution along the fiber direction of propagation; (C) transmission spectra at different values of RI; (D) estimation of the RI sensitivity for different values of cavity length *L*. *PCF*, photonic crystal fiber; *RI*, refractive index. Source: *Image reproduced with permission. Proposed by Wang, Q., Kong, L., Dang, Y., Xia, F., Zhang, Y., Zhao, Y., ... Li, J. (2016). High sensitivity refractive index sensor based on splicing points tapered SMF-PCF-SMF structure Mach-Zehnder mode interferometer.* Sensors and Actuators B: Chemical, *225*, *213–220*.

sensitivity has been estimated as 14,314 nm/RIU, a value similar to other microstructured MZI sensors.

A different approach has been proposed by Hu et al. (2019) and Wang et al. (2016), using a structure in which a photonic crystal fiber (PCF) is spliced to the two SMFs to form the interferometer cavity. The first work proposes an SMF-PCF-SMS in which the sides of a PCF are etched and the holes of the fiber collapsed at the two splicing regions. In the work of Want, shown in Fig. 6.9, the SMS-PCF splices are tapered, achieving a partial collapse of the air holes of the PCF. The electric field distribution simulated along the fiber, shown in Fig. 6.9B, shows that the fiber propagation along the main direction (solid core of the PCF) overlaps to the multiple paths of light around the sides hole, with the path closest to the core carrying the higher intensity. As a result, this structure is more similar to a multipath transmission interferometer, as multiple paths interfere at the PCF-SMF output interface. Transmission spectra appear to have envelope with fluctuating intensity, similar to EFPI spectra in which there appear to be different interference path; however, it is possible to measure a spectral shift of the transmission peak at 1532 nm, resulting in a sensitivity of 46–224 nm/RIU depending on the cavity length.

Overall, SMS structures are suitable for splicer-based fabrication, which is possibly a scalable process. The basic SMS structure has a good sensitivity, but further manipulation can increase it to the several thousands of nm/RIU. The behavior of SMS interferometer is very dependent on the type of MMF and to the way SMF-MMF splices excite the modes in the cavity. The interferometer transmission spectra appear as either a two-path interferometer, similar to an MZI, or to a multipath interferometer when many modes propagate with different n_{eff}.

6.3.5 Tapered fiber interferometer

The process of tapering an optical fiber has been used in several applications in photonics, and has recently started to find consistent applications in biosensors. To some extent, tapering is a counterpart of chemical etching: the two processes are used to change the geometry of the fiber by thinning its diameter. While etching is a corrosive process, which erodes the outer surface of the fiber, tapering is a process that combines hot temperature, required to melt the glass, and a pulling micropositioner, which elongates the fiber, changing its diameter. Unlike etching, tapering maintains the fiber proportion between core and cladding. Hence, if we taper an SMF fiber in which the core/cladding diameters are 10/125 μm, down to 20% of the original size, the tapered fiber would have 2/25 μm diameters.

The structure of a fiber taper is shown in Fig. 6.10, along with the key definitions. The taper collapses a fiber having an original diameter into a waist region, where the minimum fiber thickness is observed; in the waist region, the two important parameters are the waist diameter, and waist length, which define the amount of collapsing of the taper. The taper lengths (left and right) define the extension of the collapsed region. When the taper has a conical

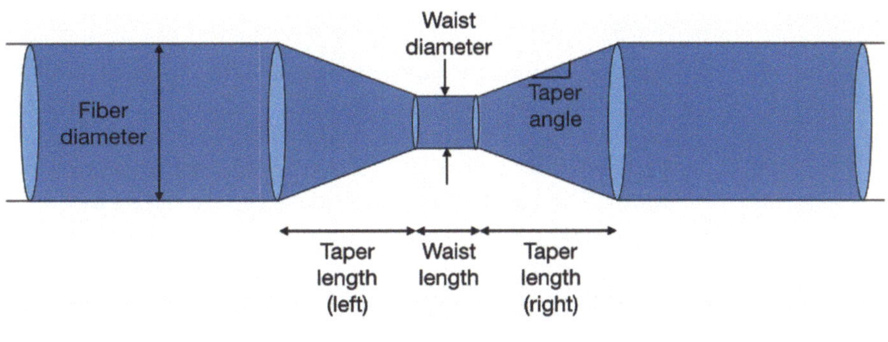

Figure 6.10 Schematic of a fiber taper, and definition of the main taper parameters.

profile, as in the figure, and therefore the fiber diameter reduces at a constant rate, we can define the taper angle, formed by the slope of the cone wall. For a fiber having diameter *d*, waist diameter *w*, and taper length *l*, the taper angle is $\theta = \text{atan}((d - w)/(2l))$. We can define three noteworthy architectures for tapers, which are applied to most of the designs and are usually part of the glass processing stations used to fabricate tapers: *adiabatic* tapers, in which the fiber is collapsed at a very slow rate, that is, $l >> d$ and therefore θ is a small angle (usually in the order of <2 degrees); *parabolic* taper, in which the profile follows a parabolic function; *abrupt* tapers, in which the taper length is short, usually comparable with *w*.

Fiber tapers are common in optical tweezers and as evanescent field termination of laser microscopy apparatus; for this reason, the fabrication of standard tapers is already present in many user-controllable splicing system, such as the CO_2 laser splicers such as Fujikura LZM-100, which has a whole automated routine on adiabatic and parabolic tapers that can work down to $w = d/10$ (i.e., a 10-fold reduction of diameter) (LaserFocusWorld, 2019). Tapers fabricated with a CO_2 splicer are very accurate, as the heating and pulling splicer parameters are automatically derived from the taper waist diameter, waist length, and target taper length; hence, the fabrication process is very robust. Tapers with lower diameter are usually fabricated by means of a heat and pull process, in which the fiber is heated with a furnace or an oxygen flame while a micropositioner is controlled by a translation stage motor, pulling the fiber away from the heat source. This process, more artisanal, allows achieving waist diameters even down to $\sim d/100$, but the fabrication is very delicate and the resulting fiber can be too fragile to sustain mechanical stress, such as the processes for thin film coating used for functionalization and biorecognition.

Tapered fiber interferometers make use of a fiber taper as a building block for a cavity or evanescent field sensor, with spectra resulting from the process that appear similar to the previously treated devices. We can identify two approaches for taper-based interferometer: a first approach uses a fiber with a very low waist diameter (Huang et al., 2015), with the sides of the waist region acting as the sides of a cavity; the second approach (Tian et al., 2008) makes use of two concatenated tapers, each acting as the reflective element of a cavity.

The first approach was proposed by Huang et al. (2015), fabricating a taper with waist diameter 7.5 μm, waist length 1.4 cm, and taper length of 0.4 cm on each side. The taper was fabricated with the flame-heat technique, placing both sides of a fiber into a micropositioner and applying a flame with 5 mm width. The taper acts as a modal interferometer: as the fiber is tapered down, the several modes interfere causing the spectral fringes. The taper is optimized to work with the fundamental mode and second-order mode, hence with an FSR similar to the previously described two-mode interferometer. The spectral fringes obtained are in the order of 10 dB contrast ($\upsilon \sim 0.8$), hence the interferometer has a high finesse. The FSR is about 25 nm at 1550 nm wavelength, and it is also expressed as $FSR = \lambda^2/(L\Delta n)$ where $L = 1.4$ cm and $\Delta n \sim 0.07$ is the difference in effective RI between the first and second-order mode. The structure, functionalized for biosensing, has sensitivity around 5000 nm/RIU and works as a transmission interferometer.

The second approach leads to a lower sensitivity, as the sensor behaves as an FPI, having two separate mirrors forming a cavity. With respect to an ideal FPI, since mirrors are replaced by tapers, the fringes are less prominent due to the inherent diffusiveness of tapers, and sensitivity values are in the order of tens of nm/RIU as for typical FPI and EFPI structures. The work of Tian et al. (2008) reports an interferometer fabricated with two concatenate tapers, both fabricated with a fusion splicer. Both tapers have a thin waist, with 40 μm waist diameter ($w/d = 0.32$) and 707 μm taper length regions. The distance between the tapers varies between 24 and 55 mm. The resulting interferometer has FSR $\sim$10 nm at 1550 nm, contrast of about 10 dB, and sensitivity of -9.4 to -17.1 nm/RIU depending on the distance between the concatenated tapers.

Tapers fabricated with $w/d > 0.2$ are in general quite robust, and therefore suitable for in situ application where the fiber has sustain certain amounts of mechanical stress. Thin tapers appear to be very fragile, but their sensitivity is generally superior and therefore is more suitable for low limits of detection.

6.3.6 Sagnac loop birefringence interferometer

The Sagnac, or loop, interferometer is used in several applications thanks to its high precision and sensitivity, which generate interferometric spectra with high fringe visibility (Culshaw, 2005). The intrinsic precision of the Sagnac method derives from the loop structure: rather than having two or more optical paths propagating in different directions or rebounding within a cavity, in the Sagnac ring the paths are the two counterpropagating waves traveling into the same fiber, which means that any effect occurring on the fiber applies to the both waves. As in other interferometers, several methods have been implemented in order to convert a change of the surrounding RI into a wavelength shift, exploiting the fiber properties. The peculiarity of the Sagnac loop is that it allows generating clean spectra with high contrast; however, it is not a great RI sensor in its basic scheme of Fig. 6.1C, because an RI change would affect both paths of the interferometer, hence having a lower sensitivity. The other difference between Sagnac loops and the previous interferometers is that, while reflection interferometers (EFPI, spherical resonators) are naturally working in reflection, and transmission interferometers (SMS, MZI, microcavities) can be turned into a reflective probe by applying a mirror at the output, the structure of the Sagnac loop requires that the two sides of the sensing region are both connected to the interrogation device, hence it is mainly suitable as a benchtop device, rather than as a probe with capability to operate in vivo.

The modern biosensors working on Sagnac loop exploit in general the polarization properties of the fiber, operating with fibers having high birefringence (Gao et al., 2017), or asymmetrical microfabrication that introduces a birefringence effect (Li, Nguyen, Zhao, Ebendorff-Heidepriem, & Warren-Smith, 2018), or polarization-maintaining fibers with intrinsic birefringence effect (Wu, Zhao, Xu, & Li, 2018). The formal definition of birefringence is: a property of the material having RI that depends on the polarization of the traveling waves. In an optical fiber, this results in the two principal states of polarization (slow axis, fast axis) having a different effective RI. In this case, a light beam that contains both polarization term, traveling through a Sagnac loop, would form interference fringes caused by the difference of n_{eff} of the two main polarization states. While birefringence is a property common to all fibers, high-birefringence fibers or devices enhance this effect, usually through asymmetrical fiber designs that enhance the difference in propagation speed between slow and fast axis of the fiber. By using the birefringence effect in a fiber loop, and using fabrications that expose the propagating light to the outer RI, usually tapering, etching, or fiber ablation, it is possible to obtain a high-finesse and high-sensitivity RI-sensing interferometer, suitable for biosensing.

The work presented by Gao et al. (2017) uses a tapered high-birefringence fiber in a Sagnac loop, with a polarization controller. The light is split into 2 branches through a 50/50 splitter; each clockwise and counterclockwise wave travels through the loop, and runs once across the polarization controller. The polarization controller allows rotating the polarization of the incoming light, hence ensuring that both the horizontal and vertical polarizations of the fiber are excited. The sensing region is a fiber with high birefringence, in which the n_{eff} difference between slow and fast axis is around 0.001; the fiber has an elliptical shape with axes 125 μm (similar to a standard SMF) and 55 μm. In order to make the fiber sensitive to the surrounding RI, the fiber is tapered down to 5.2 μm diameter on the larger axis, and 2.3 μm diameter on the smaller axis. The resulting spectrum has FSR = 120 nm and FWHM = 0.24 nm, hence the finesse is equal to $F = 500$. The sensitivity of the Sagnac interferometer is 13,488 nm/RIU.

A similar setup, but with a different fiber fabrication, was proposed by Li et al. (2018), and it is shown in Fig. 6.11. The setup is a Sagnac loop, with a polarization controller that excites both polarization. The sensing region is an exposed-core fiber. This fiber is a 125 μm diameter microstructured fiber having three cores, one of which is exposed to the outer RI through a microfabrication, as shown in Fig. 6.11B microscopic view. The asymmetry introduced with this design introduces a birefringence of 7.461×10^{-5}, which triggers the RI-sensitive behavior of the Sagnac loop. Through this fabrication, the analyte is

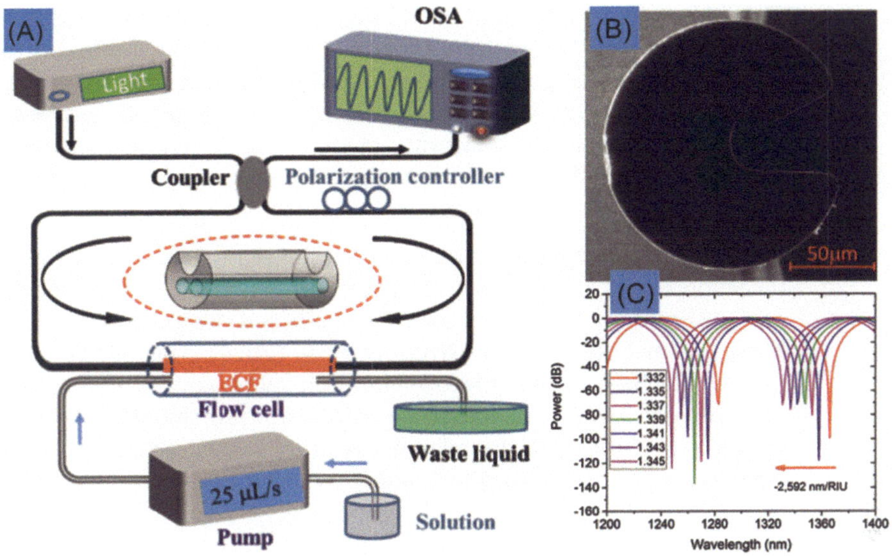

Figure 6.11 Biosensor using a core-exposed fiber in a loop configuration. (A) Schematic of the setup; (B) microscopic view of the core-exposed fiber; (C) interferometer spectra for different values of RI, and sensitivity estimation −2592 nm/RIU. *RI*, refractive index. Source: *Image reproduced with permission. Proposed by Li, X., Nguyen, L. V., Zhao, Y., Ebendorff-Heidepriem, H., Warren-Smith, S. C. (2018). High-sensitivity Sagnac-interferometer biosensor based on exposed core microstructured optical fiber.* Sensors and Actuators B: Chemical, 269, *103–109.*

directly introduced in the suspended core of the fiber, hence the design yields a high sensitivity of 2592 nm/RIU. The spectral fringes are very deep, over 60 dB, and the interferometer has a finesse value similar to the previous design of Gao et al. A similar interferometer was proposed by Wu et al. (2018), replacing the fiber link of the Sagnac loop with a polarization-maintaining fiber, which does not require a fiber microfabrication in order to trigger the interferometric effect.

6.4 Discussion

Interferometry is a powerful technique for biosensing, leading to high RI sensitivity values, which can easily achieve hundreds or thousands of nm/RIU figures. The essence of fiber-optic biosensing interferometers is to replicate one of the main schemes (MZI, Michaelson, FPI, or Sagnac) within an optical fiber, compacting the optical paths that characterize the interferometric behavior into a single fiber or microfiber. The methods for obtaining this two- or multipath interference vary, and usually involve a microfabrication, which can commonly done with a splicer, such as modern CO_2 splicing stations, or through chemical wet-etching.

The common denominator of interferometers is that, unlike gratings or SPR sensors, their spectra are truly broadband and the FSR is often in the order of hundreds of nanometers. As such, interferometry is mainly an alternative to grating or SPR-based sensors from the application point of view: while gratings have a generally lower sensitivity, but work as a compact probe suitable for multiplexing, interferometers instead work better as a high-sensitivity benchtop device with low limit of detection.

However, the interest in probe-based interferometers capable of working in reflection, such as spherical resonators, is high; with such devices, we can achieve both high sensitivity and a probe-based design, also suitable for multiplexing with system such as Ayupova et al. (2020). This interferometer typologies do not have a clear spectra with high values of fringe visibility, but rather have a spectra with multiple low-contrast fringes, shifting with the RI. In this case, the key to enable the reliable use of these devices is the possibility to use advanced signal processing techniques to better interrogate the device.

References

Ayupova, T., Shaimerdenova, M., Korganbayev, S., Sypabekova, M., Bekmurzayeva, A., Blanc, W., ... Tosi, D. (2020). Fiber optic reflector-less refractive index distributed multi-sensors by scattering-level multiplexing with MgO nanoparticle-doped fibers. *IEEE Sensors Journal, 20*(5), 2504–2510.

Culshaw, B. (2005). The optical fibre Sagnac interferometer: An overview of its principles and applications. *Measurement Science and Technology, 17*(1), R1.

Fricke T. (2010). *Solving an optical cavity using scattering transfer matrices.* Tutorial link: http://www.phys.lsu.edu/~tfricke/notebook/2010/08/29/Tmatrix.pdf

Gao, S., Sun, L. P., Li, J., Jin, L., Ran, Y., Huang, Y., & Guan, B. O. (2017). High-sensitivity DNA biosensor based on microfiber Sagnac interferometer. *Optics Express, 25*(12), 13305–13313.

Hu, J., Fu, D., Xia, C., Long, S., Lu, C., Sun, W., & Liu, Y. (2019). Fiber Mach–Zehnder-interferometer-based liquid crystal biosensor for detecting enzymatic reactions of penicillinase. *Applied Optics, 58*(17), 4806–4811.

Huang, Y., Tian, Z., Sun, L. P., Sun, D., Li, J., Ran, Y., & Guan, B. O. (2015). High-sensitivity DNA biosensor based on optical fiber taper interferometer coated with conjugated polymer tentacle. *Optics Express, 23*(21), 26962–26968.

LaserFocusWorld (2019). *Fiber optics: CO_2 laser technology increases the flexibility of fiber end cap splicing and fiber array assembly.* Link: https://www.laserfocusworld.com/fiber-optics/article/14071886/co2-laser-technology-increases-the-flexibility-of-fiber-end-cap-splicing-and-fiber-array-assembly

Li, X., Nguyen, L. V., Zhao, Y., Ebendorff-Heidepriem, H., & Warren-Smith, S. C. (2018). High-sensitivity Sagnac-interferometer biosensor based on exposed core microstructured optical fiber. *Sensors and Actuators B: Chemical, 269*, 103–109.

Li, Z., Liao, C., Chen, D., Song, J., Jin, W., Peng, G. D., ... Wang, Y. (2017). Label-free detection of bovine serum albumin based on an in-fiber Mach-Zehnder interferometric biosensor. *Optics Express, 25*(15), 17105–17113.

Liu, Y., Wu, G., Gao, R., & Qu, S. (2017). High-quality Mach–Zehnder interferometer based on a microcavity in single-multi-single mode fiber structure for refractive index sensing. *Applied Optics, 56*(4), 847–853.

Martinez, A., Griol, A., Sanchis, P., & Marti, J. (2003). Mach–Zehnder interferometer employing coupled-resonator optical waveguides. *Optics Letters, 28*(6), 405–407.

Olivero, M., Vallan, A., Orta, R., & Perrone, G. (2017). Single-mode–multimode–single-mode optical fiber sensing structure with quasi-two-mode fibers. *IEEE Transactions on Instrumentation and Measurement, 67*(5), 1223–1229.

Poeggel, S., Tosi, D., Fusco, F., Ippolito, J., Lupoli, L., Mirone, V., ... Lewis, E. (2014). Fiber-optic EFPI pressure sensors for in vivo urodynamic analysis. *IEEE Sensors Journal, 14*(7), 2335–2340.

Song, B., Zhang, H., Liu, B., Lin, W., & Wu, J. (2016). Label-free in-situ real-time DNA hybridization kinetics detection employing microfiber-assisted Mach-Zehnder interferometer. *Biosensors and Bioelectronics, 81*, 151–158.

Tian, Z., Yam, S. S., Barnes, J., Bock, W., Greig, P., Fraser, J. M., ... Oleschuk, R. D. (2008). Refractive index sensing with Mach–Zehnder interferometer based on concatenating two single-mode fiber tapers. *IEEE Photonics Technology Letters, 20*(8), 626–628.

Tosi, D. (2016). Simultaneous detection of multiple fiber-optic Fabry–Perot interferometry sensors with cepstrum-division multiplexing. *Journal of Lightwave Technology, 34*(15), 3622–3627.

Udd, E. (1995). An overview of fiber-optic sensors. *Review of Scientific Instruments, 66*(8), 4015–4030.

Udd, E., & Spillman, W. B., Jr (Eds.), (2011). *Fiber optic sensors: An introduction for engineers and scientists*. John Wiley & Sons.

Ulaby, F. T., Michielssen, E., & Ravaioli, U. (2010). *Fundamentals of applied electromagnetics* (6th ed.). Boston, MA: Prentice Hall.

Wang, Q., Kong, L., Dang, Y., Xia, F., Zhang, Y., Zhao, Y., ... Li, J. (2016). High sensitivity refractive index sensor based on splicing points tapered SMF-PCF-SMF structure Mach-Zehnder mode interferometer. *Sensors and Actuators B: Chemical, 225*, 213–220.

Wu, B., Zhao, C., Xu, B., & Li, Y. (2018). Optical fiber hydrogen sensor with single Sagnac interferometer loop based on vernier effect. *Sensors and Actuators B: Chemical, 255*, 3011–3016.

7 Low-cost biosensors

7.1 Principles of intensity-based detection

7.1.1 Sensing architectures

Most of the architectures for low-cost biosensing operate under the approaches shown in the schematic of Fig. 7.1. The two approaches are different in terms of optical source used in the setup, and in the role of the sensing unit. The first method is particularly effective when the sensing device is a lossy element, characterized by a wide-band spectrum, that is, the attenuation through the sensing element is almost flat in wavelength. For example, it can be applied to tightly bent fibers (Sakai & Kimura, 1978), which have a loss that depends on the external refractive index (RI) and on the bending radius, or when the analyte itself is a liquid having a specific absorption spectrum, in a setup that mimics optical absorption (or transmission) spectroscopy. The second approach is effective on sensors that have a wavelength-selective pattern, with a quite broad spectrum; this is the case of surface plasmon resonance (SPR) sensors, in which the transmission spectrum is several nanometers wide and shifts as a result of external RI change. The light source is a laser, having output wavelength that matches the inner part of the sensor spectrum. As the spectrum shifts, the laser intercepts a different portion of the spectrum of the sensor, which then modulates the transmitter intensity. Both systems are designed to use a simple photodetector as a receiving unit, which integrates the spectral intensity over its bandwidth, rather than a spectrometer that samples the spectrum over a broad band.

7.1.2 Theoretical considerations

Consider a broadband source such as a light emitting diode (LED), superluminescent light emitting diode (SLED), or amplified spontaneous emission transmitter having spectral intensity $I(\lambda)$, where λ is the wavelength; the input power is equal to

$$P_{in} = \int_{\lambda_1}^{\lambda_2} I(\lambda) d\lambda \tag{7.1}$$

Optical Fiber Biosensors.
DOI: https://doi.org/10.1016/B978-0-12-819467-6.00007-X

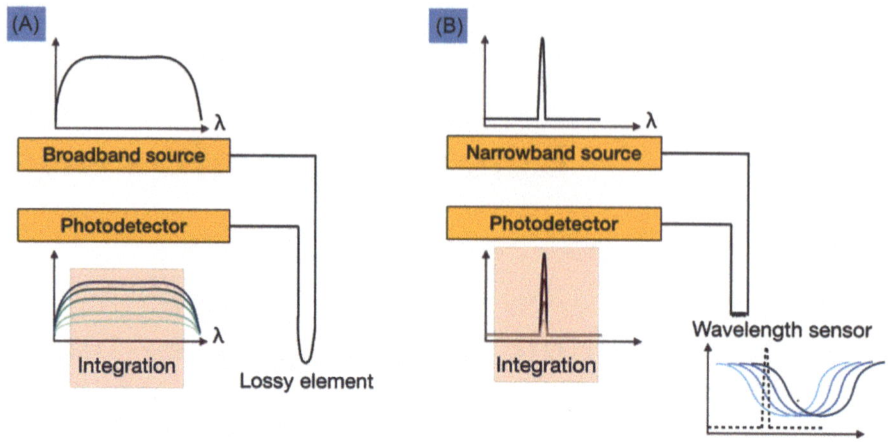

Figure 7.1 Schematic of the main intensity-based detection schemes. (A) Broadband source scheme, using a lossy element (such as a bent fiber) as a sensor, which modulates the light at the detector. (B) Narrowband source setup, in which a wavelength-selective sensor (such as a surface plasmon resonance sensor) modulates the intensity of a laser transmitter.

where λ_1 and λ_2 are the bandwidth limits of the photodiode. The sensor is a lossy element, having attenuation $A(n_{ext})$, where n_{ext} is the external RI. Consider also that the losses of the fiber link is L. The power detected at the receiver is equal to:

$$P_{\text{out}} = \int_{\lambda_1}^{\lambda_2} I(\lambda)A(n_{\text{ext}})L \quad d\lambda = A(n_{\text{ext}})LP_{\text{in}} \tag{7.2}$$

and therefore the output power is proportional to the attenuation of the sensor, through a constant (transmitted power multiplied by the insertion loss of the fiber link). In this setup, we rely on a sensing element with a high capability of converting a change of RI surrounding the fiber into a significant loss.

In a laser-based system, we can approximate the laser spectrum as a delta function:

$$P_{\text{in}} = P_L\delta(\lambda - \lambda_L) \tag{7.3}$$

where λ_L is the laser emitting wavelength and P_L is the laser power. The sensor has a wavelength selective spectrum $S(\lambda)$, which shifts by the wavelength quantity $\Delta\lambda$ when exposed to an RI change; we can define, as in the previous setup, L as the link loss on the fiber.

The power at the receiver is:

$$P_{\text{out}} = \int_{\lambda_1}^{\lambda_2} P_L\delta(\lambda - \lambda_L)S(\lambda - \Delta\lambda)Ld\lambda = P_LS(\lambda_L - \Delta\lambda)L \tag{7.4}$$

which is a response similar to Eq. (7.2). Both sensors provide a similar response, in which the output power variations are proportional to the capability of sensing element to modulate the intensity as a function of RI.

7.1.3 System considerations

The intensity-based setups have two main drawbacks with respect of the setups capable of resolving the wavelength, which will be treated in the next chapter. The first implication is due to the sensing element, which does not return a linear response. For example, a broadband setup which uses a lossy bent fiber as a sensing element has losses that are increasing with the RI change with an exponential pattern. On the other side, laser-SPR sensors sketched in Fig. 7.1B have a specific working range, and when the laser falls outside of the SPR bandwidth the response is null. Depending on the working range of the sensor, several strategies can be employed. In case of a small RI change, such as biosensors working close to the limit of detection, we can linearize the response of the sensor as in the small-signal analysis, quite popular in electronics (such as the analysis of transistors). For laser-based systems, it is a good practice to align the laser wavelength to the Q-point of the spectrum, as shown in Fig. 7.2. By tuning the laser at the Q-point, either on the left or on the right side of the spectrum, we observe the maximum variation of the intensity for a given spectral shift. Moving away from the Q-point, the sensitivity decreases, until the laser line falls off the spectrum and the sensitivity drops to low values. Both sides of the sensor spectrum can be used; on the left side, for a transmission sensor having a spectral dip (such as SPR or LPG sensors), we observe a positive sensitivity (i.e., a positive shift yields an increase of intensity), while on the right side we observe a negative sensitivity.

The second drawback of the intensity-based sensors requires, in general, a careful design of the whole sensing system. We have observed that in both broad and narrow optical sources, the detected power is proportional to both the

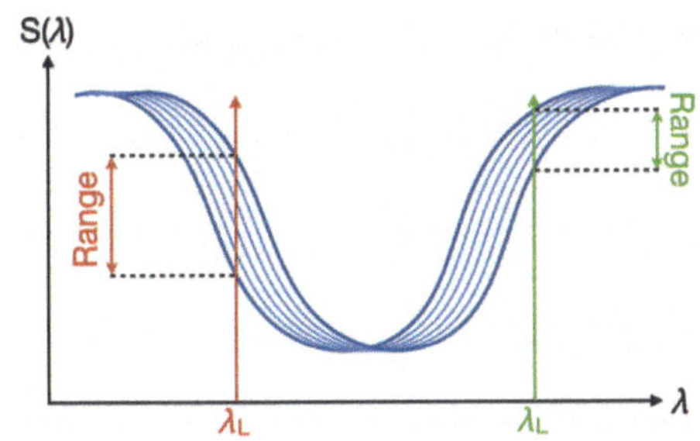

Figure 7.2 Calibration of a laser intensity-based setup. By tuning the laser wavelength at the Q-point (red case), we can expand the dynamic of the system and have the maximum change of intensity for a corresponding spectral change. By moving away from the Q-point, the sensitivity drops, as the output power has a lower variation in correspondence to the same spectral shift.

source power, and to the link losses, that is the insertion loss of all components of the system. For sensors operating over a long term, we cannot guarantee that the two terms are constant and never vary over time; for example, fibers might be squeezed or slightly bent away from the sensing point or can have a temperature-dependent loss, or the light source can slightly change the emitted power over time due to some fluctuations of the thermo-electric controller (TEC). This is the main weakness of the system, as it is hard to compensate with a perfect system: the addition of redundant channels introduces new components that are themselves cause of intensity fluctuations (e.g., the splitting ratio of a splitter has a temperature dependence).

Several techniques have been designed to compensate for the fluctuations of components in intensity-based sensors, each accomplishing the task with partial success (in general, an acceptable compensation of the transmitter fluctuations) and several degrees of limitations (the addition of other components, which are themselves subjected to fluctuations). We report, in Fig. 7.3, two schematics that are designed to improve the robustness of broadband intensity-based, which can be applied to laser-based systems in a similar manner. The first scheme is the simplest one and is designed to compensate the fluctuations of the light source (Perrone & Vallan, 2008); it is particularly common in SLED-based systems as this type of source provides an output that can significantly vary (power fluctuating by several %) over time. The light source is split between a reference arm and a sensing arm. The light collected by the photodetector connected to the sensing arm is then normalized by the power collected through the reference channel. Thus if the input power P_{in} varies, the same fluctuation occurs in both channels, and the normalization cancels it out. By properly designing the system, for example placing the reference and

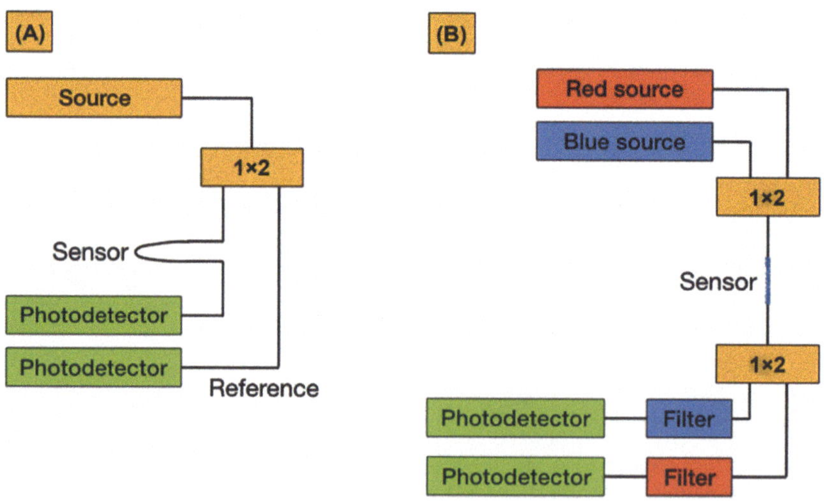

Figure 7.3 Methods for compensation of power fluctuations in intensity-based sensors. (A) Two-channel system based on splitting the laser source to sensor and reference arms and (B) two-wavelength system based on wavelength-selective filters.

sensing fiber in proximity of each other, it is also possible to partially mitigate the change of the fiber link loss *L*. However, the system now introduces new components, such as a 1×2 splitter, which are also subjected to variations over time.

The second system, shown in Fig. 7.3B, uses a two-wavelength setup (Vallan, Casalicchio, Olivero, & Perrone, 2012); it is quite common in visible light sensing system, using two sources operating in two wavelength ranges and a sensor that has a spectral response at only one of the two wavelength. In the example of the figure, the sensor operates in the blue range, and two sources (blue and red) are used. Both sources are coupled into the sensing fiber and are separated using a splitter at the detector. By using a wavelength filter (which is an easy implementation at visible wavelengths), it is possible to separate the two channels and perform a normalization. In this case, we can normalize the fiber link losses, since the loss is experienced by both red and blue channels, but only the blue channel experiences the intensity modulation at the sensing point. The drawback of this setup is that it does not compensate the fluctuations of the sources. Overall, it is possible to combine the two setups, with a three- or four-channel system; however, the redundant component introduce also possible fluctuations and therefore yield uncertainty to the system.

The drawbacks of the intensity-based system are intrinsic in the approach used, which is inherently low cost and with a high sensitivity, but the lack of robustness and long-term stability causes systematic errors in the sensing system. By properly designing the fiber link, and mitigating part of the errors, it is still possible to achieve designs having respectable performance and great affordability.

7.1.4 Devices and fibers for intensity-based setups

Many of the biosensors described in the previous chapters are inherently based on single-mode fibers (SMFs), as they resonate at a specific wavelength that depends on the effective RI of the mode, in intensity-based sensor architectures that achieve low-cost figure and simple systems, multimode fibers (MMFs) are typically used and the wavelength of operation is shifted toward the visible range.

The use of an MMF, having dimensions larger than an SMF, has two key advantages in system based on light intensity detection. At first, having a larger core and therefore a larger acceptance angle, it is much easier to couple light from the optical source into the fiber. An SMF-28 fiber has numerical aperture $(\mathrm{NA}) = 0.14$, which means the half-angle of acceptance is $8°$; the MMF reported by Bremer and Roth (2015) has $\mathrm{NA} = 0.48$, and the half-angle of acceptance is $29°$. Many systems have been reported using plastic optical fibers (POFs), which also have NA of 0.48 in typical conditions. MMFs have also larger core; intensity-based sensors can make use of standard telecom MMFs having core/cladding diameter of $62.5/125\,\mu\mathrm{m}$, up to POFs having $980/1000\,\mu\mathrm{m}$

dimensions. The combination of larger NA and larger core makes it straightforward to couple light from the source to the fiber, which is essential when using LED incoherent sources, which have a wide angle of emission; this ease of interconnection facilitates low-cost sensing. The second advantage is that the larger dimensions, and the strong multimodality of the sensing structures, facilitate the fabrication of lossy structures for sensing. Particularly when broadband sources are employed, the sensor devices are designed to modulate the light losses; having fibers with a large core enables the easy and RI-dependent fabrication of lossy devices (such as fiber bending patterns, etching or polishing of fibers) which would be hard on an SMF fiber.

Intensity-based sensors are typically designed to operate at visible wavelengths, which have significant advantage in terms of operativity and affordability. Since fibers have a lower *V* number at visible rather than at infrared wavelengths, they support more modes and therefore the intensity modulation process is typically more effective. At visible wavelengths, it is possible to exploit inexpensive LED as light sources, and silicon photodetectors as receivers; both components are significantly cheaper than their infrared counterparts. Standard cameras can also be used as detectors or spectrometers in the visible range. In addition, having the possibility to see the light makes it easier to design the sensors in the laboratory and prototype the devices.

7.2 U-bent fiber sensors

A low-cost and scalable approach for sensing is the use of an U-bent fiber structure, which can be used as a stand-alone sensor or in conjunction with an SPR sensor for enhanced sensitivity. In an U-bent fiber sensor, a fiber (usually POF or glass MMF) is bent around a tight angle. The structure of a common U-bent fiber sensor and the geometrical properties are shown (Danny, Raj, & Sai, 2018). An U-bent fiber probe is constituted by a stripped fiber (the protective jacket has to be removed) having radius ρ, bent through a 180° turn on a radius *R*. When immersed in a liquid having a specific RI, the input rays can either be converted to evanescent waves, and leave the structure, or be partially reflected within the fiber and partially transmitted through, or totally reflected internally within the fiber itself. POFs are particularly effective for this sensing system, since standard POFs have a very thin cladding compared to the core (the cladding is a perfluorinated 20 μm circular crown, around a core having 490 μm radius), the surface of interaction of a POF is much larger. The amount of light transmitted through the U-bend is equal to the sum of the totally internal reflected light, and the portion of light partially reflected that still satisfies the guidance condition. The simulation performed in Danny et al. (2018) aims, through a Monte Carlo algorithm, at calculating the amount of light transmitted through the U-bend for a specific fiber geometry and for a specific input configuration.

When the external RI increases, the contrast between the core and outer refractive indices reduces, causing a diminution of the light confinement, and therefore an increase of evanescent light. Hence, the losses of the U-bent probe increase with a change of RI, and this can be monitored with a setup similar to Fig. 7.1A, by measuring the losses through the bent region. The sensitivity and losses are controlled by the bending radius by reducing R, and therefore having a tighter bending, the relative angle between the input light and the fiber wall reduces, causing a reduction of the incident light and therefore a higher amount of evanescent light. The simulations of Fig. 7.4B and C show the specific pattern: given a specific value of RI, the sensitivity (normalized values in the figure) has a plateau for R/ρ values up to 20, and diminishes for higher values as the fiber becomes less curved.

The work of Rodrigues, Lopes, Franco, Werneck, and Allil (2017), reproduced in Fig. 7.4, shows an example of U-bent fiber application that employs a POF with 0.98 mm core radius, for *Escherichia coli* bacteria detection. The system is

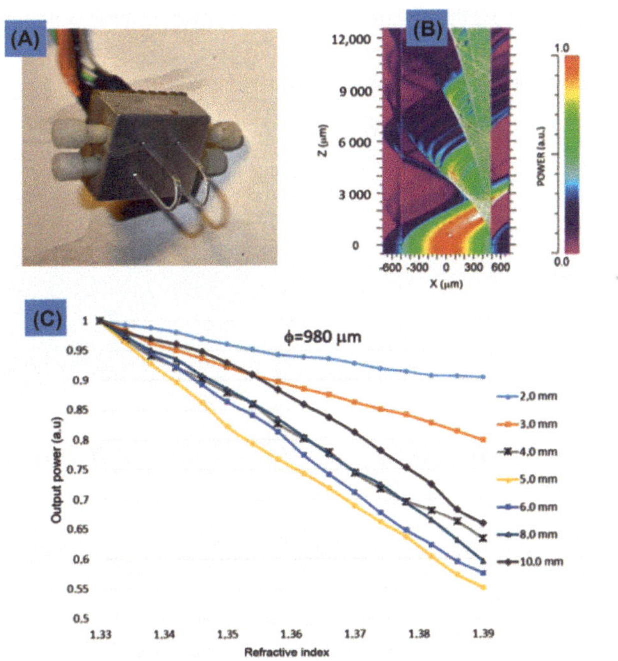

Figure 7.4 Design of an U-bent fiber probe based on a POF for *Escherichia coli* detection. (A) Photograph of the packaged sensor; (B) electric field intensity distribution within the U-bent part of the fiber; and (C) output power measured for different values of RI and different values of bending radius. Source: *Image adapted from Rodrigues, D., Lopes, R. N., Franco, M. A., Werneck, M. M., & Allil, R. C. (2017). Sensitivity analysis of different shapes of a plastic optical fiber-based immunosensor for* Escherichia coli*: Simulation and experimental results.* Sensors, *17(12), 2944, reproduced with permissions.*

packaged in a miniature probe and detects the intensity change as a function of the RI, showing the maximum response for a 5 mm bending radius (where the maximum RI dependency is observed).

The work of Gowri and Sai (2016) shows the application of an U-bent fiber setup to a localized SPR biosensor; the work is reported in Fig. 7.5. The setup is based on a green LED, simply coupled into the fiber through an objective, and a spectrometer for detection. However, since the light intensity is detected at one wavelength (560 nm), the setup is substantially equivalent to the broadband scheme of Fig. 7.1A, as the spectrometer does the function of a silicon photodiode. The fiber used in the setup is a polymethyl methacrylate POF (Mitsubishi SK10, SK20, SK30, SK40) with fiber diameter equal to 250, 500, 750, and 1000 μm). The sensor has been bent according to an U-curve pattern, and maintained in hot air in a capillary to maintain the bending shape consistently. Then the fiber cladding has been removed by chemical etching (ethyl acetate), and subsequently functionalizing the fiber surface with hexamethylenediamine, with subsequent deposition of gold nanoflowers. As a result, the sensor behaves as an U-bent fiber, with an enhancement of the losses due to the localized SPR occurring at the center of the bending region; this effect can be visible in the photograph of Fig. 7.5B, where the light evanescent in the bending region is well visible.

Fig. 7.5C shows the experimental results of the U-bent probe for different values of RI, bending diameter, and fiber size. The charts report, for RI values

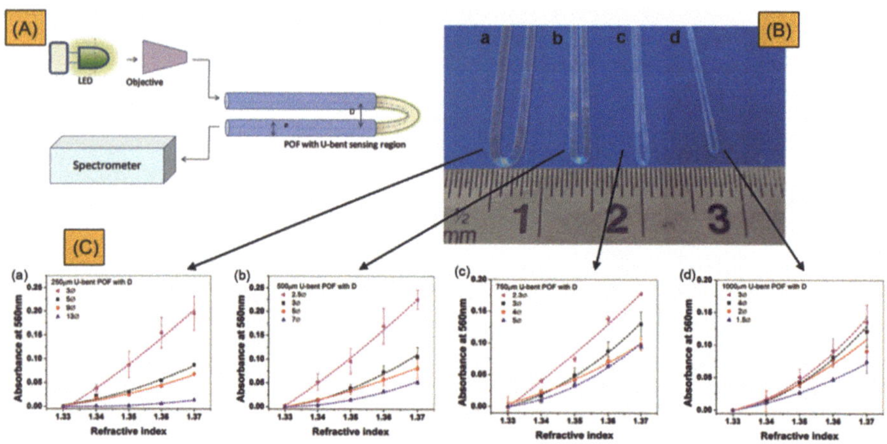

Figure 7.5 Design of an U-bent fiber probe with different fiber types. (A) Experimental setup; (B) photograph of probes having different fiber diameter (a: 1000 μm; b: 750 μm; c: 500 μm; d: 250 μm); and (C) change of light intensity (measured at 560 nm on the spectrometer), for different values of RI between 1.33 and 1.37, for different value of fiber diameter (∅) and fiber bending radius (*D*). Source: *Image from Gowri, A., & Sai, V. V. (2016). Development of LSPR based U-bent plastic optical fiber sensors.* Sensors and Actuators B: Chemical, 230, *536–543, reproduced with permission.*

within 1.33 and 1.37, the losses (i.e., increase of absorbance) measured for each fiber. As expected by increasing the RI, there is an increase of losses, which augment by 5%–25% depending on the sensitivity, as a consequence of reduction of light confinement. We observe that for each fiber size, the fiber having tighter bending diameter exhibits the higher sensitivity (highest slope of the absorbance vs RI function), while for the larger bending diameter the sensitivity reduces. We observe, however, that the opposite trend exists for uncertainty, which is very robust (low uncertainty) for wider curving and is very large for fibers having a tight turn. By changing the fiber diameter, the pattern of losses maintains a similar trend, hence suggesting that the use of larger fibers achieves similar performance but with an easier light coupling process. The sensitivity of the device ranges from 0.4 to 5.6 RIU, measured as the ratio between the absorbance change (the reciprocal of light losses) over the RI change, upon linearizing the relationships of Fig. 7.5C.

Zhang et al. (2017) reported a similar result, on a POF having 1000 μm diameter, coated with a compound of graphene and silver nanoparticles. The device is based on a wide bending diameter of 5 mm (hence $R/\rho = 50$) and records the localized change of SPR by detecting the intensity of the signal in the SPR region. Similar considerations have been reported by Satija et al., who investigated the (Satija, Punjabi, Sai, & Mukherji, 2014) optimal design of gold nanoparticle-coated POF–SPR sensors based on an U-bent pattern, concluding that the sensitivity does not have a great dependence on the fiber size, but rather on the bending tightness and on the type of gold coating.

Overall, the U-bent sensor is an excellent low-cost tool for RI sensing and biosensing because it is simple to design with commercial POFs (including the telecom POF having 980/1000 μm, core/cladding diameter, which are commercially available in most electronic stores) and can use simple LEDs and silicon photodiodes or low-cost spectrometers as detector. Uncertainty and long-term stability are the two main weaknesses of this system, since POFs propagate millions of modes, it is relatively easy to get a high sensitivity but in practical operation, the robustness of the system is hard to achieve over a long term.

7.3 Surface-modified plastic optical fiber sensors

POFs are a good platform for low-cost sensing, thanks to their large core size that facilitates the coupling of evanescent waves; the possibility to modify the surface of a POF allows the fabrication of sensors that detect superficial RI change through SPR phenomenon.

Cennamo, Massarotti, Conte, and Zeni et al. (2011) presented a system for SPR sensing on a POF, based on the manipulation of the fiber surface. The schematic of the sensor is shown in Fig. 7.6. The fiber used in this work is

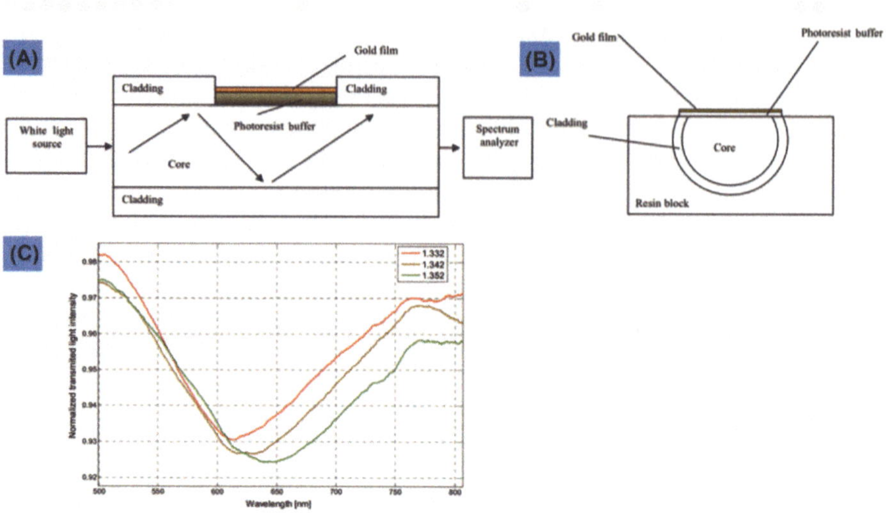

Figure 7.6 Design of an surface plasmon resonance (SPR) sensor on a plastic optical fibers with removed cladding. (A) Experimental setup; (B) schematic of the cross section of the sensor; and (C) SPR spectra acquired in the visible range, for different values of RI. Source: *Image from Cennamo, N., Massarotti, D., Conte, L., & Zeni, L. (2011). Low cost sensors based on SPR in a plastic optical fiber for biosensor implementation.* Sensors, *11(12), 11752–11760.*

a standard 980/1000 μm POF fiber having the cladding removed along half of the fiber cylindrical surface. Through spin coating, a layer of photoresist (Microposit S1813) has been deposited on the fiber, and then a gold layer has been sputtered on the outer surface to form the SPR structure. The sensor hence works as a multilayered coating structure, on a portion of the fiber. The same structure has been reported in Cennamo, Massarotti, Galatus, Conte, and Zeni (2013) and Cennamo et al. (2014), adjusting the formation of the coating.

The result of experimental characterization is shown in Fig. 7.6C, showing the SPR transmission spectra at different RI values. Spectra appear similar to the standard SPR phenomena in glass fibers, hence it can be exploited by either interrogating the wavelength shift of the transmission dip or by interrogating the amplitude change at the Q-point (710 nm, on the right side of the spectrum) for a simpler and low-cost sensing format. At the Q-point, the power transmitted through the sensor changes by 1% for an RI change of 0.01 RIU.

7.4 Smartphone-based fiber optic sensors

The advent of smartphones, as ubiquitous devices, and the increase development of Internet of things have driven a large effort in researching sensing and detection architectures that can make use of the several on-board devices, which can be either part of a sensing scheme or can be supporting devices. If we compare the schematic of Fig. 7.1A, based on an LED source and an intensity detector, with a smartphone, we observe that the front-end of the minimal sensing architecture is already present on a phone. The flashlight is a wide-band LED, which covers the visible spectrum; the latest generation of phones mounts wide-angle flashlights that combine a blue LED (GaN or InGaN) and a wide-spectrum green LED (Ce:YAG) that covers the green and part of the red spectrum; thus the whole 420–710 nm is covered by the light source on the phone. As a detector, smartphones use a camera, up to 16 megapixels (MP) for the latest versions, which works as a pixel-based spectrometer, usually having a peak of response at green wavelength and also covering the 410–690 nm range, matching the range of the light transmitter. Hence, a smartphone embeds the minimal source-detector architecture at visible wavelengths for a fiber-optic sensing system; besides, developers can make use of the other devices (e.g., global positioning system for geolocalization or the inner temperature sensor for thermal compensation). Mobile applications can be developed, which can access the devices of the phone through advanced programmable interfaces and can perform data analysis and computation task, for example, calculating the integral of light intensity or computing the wavelength shift estimation. In medicine, the possibility of performing sensing and analysis through a phone, as opposite as through a stand-alone system, can enable significant advantages such as online and continuous monitoring, telemedicine, and bringing several healthcare functions to remote places or remote workers that are not in proximity of hospital facilities.

Over the course of the year, several optical sensors for smartphones have been developed, using the built-in LED and camera and adding an external optical device that embeds spatial filters, lenses, pin-holes, or diffractive elements to enable functions such as blood analysis, biosensing, water analysis, and other types of detection associated with biosensors and chemical sensors.

Building on these results, there has been also a substantial recent research on fiber optic sensors for smartphones, which mount all the front-end of the system on the phone, with minimal use of external devices, but in which the sensing probe(s) are located within an optical fiber, and therefore at far distance (up to several meters) from the phone itself; this architecture has the goal of combining the remote sensing feature of fiber optic sensors with the ease of implementation. Clearly, as the flashlight is a wide-angle source, and the camera has a high angle of acceptance, the systems are designed to work on MMF, usually large-core glass fibers or POFs. Two approaches have been implemented, achieving a true fiber-optic smartphone sensing system. A first method, similar to Fig. 7.1A, makes turns the camera into an intensity detector, mimicking the use of a photodiode, integrating the power detected by the camera on multiple pixels. The alternative method makes use of the camera as a spectrometer, hence doing a spectral analysis with the possibility to estimate the wavelength shift. This method appears more similar to the other fiber-optic sensors and can work with SPR, but it requires the use of additional devices (in particular, a diffractive element that can spread the wavelengths over the spectrometer pixels) that are not present on the smartphone and therefore require specific mounts.

The first approach has been reported in Sultangazin et al. (2017) for chemical analysis and Aitkulov and Tosi (2019a, 2019b) for breathing analysis. The first system was reported in 2017, and the approach is shown in Fig. 7.7, and optimized for chemical analysis. The fiber used in experiments is a POF, having the same size (980/1000 μm) and NA (0.48) of the POFs described in the previous system. The phone is a Samsung Galaxy S6 Edge, with a 16 MP rear camera. The light from the flashlight is coupled to the POF link, which terminates at the rear camera of the phone, which detects the light intensity. The only external device is a 3D-printed connector, optimized for the specific phone, which has two cylindrical outlets designed to host the POF, controlling the amount of coupled light by selecting a calibrated displacement between the flashlight and the lead-in side of the fiber. The sensor region has been designed by stripping and Ag coating a portion of the fiber, which allows to detect hydrogen sulfide (H_2S) by exploiting the formation of silver sulfide at the boundary with the coating: through the reaction $2Ag^+ + S^- \rightarrow Ag_2S + 2e^-$, the presence of high-brilliance Ag_2S causes a significant drop of the transmission through the sensing region. The detection is performed by calculating the intensity of the mutual correlation between the reference image (at the start of the experiment), and the measured image, for a specific value of camera ISO as shown in

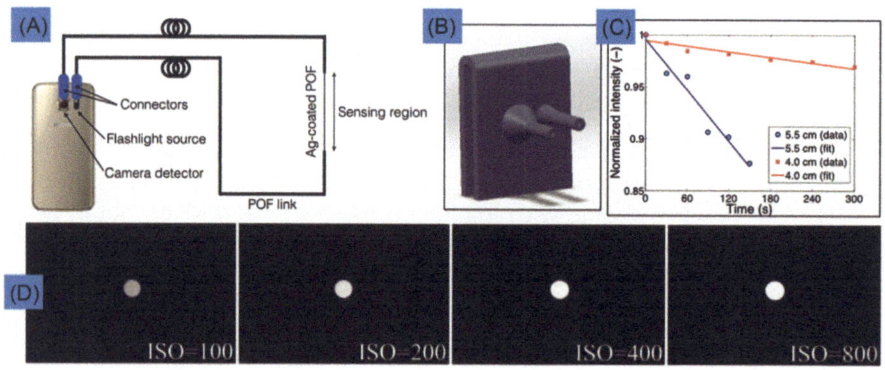

Figure 7.7 Smartphone-POF sensing system for chemical analysis. (A) Schematic of the smartphone-POF sensing system; (B) model of the connector used for coupling the light from the flashlight to the POF and from the POF to the camera; (C) experimental data, reporting the normalized intensity value over time upon exposure to hydrogen sulfide; and (D) image detected on the camera for different values of camera ISO. *POF, plastic optical fibers.* Source: *Image from Sultangazin, A., Kusmangaliyev, J., Aitkulov, A., Akilbekova, D., Olivero, M., & Tosi, D. (2017). Design of a smartphone plastic optical fiber chemical sensor for hydrogen sulfide detection.* IEEE Sensors Journal, 17 *(21), 6935–6940, reproduced with permission.*

Fig. 7.7D. An app has been developed in Java for operating the whole sensor; the app turns on the flashlight and the camera disabling the self-aligning features (that would change the amount of input light), detects a video or a series of image, and computes the 2D correlation between the reference and detected image (such feature enable to correct for the slight movements of the phone that might cause a misalignment of the image).

The smartphone-POF architecture has been subsequently expanded in Aitkulov and Tosi (2019a) and Aitkulov and Tosi (2019b), as shown in Fig. 7.8. The smartphone used in this experiments is a Redmi Note4, running on Android 7 operative system. Having a flashlight LED and a camera positioned in the center of the phone has allowed a reduction of the footprint of the connector, which has been mounted on the side of the phone and allows handheld operation during the measurement of the intensity change. A further improvement has

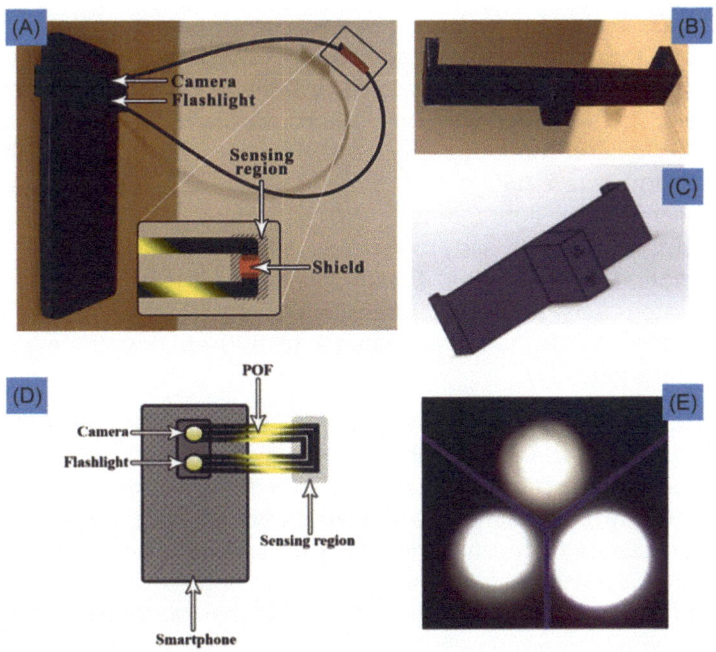

Figure 7.8 Smartphone-POF sensing system for breathing analysis. The image shows the prototype for single fiber (Aitkulov & Tosi, 2019a) and for multifiber (Aitkulov & Tosi, 2019b). (A) and (B) Single-fiber system; (C)–(E) multifiber system according to camera-division multiplexing. (A) Photograph of the sensing system and schematic of the sensing region. (B) Photograph of the single-fiber connector. (C) Sketch of the multifiber connector hosting three fibers. (D) Schematic of the camera division multiplexing scheme. (E) Image detected by the camera in a three-fiber system, blue line shows the spatial division lines. *Source: From A. Aitkulov, D. Tosi, "Optical fiber sensor based on plastic optical fiber and smartphone for measurement of the breathing rate,"* IEEE Sensors Journal, *19, 9, pp. 3282–3287, 2019a; A. Aitkulov, D. Tosi, "Design of an all-POF-fiber smartphone multi-channel breathing sensor with camera-division multiplexing,"* IEEE Sensors Letters, *3, 5, 2019b. doi:10.1109/LSENS.2019.2912982, reproduced with permission.*

been reported in 2019 in Aitkulov and Tosi (2019b); in this work, the connector has been remodeled to host three fibers and demonstrate the possibility to detect multiple fibers simultaneously. The wide-angle of the camera, together with a careful calibration of the focus distance and the position of each POF fiber, allows distributing the LED light onto a bundle of fibers, each hosting a sensing region. This architecture, labeled camera-division multiplexing, effectively uses the camera as a spatial detector, since each fiber uses a different portion of the camera. The work by Aitkulov and Tosi demonstrates this principle with three fibers, mounted on a slim 3D-printed connector and forming an equilateral triangle. As a result, in Fig. 7.8E, we can see the spot detected by the camera for each fiber, and through a tessellation we can isolate each contribution; the cross-talk is limited to 8–15 dB.

The use of a smartphone as an intensity-based system has been demonstrated, and the system works as an all-smartphone-POF with a single external device that is attached to the body of the phone and can be customized for each shape of phone and camera. The portability of the phone is guaranteed, but the mount must ensure that the amount of light coupled in and out remains constant. At this stage, a setup that mimics a reference channel as in Fig. 7.3, whether through wavelength filters, or through an additional fiber, can extend the range of use. A very important factor is the selection of the exposure rate (ISO of the camera): at low ISO, the image is not saturated and therefore the light intensity is almost proportional to the optical power at fiber output, but the system is more susceptible to power fluctuations due to motions of the phone. At high ISO values, the image is saturated, making the system very stable but insensitive to power variations. In the works hereby presented, the ISO has been set to 800 for best trade-off between stability and sensitivity.

The second approach, reported by Bremer and Roth (2015) and shown in Fig. 7.9, turns the smartphone into a spectrometer, and therefore enables the full spectral detection. The sensor is an SPR probe, fabricated on a standard MMF (400 μm core diameter and plastic cladded silica fiber, with NA = 0.480). The SPR surface has been fabricated by removing the fiber cladding, and depositing a silver coating around the surface. The light source has been coupled to the MMF; compared to the POFs, since the fiber has a smaller core, the coupling has been facilitated by polishing the fiber at a 45 degree angle. At the detector, we observe the main difference with the previous setup: a diffraction grating has been mounted between the fiber end (also polished at a 45 degree inclination) and the camera; this way, the different wavelengths are diffracted onto the different pixels of the camera. This is a similar principle of the Kretschmann SPR, whereas a white light source, p-polarized, is incident upon the SPR film and light is collected through a prism or diffractive element. The prototype of Bremer and Roth demonstrates the principle, by gluing the fiber onto the smartphone case and mounting the SPR in a plastic case for in-liquid detection.

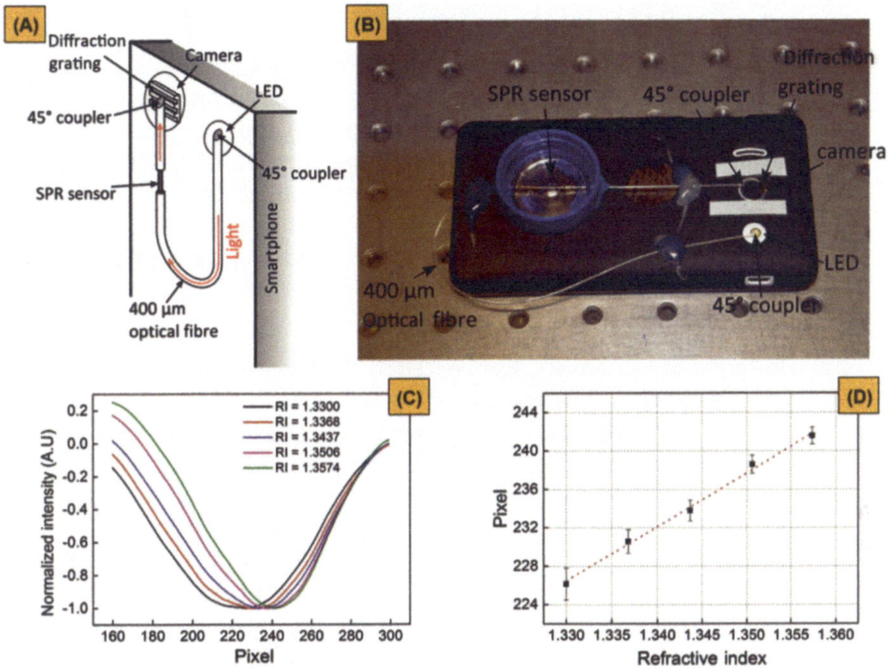

Figure 7.9 Smartphone-SPR sensor on multimode fiber. (A) Sketch of the setup; (B) photograph of the optical fiber sensor; (C) spectra of the SPR sensor, for different values of RI; and (D) evaluation of the sensitivity through the estimation of the wavelength dip as a function of RI. Source: *Reprinted/Adapted with permission from © The Optical Society. Bremer, K., & Roth, B. (2015). Fibre optic surface plasmon resonance sensor system designed for smartphones.* Optics Express, *23(13), 17179–17184.*

By controlling the flashlight and the camera through a video app, the intensity on a pixel line can be detected, and it corresponds to the SPR transmission spectrum. This is shown in Fig. 7.9D for different RI values. As a result, the sensitivity can be expressed as 546.4 pixels/RIU up to 1678 pixels/RIU depending on the camera resolution.

The system of Bremer and Roth has the advantage of a high sensitivity and maintains the wavelength shift detection method that is very efficient on SPR sensing. That allows a better compensation of power fluctuations on the device that can be more effectively mitigated as the spectral shifts can be decoupled from the intensity change. The disadvantage is that the architecture is much more complicated, requiring additional devices that cannot be placed on an external mount, as on the previous system, but rather at close contact with the camera, diminishing the portability in handheld use. In particular, since the distance between the diffractive element and the camera has to be calibrated, which requires an external mount that hosts the device and the fiber, rather than the fiber only as in an intensity-based system.

7.5 Smart textiles

Low-cost sensors, based on MMFs and on a simplified and portable architecture, have been applied to wearable sensors (Massaroni, Saccomandi, & Schena, 2015). The research in this area has aimed to apply fiber optic sensors to the field of smart textiles, which integrate sensors into clothing fabric to achieve a wearable and online sensing. Several works have reported the application of sensors, based on a macrobending approach applied to POF fibers, to detect cardiorespiratory patterns; among others, the European project OFSETH (Ofseth, 2006) studied the incorporation of fiber optic fiber Bragg grating (FBG) and intensity sensors for smart textiles.

In terms of biosensors, Esmaeilzadeh et al. reported a fiber-optic sensors based on SPR for dew monitoring, which is incorporated in a tissue and designed for sweat analysis (Esmaeilzadeh, Rivard, Arzi, Legare, & Hassani, 2015); the photograph and cross section of the sensor are reported in Fig. 7.10. The sensor proposed in this work detects humidity and is integrated into wool fabrics in one of the most interesting packaging form factors presented so far with optical fibers; it detects condensation and water evaporation, and is a milestone toward sweat analysis, which is addressed in modern biosensors (Jadoon et al., 2015). The sensor cross section shows the propagation of light into the fiber core and the interaction with the SPR gold layer. The result presented in this work is an important building block for fiber-optic smart textiles, which are capable of analytical detection in real time in fabric that are permanently worn.

7.6 Laser-based systems

The previous sensing methods have been optimized for MMFs, exploiting loss-dependent or spectral-shift sensors that can be detected through intensity

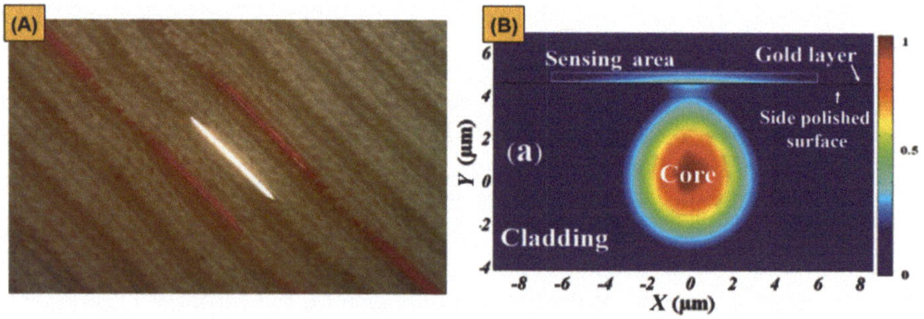

Figure 7.10 Fiber optic SPR dew sensor incorporated in a textile. (A) Photograph of the sensor, illuminated into the textile and (B) cross section of the fiber-SPR sensor. Source: *Reprinted/Adapted with permission from © The Optical Society. Esmaeilzadeh, H., Rivard, M., Arzi, E., Legare, F., & Hassani, A. (2015). Smart textile plasmonic fiber dew sensors.* Optics Express, *23(11), 14981–14992.*

analysis. Using a laser-based setup, as in Fig. 7.1B, it is possible to interrogate a device such as an FBG or an interferometer. Three main approaches have been reported so far and are sketched in Fig. 7.11, showing both the schematic of the setup and the working principle applied to the spectrum of an FBG; the same principle can be applied to any narrow-band reflector, such as an etched FBG, a tilted FBG, an etched-tilted FBG, or a narrowband interferometer.

The approach reported by Tosi et al. (2008) makes use of a single laser, to interrogate an FBG in reflection, following the approach in Eqs. (7.3) and (7.4). The laser is designed to have an emission wavelength in proximity of the Bragg wavelength of the FBG; a TEC is used to adjust the laser wavelength λ_L and the transmitted power, selecting the working point of the device. To protect from the backreflections, the laser is followed by an isolator. As the FBG spectrum shifts, the reflectivity of the grating at the laser wavelength varies, causing a change of the output power at the photodetector, which is a simple InGaAs fiber-coupled p-i-n photodiode for infrared operation. Since the output of the photodiode is a photocurrent, to operate with a data acquisition board, it is necessary to convert the current into voltage; this is performed through a transimpedance amplifier based on an electronic operational amplifier. The system

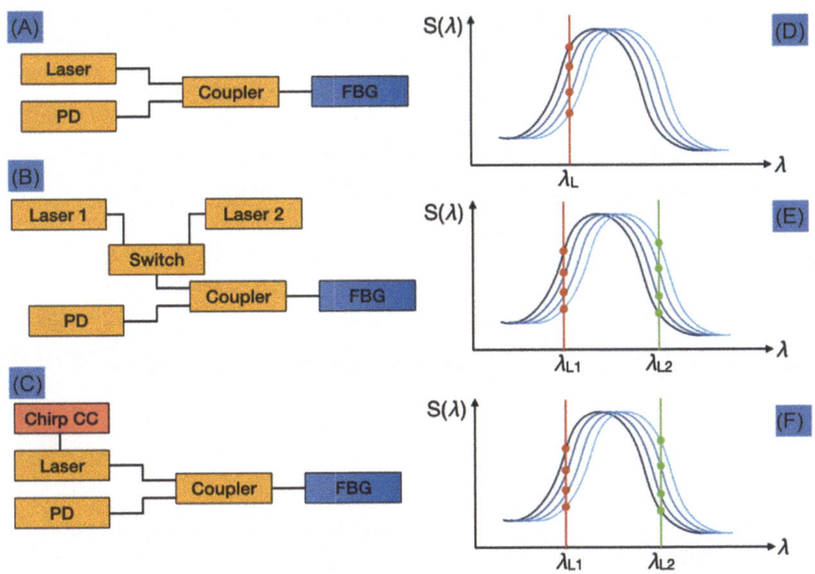

Figure 7.11 Schematic of low-cost laser-based intensity detection of FBG sensors, utilizing a laser–photodetector (PD) pair. (A) Single-laser system as described in Tosi, Olivero, and Perrone (2008, 2009). (B) Two-wavelength, two-laser system as described in Wilson, James, and Tatam (2001) and Cheng and Xia (2016). (C) Two-wavelength system based on a single chirped laser as described in Ouellette, Li, Ou, and Albert (2020). (D)–(F) Working principles of the three interrogation schemes applied to the spectrum of a reflective element.

has the advantage of simplicity but the fluctuations of the laser power are not compensated, and the addition of a reference channel can only partially mitigate the issue. For this reason, the system is mainly used for the interrogation of rapid changes of FBG wavelength (Tosi et al., 2009).

However, the methods proposed in Wilson et al. (2001), Cheng and Xia (2016), and Ouellette et al. (2020) utilize a similar approach, but make use of two wavelengths, and interrogate an FBG (Wilson et al., 2001) or a tilted FBG (Ouellette et al., 2020). The two approaches are based on the same principle of operation, consisting at having two wavelengths λ_{L1} and λ_{L2} and detecting the FBG reflectivity at two wavelengths instead of one, allowing to normalize for the laser transmitted power. Consider an FBG having a spectral envelope that can be approximated as a Gaussian function, having standard deviation σ, maximum reflectivity R, and Bragg wavelength λ_B:

$$S(\lambda) = Rexp\left[\frac{(\lambda - \lambda_B)^2}{2\sigma^2}\right] \tag{7.5}$$

Then the power detected at the wavelengths λ_{L1} and λ_{L2} is equal to:

$$P_1 = P_L TRexp\left[-\frac{(\lambda_{L1} - \lambda_B)^2}{2\sigma^2}\right] \tag{7.6}$$

$$P_2 = P_L TRexp\left[-\frac{(\lambda_{L2} - \lambda_B)^2}{2\sigma^2}\right]$$

where P_L is the power transmitted by the laser and T is the factor that takes into account all the losses on the fiber link (e.g., losses of the couplers and fibers). It is shown in Chapter 3 that gratings have very narrow bandwidths, usually up to 0.3 nm; when interrogating tilted FBGs, the cladding modes have bandwidth in the order of ~0.1 nm. Hence, when aligning the wavelengths in proximity of the FBG bandwidth, the wavelength difference is a very small factor: $\delta = (\lambda_{L2} - \lambda_{L1}) \ll \lambda_B$. Consider now the power difference $(P_2 - P_1)$:

$$P_2 - P_1 = P_L TR\left\{exp\left[-\frac{(\lambda_{L2} - \lambda_B)^2}{2\sigma^2}\right] - exp\left[-\frac{(\lambda_{L1} - \lambda_B)^2}{2\sigma^2}\right]\right\} \tag{7.7}$$

and since $(\lambda_{L1} - \lambda_B)$ and $(\lambda_{L2} - \lambda_B)$ are small, we can expand Eq. (7.7) using Taylor series:

$$P_2 - P_1 \cong -2P_L TR\frac{\delta}{\sigma^2}(\lambda_{av} - \lambda_B)\left\{exp\left[-\frac{(\lambda_{av} - \lambda_B)^2}{2\sigma^2}\right]\right\} \tag{7.8}$$

where $\lambda_{av} = (\lambda_{L1} + \lambda_{L2})/2$ is the average of the two laser wavelengths. A similar analysis can be repeated for the power sum $(P_2 + P_1)$. Then, if we normalize the difference of the two power levels by the sum of the power, we can cancel the Gaussian term out, maintaining only the linear term (Ouellette et al., 2020):

$$\eta = \frac{P_2 - P_1}{P_2 + P_1} = \frac{\delta}{\sigma^2} \quad (\lambda_{av} - \lambda_B) \tag{7.9}$$

With this result, obtained for a Gaussian-shaped spectrum, we have achieved two targets. At first, the term η does not contain the laser power P_L and the loss term T, as they are normalized out. Hence, eventual power fluctuations occurring in the fiber links can be mitigated, as they would affect both the P_1 and P_2 terms proportionally. Second, a shift of the Bragg wavelength $\lambda_B \rightarrow \lambda_B + \Delta\lambda$ would cause a linear variation of η, hence there is a linear relationship between wavelength shift and normalized output power. Although obtained for a Gaussian-shaped spectrum, this results can be easily extended to all FBG and tilted fiber Bragg grating (TFBG) types, since their spectrum resemble a Gaussian shape, and as shown by Ouellette et al., the linearity of the η term with the wavelength shift is >0.99 for FBG and TFBGs, by properly selecting two wavelengths that lie on the two sides of the spectrum of the grating as shown in Fig. 7.11.

This interrogation method, labeled dual differential wavelength detection, can be implemented in various ways, varying the number of lasers and photodetectors. The first work, proposed by Wilson et al. (2001) and sketched in Fig. 7.11B, uses two distinct lasers and one photodiode. The lasers are connected to a switch, and the rest of the setup is similar to the previous setup. When the switch is connected to the reference position, the photodiode acquires the P_1 term at λ_{L1} wavelength; as the switch commutes, the second power level is detected. Through the synchronization of the photodiode and the switch controller, the system can operate the FBG interrogation. The drawback is that the system requires two separate lasers, each controlled by a TEC; hence, the source needs to be duplicated. In this system, it is not possible to assign one TEC to two lasers, since each source requires to be tuned; hence, the two temperature controllers that tune the laser wavelength operate at different values. In addition, an intensity drift occurring to one laser would not occur on the second laser, hence the normalization term η does not cancel out power fluctuations.

The recent work by Ouellette et al. (2020) proposes the use of a single laser source, controlled by one TEC; overall, the schematic is similar to Tosi et al. (2008). The two-wavelength setup is arranged through the current controller of the laser, which is modulated by a chirped function. The current jitter acting on the laser causes a frequency chirp, which results in a change of the emitted laser wavelength over time; the results reported in this work achieve $\delta = 232$ pm for a 100 μm modulation, which is compatible with the bandwidth of most FBGs and TFBGs. The solution demonstrated in this work achieves both a perfect (nominal) normalization of the laser power and of the fiber losses, as well as a linear relationship between η and $\Delta\lambda$, and has the key advantage of using a single laser and a single photodiode. The main weakness is the robustness, as the chirp functions are significantly temperature dependent, and the experimental results show the presence of significant oscillations as the TFBG changes reflectivity level. The entire complexity of this system lies within the TEC, which is designed to deliver a temperature and current modulation pattern stable over time, and maintain its wavelength chirp.

7.7 Conclusions

This chapter presented several methods to achieve a low-cost sensing unit for biosensors. The effort in reducing the cost of sensing device, and enhance portability for operation, requires using methods in which the sensing element modulates the intensity of light transmitted through the fiber optic system. This can be achieved either by using MMFs, and sensors having lossy response of wide-bandwidth SPR, or by using a laser source and photodetector. In both cases, the access to the full spectrum of the sensor is denied, since that would require a spectrometer or optical spectrum analyzer, or even more expensive setups, which are not compatible with this typology of systems. In terms of fibers, largely MMFs (such as POF) have been used, and functionalized in a similar way to more traditional types of sensors.

The possibility to integrate sensors into smartphones or wearable devices, and exploit their features (such as the presence of light sources or detector, of the contact with sensing points placed on the skin) is attractive, and it is expected that the next generation of fiber optic sensors will devote significant effort in downscaling the size and power consumption of the sensing units, from benchtop to handheld. It is, however, true that most of these setups have lower stability and performance than their counterparts that resolve optical spectra, or even optical spectra in each location, therefore a tradeoff between cost and performance is still existing.

The typology of sensors also affects cost and portability. Since spectrometers are based on diffractive elements, resolving narrow wavelength range requires a long optical path. For this reason, coarse spectrometers having wide spatial resolution can be packaged in a small form factor, of few centimeter each size. However, sensors such as FBG or some interferometers require a denser wavelength grid, and therefore spectrometers employed for such detection cannot be shrunk to the same size but are much larger in terms of size.

References

Aitkulov, A., & Tosi, D. (2019a). "Optical fiber sensor based on plastic optical fiber and smartphone for measurement of the breathing rate. *IEEE Sensors Journal, 19*(9), 3282–3287.

Aitkulov, A., & Tosi, D. (2019b). Design of an all-POF-fiber smartphone multi-channel breathing sensor with camera-division multiplexing. *IEEE Sensors Letters, 3*(5). Available from https://doi.org/10.1109/LSENS.2019.2912982.

Bremer, K., & Roth, B. (2015). Fibre optic surface plasmon resonance sensor system designed for smartphones. *Optics Express, 23*(13), 17179–17184.

Cennamo, N., Alberti, G., Pesavento, M., D'Agostino, G., Quattrini, F., Biesuz, R., & Zeni, L. (2014). A simple small size and low cost sensor based on surface plasmon resonance for selective detection of Fe (III). *Sensors, 14*(3), 4657–4671.

Cennamo, N., Massarotti, D., Conte, L., & Zeni, L. (2011). Low cost sensors based on SPR in a plastic optical fiber for biosensor implementation. *Sensors, 11*(12), 11752–11760.

Cennamo, N., Massarotti, D., Galatus, R., Conte, L., & Zeni, L. (2013). Performance comparison of two sensors based on surface plasmon resonance in a plastic optical fiber. *Sensors, 13*(1), 721–735.

Cheng, R., & Xia, L. (2016). Interrogation of weak Bragg grating sensors based on dual-wavelength differential detection. *Optics Letters, 41*(22), 5254–5257.

Danny C.G., Raj M.D., Sai V. (2018). Ray optics model for light attenuation in U-bent fiber optic sensors. In *Proceedings of the IEEE sensors* (pp. 1–4). October 28–31, IEEE.

Esmaeilzadeh, H., Rivard, M., Arzi, E., Legare, F., & Hassani, A. (2015). Smart textile plasmonic fiber dew sensors. *Optics Express, 23*(11), 14981–14992.

Gowri, A., & Sai, V. V. (2016). Development of LSPR based U-bent plastic optical fiber sensors. *Sensors and Actuators B: Chemical, 230*, 536–543.

Jadoon, S., Karim, S., Akram, M. R., Khan, A. K., Zia, M. A., Siddiqi, A. R., & Murtaza, G. (2015). Recent developments in sweat analysis and its applications. *International Journal of Analytical Chemistry, 2015*, 164974.

Massaroni, C., Saccomandi, P., & Schena, E. (2015). Medical smart textiles based on fiber optic technology: An overview. *Journal of Functional Biomaterials, 6*(2), 204–221.

Ofseth. (2006). OFSETH project, FP6-IST-2005–027869. <http://www.ofseth.org/>.

Ouellette, F., Li, J., Ou, Z., & Albert, J. (2020). High-resolution interrogation of tilted fiber Bragg gratings using an extended range dual wavelength differential detection. *Optics Express, 28*(10), 14662–14676.

Perrone, G., & Vallan, A. (2008). A low-cost optical sensor for noncontact vibration measurements. *IEEE Transactions on Instrumentation and Measurement, 58*(5), 1650–1656.

Rodrigues, D., Lopes, R. N., Franco, M. A., Werneck, M. M., & Allil, R. C. (2017). Sensitivity analysis of different shapes of a plastic optical fiber-based immunosensor for *Escherichia coli*: Simulation and experimental results. *Sensors, 17*(12), 2944.

Sakai, J. I., & Kimura, T. (1978). Bending loss of propagation modes in arbitrary-index profile optical fibers. *Applied Optics, 17*(10), 1499–1506.

Satija, J., Punjabi, N. S., Sai, V. V., & Mukherji, S. (2014). Optimal design for U-bent fiber-optic LSPR sensor probes. *Plasmonics, 9*(2), 251–260.

Sultangazin, A., Kusmangaliyev, J., Aitkulov, A., Akilbekova, D., Olivero, M., & Tosi, D. (2017). Design of a smartphone plastic optical fiber chemical sensor for hydrogen sulfide detection. *IEEE Sensors Journal, 17*(21), 6935–6940.

Tosi, D., Olivero, M., & Perrone, G. (2008). Low-cost fiber Bragg grating vibroacoustic sensor for voice and heartbeat detection. *Applied Optics, 47*(28), 5123–5129.

Tosi, D., Olivero, M., & Perrone, G. (2009). Dynamic strain measurement system with fiber Bragg gratings and noise mitigation techniques. *Measurement Science and Technology, 20* (6). Available from https://doi.org/10.1088/0957-0233/20/6/065203.

Vallan, A., Casalicchio, M. L., Olivero, M., & Perrone, G. (2012). Assessment of a dual-wavelength compensation technique for displacement sensors using plastic optical fibers. *IEEE Transactions on Instrumentation and Measurement, 61*(5), 1377–1383.

Wilson, A., James, S. W., & Tatam, R. P. (2001). Time-division-multiplexed interrogation of fibre Bragg grating sensors using laser diodes. *Measurement Science & Technology, 12*(2), 181–187.

Zhang, C., Li, Z., Jiang, S. Z., Li, C. H., Xu, S. C., Yu, J., . . . Man, B. Y. (2017). U-bent fiber optic SPR sensor based on graphene/AgNPs. *Sensors and Actuators B: Chemical, 251*, 127–133.

8 Interrogation of sensors

8.1 Optical fiber biosensor interrogators

A common aspect of the optical biosensors described in the previous chapters is that the refractive index (RI) variation is encoded in the optical spectrum of the sensor. While each specific sensing phenomenon is characterized by different spectral characteristics, the interrogation of each optical biosensor involves detecting the reflection, transmission, or transmission–reflection spectrum and estimating the wavelength or amplitude shift (Chiavaioli, Gouveia, Jorge, & Baldini, 2017). In this section, the main types of optical fiber sensor interrogators are described, reviewing the methods and the characteristics, and then comparing the performance of some of the commercial systems that are available either as benchtop interrogators, embedding all the optical hardware, or as original equipment manufacturer (OEM) version, which allows to self-assemble the interrogator using off-the-shelf components.

8.1.1 LED-spectrometer systems

One of the most common interrogation systems for biosensors makes use of a broadband light source and a spectrometer that cover the bandwidth of the sensors under interrogation; this spectral detection system measures at a rapid speed the spectrum of the sensor without any tunable or scanning components (Tosi, 2017). The sketch of the light-emitting diode (LED)-spectrometer interrogator is shown in Fig. 8.1, for both sensors operating in reflection (or transmission–reflection) and in transmission (Chen, Liu, Yang, Wilkinson, & Zhou, 2019). The key principle of this schematic is to use a broadband light source, usually an LED when the system operates in visible wavelengths or a superluminescent LED or amplified spontaneous emission source in the infrared wavelengths, to illuminate the sensors, and then collect the reflection or transmission spectrum through a spectrometer. The LED source is controlled by a thermoelectric controller (TEC), which ensures that the control board of the LED receives a controlled power supply and that the temperature of the LED board is stabilized, to stabilize the emission properties of the source. As detector, it is possible to use a spectrometer having bandwidth matching the LED

Optical Fiber Biosensors.
DOI: https://doi.org/10.1016/B978-0-12-819467-6.00008-1

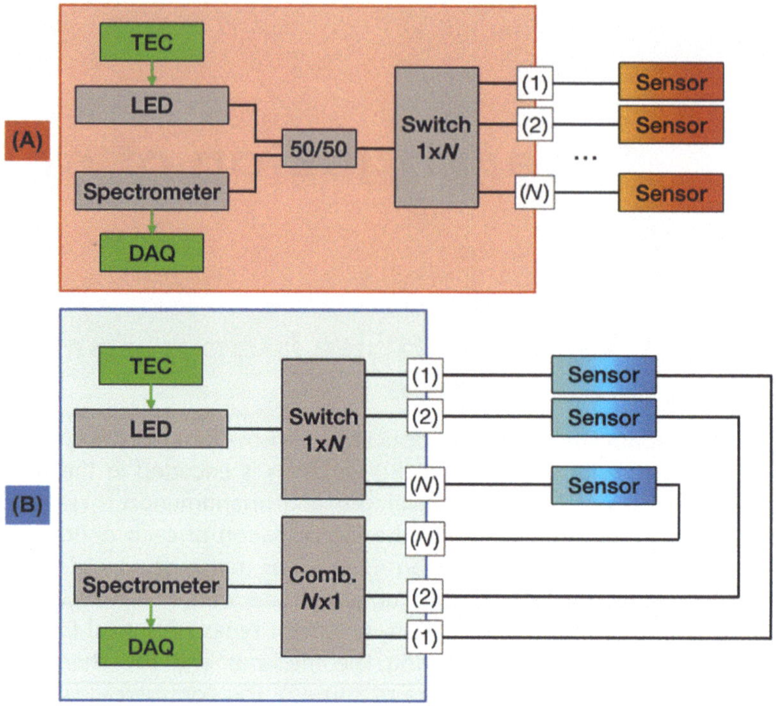

Figure 8.1 Schematic of a light-emitting diode (LED)-spectrometer interrogation system, working in reflection (A) or in transmission (B) with *N* sensors. Red and blue boxes show the hardware embodied in the interrogation unit; (1) . . . (*N*) mark the output connectors for each sensor; *black* lines = fiber connections, *green* arrows = electrical connections. *DAQ*, data acquisition; *TEC*, thermoelectric controller.

source. The performance of this interrogation method is dominated by the spectrometer, in terms of wavelength resolution, acquisition speed, and dynamic range (Poh, Adikan, & Moghavvemi, 2020). The wavelength resolution is largely depending on the detector array of the spectrometer, which determines the bandwidth and wavelength grid (usually 256–2048 pixels). Most spectrometers work at 1–5 kHz speed, and it is possible to set the integration time to optimize the performance as a function of the amount of detected power: spectrometers detect the intensity level over a defined range, typically 16 bits (65,536 levels often referred as "counts"). By changing the integration time, it is possible to raise or lower the intensity of the signal on the spectrometer; this ensures avoid spectral saturation, while maximizing the range of signal at detector. It is also possible to remove the dark level, compensating for the ripples of the light source, by calibrating the spectrometer with no sensor connected.

The LED-spectrometer system can also work by simultaneously interrogating a plurality of *N* channels, using a $1 \times N$ switch. For this task, an optoelectronic switch having N outputs and an electrical controller can be used, usually based on micro electro-mechanical system technology. Most optical switches have switching time ~ 1 ms, which is well compatible with real-time operation, as it allows a detection time $<< 1$ second even when interrogating tens of different channels. This approach that uses a switch to select one channel among many is called time-division multiplexing (TDM), since the N channels share different time slots, and each sensor is interrogated for $1/N$-th of the time (Tosi, 2017).

The setup for LED-spectrometer TDM optical interrogation systems is shown in Fig. 8.1A for sensors operating in reflection or in transmission–reflection, and in Fig. 8.1B for sensors operating in transmission. Interrogators working in reflection use a 50/50 coupler, or a circulator, to route light from the LED into the switch, and collect the reflected element with the spectrometer. The data acquisition (DAQ) unit reads data from the spectrometer and optionally can perform the control of the switch. All the hardware including LED, spectrometer, coupler, and switch are packaged inside an interrogator box, having N output connectors. Sensors can be connected to the interrogator box, one for each channel; it is possible to interrogate multiple sensors in a single channel using a wavelength-division multiplexing approach (Fallauto, Liu, Perrone, & Vallan, 2013). In a transmission-based setup, the connectors are duplicated as they need to connect both the input and the output of each sensor to the interrogator. In TDM multichannel setups, the switch is mounted on the transmission side, while a combiner N to 1 is mounted at the detector. By synchronizing the DAQ and the switch, it is possible to retrieve the spectrum of each individual sensor.

The LED-spectrometer setup is fast, low cost, and effective, and can work with any fiber type provided that all the system is cabled with the same fiber. The setup has no scanning element, and the digital sampling of the spectrum is performed directly by the detector. The spectrometer can be replaced by an optical spectrum analyzer (OSA), based either on a monochromator or on a Fourier-transform infrared reflectometer.

8.1.2 Scanning laser systems

The other main approach for the interrogation of optical fiber biosensors is based on sampling the spectrum (reflection or transmission) of each sensor wavelength-by-wavelength through a scanning laser. In this case, the photodetector integrates all over the detection bandwidth, but the light source is the scanning element. The setup is shown in Fig. 8.2 (Tosi, 2017).

The light source is a scanning laser, which sweeps a wide wavelength range where the spectral features of the sensors under test are located. To obtain a rapid scanning system, the laser is controlled by a TEC that controls the temperature of the Peltier cell of the diode and the current input to the laser board (Haber, 2017). A sweep function generator is used to provide the tuning signal

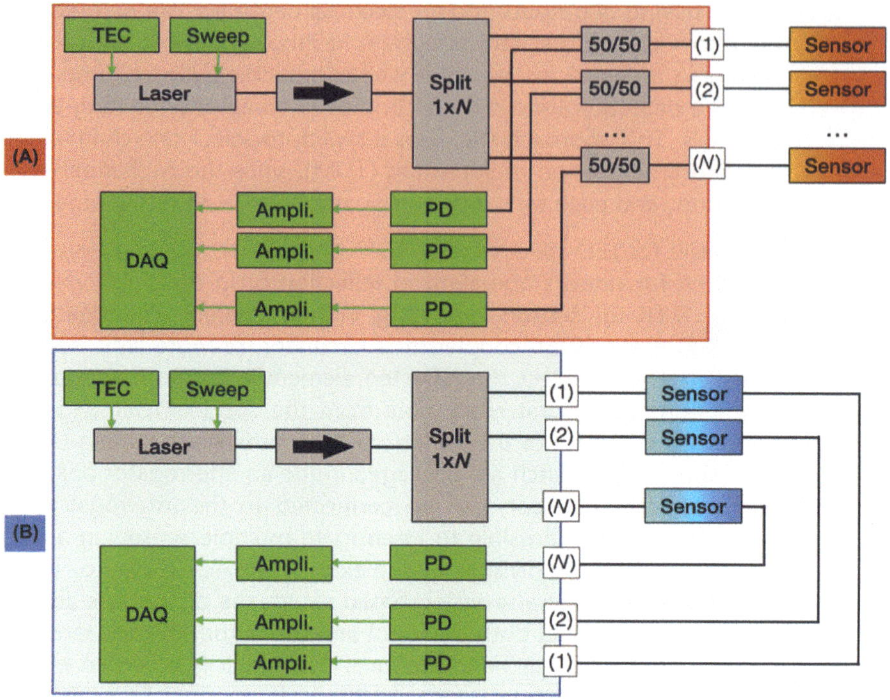

Figure 8.2 Schematic of a scanning laser-based interrogation system, working in reflection (A) or in transmission (B) with *N* sensors. Red and blue boxes show the hardware embodied in the interrogation unit; (1) . . . (*N*) mark the output connectors for each sensor; *black* lines = fiber connections, *green* arrows = electrical connections. *DAQ*, data acquisition; *PD*, photodetector; *TEC*, thermoelectric controller.

to the laser: this allows a rapid scan rate over the bandwidth of operation of the laser (several tens of nanometers). Since the laser bandwidth is much narrower than the optical spectra under analysis, this approach perform a point-by-point scan of the optical spectrum; the laser spectrum can be approximated to a delta function, then performing a digital sampling of the spectrum. As detector, it is possible to use a photodiode or any high-speed photodetector operating on the same bandwidth of the laser source. As most of this type of interrogators operate in the near infrared around 1550 nm wavelength, the most common detector is an InGaAs high-speed photodiode, followed by an amplification stage (a transimpedance amplifier followed by voltage amplifiers with variable gain). Postprocessing is performed with a DAQ unit, which collects the output of the photodetectors synchronously with the laser diode, hence reconstructing the optical spectra under analysis.

To extend the system from 1 to *N* channels, the preferable approach is to physically separate the channels, duplicating the hardware at the detection, rather than using a TDM approach. At first, since the speed of the system is dominated by the sweep function generator, the use of TDM through a switch would severely impact on the software, as it would require synchronizing the switch to the wavelength scan routine that would severely reduce the speed of detection and generate outlier measurements. Then, since the laser and its control hardware are by far the most expensive element of this setup, the physical separation of the channels into *N* optical receivers has a moderate impact on the cost of the interrogator; on the contrary, in a LED-spectrometer, the most expensive element of the system is the detection hardware.

The rest of the optical circuitry is shown in Fig. 8.2A for sensors operating in reflection or transmission–reflection sensors, and in Fig. 8.2B for sensors operating in transmission. As for the previous interrogation method, the instrument can be packaged in a single box with *N* connectors for reflection sensors, or 2*N* connectors (one for each side of the sensor) for transmission sensors. At first, the laser is protected by a strong isolator, to prevent the backreflected light to alter the laser performance. Then, a splitter 1 to *N* physically separates the channels, delivering (1/*N*)-th of the laser power to each channel. In reflection, each channel uses a 50/50 coupler or a circulator to route light to sensors and backwards to each detector; in transmission, instead the light output of the splitter is directly collected by each of the *N* photodetectors after traveling through each sensor.

The scanning laser setup operates on a very narrow wavelength resolution, hence it is compatible even with the narrowest bandwidth levels, such as the cladding modes of a tilted fiber Bragg grating (FBG) that can be detected with high precision. By physically splitting the channels, the system operates at the same rapid speed regardless of the number of sensors. The system is more expensive than an LED-spectrometer setup due to the cost of the laser and its circuitry for wavelength scanning, and has an increased power consumption which prevents, for example, battery operation.

8.1.3 Optical backscatter analyzer and optical vector analyzer

Recent works have shown the possibility of using advanced interrogators, usually employed in distributed sensing or for the analysis of optical devices, for the detection of biosensors. These instruments enable advanced capabilities: for example, the detection of very low optical intensity levels, the spatially resolved detection of the optical backreflections, or the possibility to analyze the reflected fields and therefore estimate the group delay or polarization components. These instruments are more expensive than traditional interrogators, and usually operate at lower speed (around 1 second for each detection) but still in real time; however, the increased performance and advanced capabilities are often compatible with the new generation of biosensors, simplifying the sensor fabrication and improving the performances.

The optical backscatter reflectometer (OBR) is an instrument capable of spatially resolving the reflectivity occurring in optical fibers (Froggatt & Moore, 1998), resolving reflective devices even with very weak reflectivity or the elastic back-scattering signal reflected by the fibers under test. As such, the OBR has also been documented for the interrogation of etched-tilted FBGs (Sypabekova et al., 2019), and more recently for ball resonators behaving as weak interferometers and for reflector-less biosensors (Sypabekova, Aitkulov, Blanc, & Tosi, 2020). The OBR is a polarization-resolved optical frequency-domain reflectometer, with detectors having great sensitivity, enough to resolve return loss levels around −100 dB. The most common implementation of the OBR is shown in Fig. 8.3. The light source is a tunable scanning laser, similar to the source used in Fig. 8.2; the laser continuously scans around the wavelength range on which the reflection measurement is performed. Light is then split into two branches, through a 90/10 splitter. The 90% side of the splitter is connected to the measurement branch, where the light is routed through a network of 50/50 splitters to the output fiber, while the reflected component is collected and resolved with the input light. A polarization controller (PC), followed by a polarization beam splitter (PBS), allows separating the parallel (P) and perpendicular (S) polarizations, and therefore resolving the polarization of the reflected light. The 10% branch of the splitter serves as trigger and is processed through a cascade of fiber splitters and a fiber delay line, which has the same length of the fiber under test. Photodetectors and a series of amplifiers are then used to detect the output of the measurement channels and of the trigger, reconstructing the reflected trace in time and frequency domain through an inverse Fourier transform.

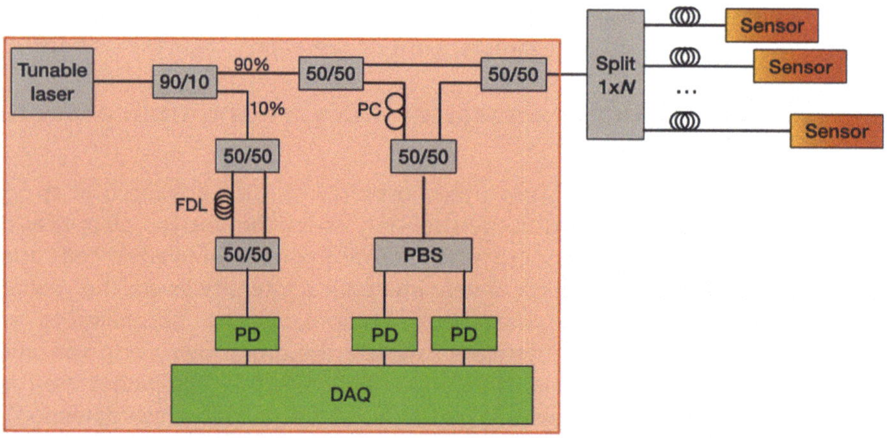

Figure 8.3 Schematic of the optical backscatter reflectometer, arranged for the interrogation of *N* multiplexed sensors operating in reflection. The *red* box shows the hardware included within the interrogation unit. *DAQ*, data acquisition; *FDL*, fiber delay line; *PC*, polarization controller; *PD*, photodetector.

The OBR is a single-fiber instrument, as the reflected light is spatially resolved through a trigger network. The extension of the OBR with a switch is possible, but the real-time operation is limited by the need to trigger each channel independently. Instead, as shown in Fig. 8.3, it is possible to extend the OBR to multiple reflectors by using a spatial division multiplexing approach (Ayupova et al., 2019): a $1 \times N$ splitter is used to separate the channels, and the diversity within each sensor is achieved by connecting into each channel a fiber delay line, different for each unit. This can be simply achieved by adding a fiber spool with different length for each channel, hence displacing each sensor at a different location along the OBR.

The OBR has a dual spatial and wavelength resolution detection method; the spatial resolution Δz is defined as the distance between the two adjacent locations that can be spatially resolved by the OBR. For an instrument operating at the wavelength λ, with a fiber having effective RI n_{eff} and with a laser scanning the wavelength range $\Delta\lambda$, the spatial resolution is $\Delta z = \lambda^2/(2n_{eff}\Delta\lambda)$. For a typical OBR, $\lambda = 1550$ nm, $n_{eff} = 1.464$, and $\Delta\lambda = 88$ nm, and therefore the spatial resolution is 9.4 μm. For measuring spectra of weak resonating sensors with the OBR, the trade-off between wavelength resolution and sensing length is imposed.

Recent works have shown the possibility of using an optical vector analyzer (OVA) (Loyez, Lobry, Wattiez, & Caucheteur, 2019), which has a similar scanning-laser circuitry of the OBR and is derived on the same Fourier transform principle. The OVA is more suited for single-sensor detection, performing a measurement of several parameters in addition to the simple reflection spectrum; light polarization can be resolved, and parameters such as group delay or polarization dependent loss can be estimated at every wavelength (Loyez, Ribaut, Caucheteur, & Wattiez, 2019). The OVA can replace an OSA or a spectrometer in terms of spectral detection, but with advanced capabilities; this has been exploited in narrow-bandwidth sensors such as plasmonic gratings or tilted FBGs for the detection of the cladding modes.

8.1.4 Commercial interrogators and performance comparison

The main commercially available interrogators and analyzers are presented in Table 8.1, reporting the main performance figures. The choice of the method for interrogation depends on the requirements in terms of performance and number of channels, and on power consumption and size requirements; however, the main factor is the type of sensor, and its spectral feature under detection, which determines the optimal interrogation system (Marin, Nannipieri, Oton, Di, & Pasquale, 2018).

Plasmonic sensors, as well as long period gratings, are characterized by wideband transmission spectral dips. For these systems, the LED-spectrometer is the preferred architecture, using single-mode fibers for the LPG and multimode

Table 8.1 Main optical fiber interrogators and spectrometers suitable for optical fiber biosensors; the table shows the main performance figures.

Manufacturer	Instrument	Type	Wavelength range (nm)	Pixels (samples)	Maximum speed (Hz)	Wavelength resolution (pm)	Fiber type	Channels	Software
Ocean Insight	Flame UV–VIS	Spectrometer	200–850	2048–3648	400	178–317	UV–VIS PVDF, 50–1000 μm core	1	OceanView
Ocean Insight	Flame VIS–NIR	Spectrometer	350–1000	2048–3648	400	178–317	VIS–NIR PVDF, 50–1000 μm core	1	OceanView
Ocean Insight	Flame Extended Range	Spectrometer	200–1025	2048–3648	400	226–402	VIS–NIR PVDF, 50–1000 μm core	1	OceanView
Ocean Insight	Flame NIR	Spectrometer	950–1650	128	400	5460	SMF, PVDF, 8 μm core	1	OceanView
Ocean Insight	HR4Pro	Spectrometer	190–1100	2048–3648	400	350–444	VIS–NIR PVDF, 50–1000 μm core	1	OceanView
Ibsen Photonics	I-MON-512 (OEM or USB)	Spectrometer	1510–1595	512	3000	166	SMF-28	1	Ibsen I-MON
Ibsen Photonics	I-MON-256 (OEM or USB)	Spectrometer	1525–1570	256	6000	175	SMF-28	1	Ibsen I-MON
Ibsen Photonics	I-MON-835 OEM	Spectrometer	810–860	1024	4000	49	SM800	1	Ibsen I-MON
Luna Inc.	Hyperion si155	FBG interrogator	1520–1680; 1500–1600; 1460–1620	20,000[a]	10, 100–1000[b]	1–3	SMF-28	1 or 4	Enlight
Luna Inc.	Hyperion si255	FBG interrogator	1500–1600; 1460–1620	20,000[a]	10, 100–1000[b]	1–3	SMF-28	4, 8, or 16	Enlight
Luna Inc.	Hyperion Single Board	FBG interrogator	1520–1680; 1500–1600; 1460–1620	20,000[a]	10, 100–1000[b]	1–3	SMF-28	1 or 4	Enlight
Luna Inc.	OBR4600	OBR	1525–1610	1024–163843	1	8–166[c]	SMF-28	1	Luna OBR4600
Luna Inc.	OVA5000	OVA	1525–1610	–	0.02–0.1	1.6	SMF-28	1	Luna OVA
Luna Inc.	OVA5013	OVA	1270–1340	–	0.02–0.1	1.6	SMF-28	1	Luna OVA
Anritsu	Ms9740B	OSA	600–1750	–	1000[c]	20–300	SMF, 50 μm/125 μm GI fiber	1	-
Yokogawa	AQ6360	OSA	1200–1650	–	NA[c]	100–2000	SMF, GI	1	AQ Viewer
Yokogawa	AQ6370D	OSA	600–1700	–	NA[c]	100–2000	SMF, GI	1	AQ Viewer
Yokogawa	AQ6373B	OSA	350–1200	–	NA[c]	10–1000	SMF, GI, Large core	1	AQ Viewer
Yokogawa	AQ6374	OSA	350–1750	–	NA[c]	50–1000	SMF, GI, Large core	1	AQ Viewer

[a] *Typical value for the number of wavelength scanning points of the interrogator.*
[b] *The 10 Hz speed refers to the spectral acquisition rate for the full spectrum. The 100–1000 Hz speed is only for dynamic tracking of FBG sensors using the on-board software.*
[c] *Depending on the wavelength range set for the measurement.*

fibers for surface plasmon resonance (SPR) sensors to obtain wider spectra. SPR sensors make use of visible or near infrared wavelengths, making use of silicon detectors, which have lower cost. LED-spectrometer systems have also the portability advantage, since they have smaller size and lower power consumption requirements; systems can be packed in small devices that embed the optical hardware, power supply, heat dissipation, and the USB output connection. Portable battery-operated systems have also been reported for remote operations. The operation with multiple channels, enabled by an optical switch, is possible provided that the sensors under analysis have similar values of reflection or transmission: this is due to the fact that, while the spectrometer is a fast detector, it is not possible to rapidly modulate the exposure time and therefore change the detector intensity scale.

Gratings, particularly etched and tilted FBGs, are usually detected through a dedicated interrogator based on a scanning laser. This method allows for the optimal detection of narrow spectra, being able to track the Bragg mode as well as cladding modes with resolution sufficient for small wavelength shift estimations. Although these sensors usually do not have high sensitivity, the accuracy of laser scanning method is extremely fine and allows for operating biosensors with small limit of detection (LoD). As these systems have physically separated channels, different types of sensors can be connected at each terminal of the interrogator, hence allowing different types of multiplexed configurations.

Interferometers usually are detected through an OSA or a spectrometer; FBG interrogators are compatible with high-reflectivity interferometers, but low-finesse interferometers pose a significant trouble in the synchronization of the sweep function generator, which is in general not compliant with sensors having a low fringe visibility. OBR and OVA interrogators are becoming increasingly effective in the interrogation of weak interferometers.

In terms of costs, LED-spectrometer systems are the most affordable; laser scanning systems are more expensive (about 4–6 times more), with OSA based on Fourier-transform infrared reflectometry having a similar cost. OVA and OBR systems are the most expensive and bulkiest interrogators, due to the increase of optical hardware and triggering functions.

8.2 Software methods for spectral analysis

8.2.1 Feature extraction methods

Optical fiber biosensors involve measuring wavelength shift variations in optical reflection of transmission spectra, having bandwidth and shape that depends on the sensing method. In this section, we address the problem of identifying and detecting the spectral changes, which is part of the data acquisition software of interrogators.

The algorithms for spectral feature identification and extractions focus on the analysis of spectral peaks or valleys, where they show the best performance. As shown in the previous chapters, with the exception of intensity-based sensors, all the biosensors based on optical fiber devices show a reflection or transmission spectrum that displays at least one spectral feature that can be interrogated. This concept is shown in Fig. 8.4, where the spectrum of a generic biosensor is shown for two different values of surrounding RI.

The spectrum $S(\lambda)$, intuitively, shows some maxima and minima that correspond to the feature under interrogation. For example, focusing on the spectral peak around 1550 nm at the center of the window, it is possible to trace the wavelength shift $\Delta\lambda$ occurring between the peak values, or the intensity change ΔS which if often reported in logarithmic units. For an unknown spectrum, to identify the best feature to be analyzed, the most common and straightforward feature detection method is to compute the absolute value of the spectral derivative, that is $|\partial S/\partial\lambda|$, which is shown in Fig. 8.4B. This function is characterized by maxima and minima that overlap to the spectral shape.

It is well known that the maxima and minima of a mathematical function correspond to the zeros of its derivative; hence, the minima of $|\partial S/\partial\lambda|$ correspond to the spectral peaks or valleys of the optical spectrum. As shown in Fig. 8.4, in a practical case, the derivative will reach a value close but not identical to zero as

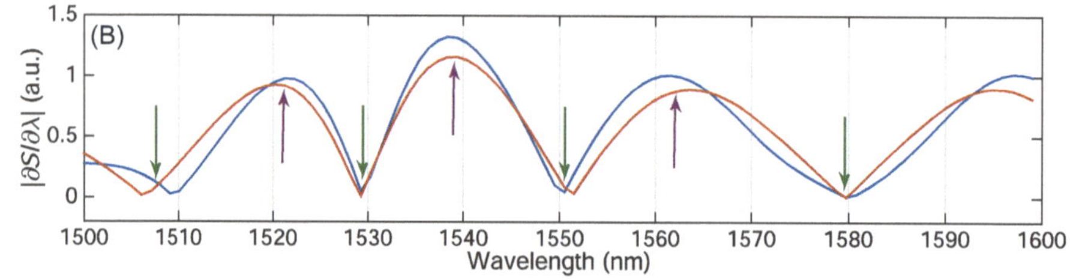

Figure 8.4 Sketch of the spectral feature extraction method. (A) Spectrum of a generic refractive index sensor for two values of surrounding RI, characterized by peaks and valleys. (B) Absolute values of the derivative of the spectrum. Minima of the derivative (*green* arrows) show the locations of spectral peaks and dips along the wavelength axis; maxima of the derivative (*purple* arrows) show the Q-point wavelengths where the spectral changes are the maximum. Peak detection methods center the analysis at the minima of the spectral derivative, on a window included between the two adjacent Q-points.

the derivative is sensitive to spectral noise and to the spectral sampling. Therefore, to identify all the peaks or valleys that occur in the spectrum, a popular approach is to run a simple optimization method that, given a starting wavelength, returns the nearest minimum. A rapid, simple, and effective approach is the Lagarias method (Lagarias, Reeds, Wright, & Wright, 1998) that works within few iterations for a one-dimensional function such as the optical spectrum, and is implemented in Matlab and Scilab (*fminsearch* command) and in LabVIEW optimization toolbox. Users can activate the *fminsearch* routine giving as input the optical spectrum, and different wavelength values as starting point, and within few steps obtain all maxima and minima of the optical spectrum.

Conversely, the peak values of $|\partial S/\partial\lambda|$ correspond to the Q-points, that is, the wavelengths at which the maximum sensitivity of the spectrum is recorded. In case $\partial S/\partial\lambda$ is positive, the spectrum transitions from a dip to a peak, while when $\partial S/\partial\lambda$ is negative, the spectrum shows the decreasing trend from a peak to a valley. Q-points are important because they surround each spectral peak providing an indicator that can reliably separate one spectral feature from the next one. For example, in the interferometer spectrum of Fig. 8.4, we can see the progression of minima and maxima of the derivative: the central peak is around 1550 nm, surrounded by the Q-points at 1539 and 1562 nm. The dips surrounding the central peaks occur at 1530 and 1580 nm, each also surrounded by Q-points.

Hence, to detect spectral features (peaks and valleys) as well as the Q-points interleaved within them, using only the Lagarias routine, it is possible to detect the features by applying *fminsearch* to $|\partial S/\partial\lambda|$ in first place, and then to apply *fminsearch* to $-|\partial S/\partial\lambda|$ to detect all the Q-points, since the minima of $-|\partial S/\partial\lambda|$ correspond to the maxima of $|\partial S/\partial\lambda|$. This step, repeated for some values of the wavelength λ, provides an estimate of the spectral features and their spectral bandwidth of a biosensor with unknown response; then, the following peak detection systems can be applied.

8.2.2 Peak detection systems

Once the spectral feature to be detected has been identified, a peak tracking method can be used to estimate the peak/dip wavelength, and therefore estimate the wavelength shift; a similar consideration can be drawn for the methods regarding the detection of intensity level. The three most effective methods for peak tracking (centroid, regression, and spline) are listed below, having different levels of suitability for each type of sensors—as described in Tosi (2017). The methods are based on treating the spectrum $S(\lambda)$ as a digital signal S_n sampled on the wavelengths λ_n, where $n=1, 2, \ldots, N$ is the digital index. Fig. 8.5 sketches the three methods for peak tracking, applied to the central peak of the spectrum shown in Fig. 8.4.

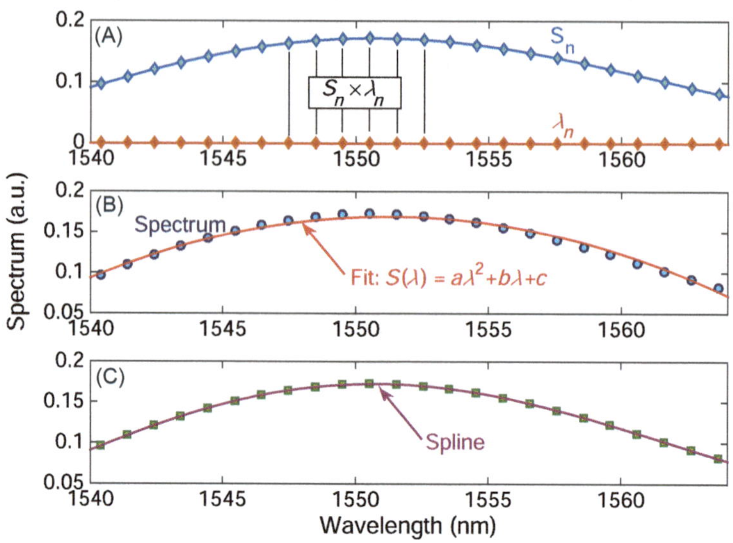

Figure 8.5
Sketch of working principles of peak tracking methods for optical fiber sensors: (A) centroid; (B) polynomial regression; and (C) spline.

8.2.2.1 Centroid

The centroid, or geometric center, is an algebraic concept that evaluates the arithmetic mean position of all the samples of the spectrum. Among reliable peak tracking methods, the centroid requires the fastest computation, as it does not involve any manipulation of the optical spectrum. The centroid wavelength λ_c of a spectral portion of N samples can be calculated from the formula:

$$\lambda_c = \frac{\sum_{n=1}^{N}(S_n \lambda_n)}{\sum_{n=1}^{N} S_n} \tag{8.1}$$

This method is visualized in Fig. 8.5A: given the spectral sampling over each wavelength, the numerator of Eq. (8.1) is computed by calculating the summation of all the spectrum-wavelength products, and it gets then normalized by the summation of all spectral values (at the denominator). It is worth noting that the centroid wavelength does not often correspond to the central wavelength of the feature; however, wavelength shifts occurring due to the concentration change of the analyte, or surrounding RI changes, cause a centroid wavelength shift that is well reproduced. The centroid algorithm works only on spectral peaks; in case of a spectral dip, it is possible to flip the spectrum (e.g., replacing S_n with $-S_n$).

8.2.2.2 Polynomial regression

The polynomial regression method, shown in Fig. 8.5B, consists on fitting the portion of the spectrum under analysis with a polynomial function. The most common method is a second-order fit, as it allows an unambiguous spectral detection:

$$S(\lambda) \approx a\lambda^2 + b\lambda + c \tag{8.2}$$

where coefficients a, b, and c can be estimated using the regression method. Most calculators perform the polynomial regression using the Vandermonde matrix method, which involves the solution of a matrix-based system using linear computation. Fig. 8.5B shows the difference between the spectrum and the polynomial fit: while the fitted data appear slightly divergent at the borders, the central part of the spectrum where the peak is located is well reproduced by the regression algorithm. Once the polynomial has been identified, we can estimate the central wavelength by estimating the maximum (or minimum, in case of a spectral valley) of the curve by imposing its derivative to zero:

$$\frac{\partial S}{\partial \lambda} = 2a\lambda + b \rightarrow 0 \tag{8.3}$$

and resolving it, we obtain the peak wavelength λ_p simply as

$$\lambda_p = -\frac{b}{2a} \tag{8.4}$$

Computationally, the second-order polynomial regression involves finding the a, b, c coefficients and then the peak wavelength is estimated as $-b/2a$; hence, wavelength shifts can be measured with this method. The approach works for both spectral peak and dips, since they both correspond to a zero in the spectral derivative. The polynomial fitting method is particularly sensitive to the selection of the spectral window to be analyzed: since the fit is more accurate at the center than on the borders of the window, the choice of a short window is preferable to improve the quality of the fit. The drawback of this method is that it works well only on symmetric spectra; while most biosensors have spectra with a symmetric shape, some interferometers (e.g., ball resonators having quasirandom spectra) and some plasmonic sensors have spectra that have a slight asymmetrical shape, which degrades the quality of the fit. To circumvent this, it is possible to use higher order polynomials, which, however, will return a plurality of peak points.

8.2.2.3 Spline

The spline method is not a peak-tracking algorithm in itself, but it used to oversample the spectrum to reconstruct all the intermediate values between each pair of adjacent pixels (deBoor, 1978); this approach is derived from interpolation in computer graphics. Once the spectrum is interpolated on a dense grid, it is possible to apply one of the previous methods (most often the centroid) to provide a fine estimate of the wavelength shift, with precision much superior to the resolution of the spectrometer or interrogator used in detection.

The spline function is a piecewise polynomial function of the third order, which interpolates the spectrum between each n and $(n+1)$ indexes. For each value of n, the spectrum is interpolated with a third-order polynomial $P_n(\lambda)$:

$$S(\lambda) \approx P_n(\lambda) = a_{n,3}\lambda^3 + a_{n,2}\lambda^2 + a_{n,1}\lambda + a_{n,0} \qquad \forall(\lambda_n \leq \lambda \leq \lambda_{n+1}) \tag{8.5}$$

The four polynomial coefficients required for each fit can be estimated imposing four conditions: polynomial fit and original spectrum coincide on the two borders λ_n and λ_{n+1}; and first- and second-order derivatives of $P_n(\lambda)$ are the same on the λ_n and λ_{n+1} points (C^2 continuity condition). In formulas:

$$\begin{cases} P_n(\lambda_n) = S_n \\ P_{n+1}(\lambda_{n+1}) = S_{n+1} \\ \dfrac{\partial P_n}{\partial \lambda}(\lambda_n) = \dfrac{\partial P_n}{\partial \lambda}(\lambda_{n+1}) \\ \dfrac{\partial^2 P_n}{\partial \lambda^2}(\lambda_n) = \dfrac{\partial^2 P_n}{\partial \lambda^2}(\lambda_{n+1}) \end{cases} \tag{8.6}$$

Imposing the conditions of Eq. (8.6) results in a linear system of equations in four variables ($a_{n,3}, \ldots, a_{n,0}$), which can be resolved using linear algebra. Once all the piecewise terms have been determined, the spectral fit can be determined on each wavelength interval:

$$S(\lambda) \approx P_1(\lambda)\Big|_{\{\lambda_1 \leq \lambda \leq \lambda_2\}} \cup P_2(\lambda)\Big|_{\{\lambda_2 \leq \lambda \leq \lambda_3\}} \cup \ldots \cup P_{N-1}(\lambda)\Big|_{\{\lambda_{N-1} \leq \lambda \leq \lambda_N\}} \tag{8.7}$$

As shown in Fig. 8.5C, unlike the polynomial fit, the spline function provides a fit that always coincides to the original spectrum on the spectrometer grid, and with smoothly shaped interpixel values. Unlike polynomial regression, which involves the solution of a nonlinear system, the coefficients of the spline are always found through a linear system that can be solved using the LU factorization through any calculator (e.g., using the *spline* command in Matlab, the *spline*-VI in Labview, or the *spline connected* chart in OriginLab).

The benefit of the spline is that, once all the interpixel values have been determined, the spectral estimates work with better accuracy. This is particularly effective on narrow-band spectra (e.g., etched or tilted FBGs) whereas the resolution of the spectrometer has the effect to undersample the detected spectra.

8.2.3 Coarse resolution methods

The previous methods are effective in detecting the spectra of most biosensors, provided that the resolution of the spectrometer allows a clear detection of the spectrum. As shown in Table 8.1, several spectrometers have resolution in the order of tens up to few hundreds of picometers, while grating-based sensors have a narrower spectrum; for example, the spectral combs of tilted FBGs have a bandwidth that is narrower than the wavelength resolution of several detectors. Several methods have been proposed to perform a detection of the optical spectrum in these conditions of coarse sampling; the key is moving away from the traditional wavelength or amplitude tracking, and move the analysis to a different domain using a linear transform operator (Tosi, 2017); in this case, the output of the algorithm is not directly related to the spectral shape or shift, but it is still an RI-dependent parameter that can serve as tracking method.

One of the most effective methods is the Karhunen-Loeve Transform, which can be applied to FBG sensors (Shaimerdenova, Bekmurzayeva, Sypabekova, & Tosi, 2017). It is a sequence of calculations similar to the principal component analysis that determines a sensor output that changes as a function of the RI. The method can be applied only with coarse wavelength grids and does not return an output that is linearly increasing with the RI, but it is effective in demodulating gratings at the limit of the sampling criteria. Another method is based on the fast phase correlation (Lamberti, Vanlanduit, De Pauw, & Berghmans, 2014), which performs a Fourier transform of a portion of the spectrum and subsequently performs a sequence of estimates of its phase term, converging to a wavelength shift estimate. A similar method makes use of discrete wavelet transform: after selecting a wavelet and performing a transform of the spectrum, the wavelet coefficients are combined to provide an estimate of the wavelength shift.

8.2.4 Toward a standard algorithm for interrogation

In summary, we can now outline a standard interrogation method for optical fiber biosensors; we propose an algorithm that works for most optical sensors (SPR, interferometers, gratings, tapers, LPGs, and many other typologies of sensors that induce a RI-dependent wavelength shift). The pseudocode of the algorithm is listed in Table 8.2.

The method is based on the previously described building blocks. The estimation of the $|\partial S/\partial \lambda|$ minima is useful to determine the location of the wavelength peaks and valleys, while the minima of $-|\partial S/\partial \lambda|$ show the position of Q-points. A good choice of each spectral window for analysis is half-way between the peak location and the adjacent Q-points on each side: this choice narrows the spectrum to a range that can be efficiently processed with the peak tracking methods, while having enough samples to run the next routine. The next step is to apply the peak detection on each feature: first, we can implement a spline that upsamples the spectrum with more values that can improve the peak detection, and then apply a peak detection method (centroid or polynomial fit). When all peaks have been tracked, we can compute the sensitivity to RI or to the concentration, and select the best performing spectral feature.

The algorithm proposed in Table 8.2 is designed to be implemented in Matlab, LabVIEW, C/C + +, or several other programming language that handle the spectral analysis; several works also show the implementation of peak tracking on field-programmable gate array technology used as a computational unit for detection and peak tracking (Yamaguchi, Ishihara, & Shinoda, 2019).

Table 8.2 Pseudocode of the algorithm proposed for spectral interrogation of optical fiber biosensors.

Step	Pseudocode
1	Estimate the spectral peaks and Q-points
	Compute $\lvert\partial S/\partial\lambda\rvert$
	for k scrolling from 1 to N
	Apply *fminsearch* to $\lvert\partial S/\partial\lambda\rvert$ with λ_k start; obtain the k-th peak
	Apply *fminsearch* to $-\lvert\partial S/\partial\lambda\rvert$ with λ_k start; obtain the k-th Q-point
	Sort the peak locations $\lambda_{P,1}, \lambda_{P,2}, \ldots, \lambda_{P,K}$
	Sort the Q-point locations $\lambda_{Q,1}, \lambda_{Q,2}, \ldots, \lambda_{Q,K}$
2	Select the spectral windows for analysis
	For each $k = 1,\ldots, K$
	Select the window within $[\lambda_{P,k}-(\lambda_{P,k}-\lambda_{Q,k})/2]$ and $[\lambda_{P,k}+(\lambda_{Q,k+}1 - \lambda_{P,k})/2]$
3	Detect each wavelength shift
	Apply spline to $S(\lambda)$
	Estimate centroid wavelength λ_c on spline-sampled spectrum
	Evaluate the wavelength shift $\Delta\lambda$ from reference condition
4	Select spectral feature
	Compare all the sensitivity values $\Delta\lambda/\Delta n$
	Select most sensitive peak/valley for detection

8.3 Characterization of optical fiber biosensors

The characterization of an optical fiber biosensor can be separated into two steps:

1. Calibrate the sensor response against a change of a known RI, using the sensor as an environmental, nonspecific detector; this step is important both to define the spectral feature that yields the best detection suitability and also to test the behavior of the sensor in a known context, with an available reference method (Chiavaioli et al., 2017)
2. Calibrate the sensor response to the measurand analyte, evaluating the main performance figures for the target application; this allows the evaluation of LoD, response time, and other important figures as discussed in Chapter 2, Principles of fiber optic sensors (Socorro-Leránoz, Santano, Del Villar, & Matias, 2019).

The measurement of the wavelength shift as a function of the surrounding RI provides the key information regarding the sensitivity of the sensor. While we cannot estimate from this response the selectivity or the specific sensitivity to the analyte concentration, as they are analyte-dependent, the RI calibration curve serves the purpose of quantifying the sensitivity of the sensing method and comparing it with other known techniques, and estimating the optical resolution of the method, which depends only on the detection and interrogation method.

The most common method for RI calibration consists in immersing the sensor in a well calibrated mixture of water and another soluble component (e.g., sucrose, ethanol). By varying the concentration of sucrose in water, it is possible to obtain small changes of RI: a popular online resource for this analysis is RefractiveIndexInfo (https://refractiveindex.info), which lists the RI values for several water mixtures. For optical fiber biosensors operating in the infrared, sucrose/water mixes result in an RI change estimated as 1.85×10^{-3} for each 1% of sucrose in water at low concentration. This method can be used to obtain RI changes usually in the order of 10^{-4} to 10^{-2} RIU, which are used to calibrate both high-sensitivity sensors (e.g., SPR, interferometers) and gratings that have a lower sensitivity. The derivative of the wavelength/RI curve reports the sensitivity of the method, and it can be obtained by simply implementing a linear regression.

As a metric to evaluate the quality of the RI response, and therefore evaluate whether the response of the sensor is accurate compared to its reference, the key parameter is the coefficient of determination (R^2). The R^2 metric has progressively replaced other uncertainty-related metrics, and it can be applied directly on the wavelength shift versus RI calibration. Given that the wavelength shift measured by the interrogation system is $\Delta\lambda_{meas,i}$, where $i = 1, \ldots, D$ is the index of each data point (usually $D = 5-10$ data points for the RI calibration), and $\Delta\lambda_{fit,i}$ is the linear fit obtained with regression method for each data point, the R^2 metric provides a method independent formula for estimating the quality of the fit:

$$R^2 = 1 - \frac{\sum_{i=1}^{D} \left(\Delta\lambda_{meas,i} - \Delta\lambda_{fit,i}\right)^2}{\sum_{i=1}^{D} \left(\Delta\lambda_{meas,i} - \Delta\lambda_{av}\right)^2} \tag{8.8}$$

where $\Delta\lambda_{av} = 1/D \left(\sum_i \Delta\lambda_{meas,i}\right)$ is the average measured wavelength shift. This process is shown in Fig. 8.6, for a generic sensor. The measured data points ($\Delta\lambda_{meas}$) for each value of RI are acquired through the calibration process, and the average wavelength shift ($\Delta\lambda_{av}$) is simply calculated as the mean of the wavelength shifts. A linear fit allows estimating the sensitivity to 113.68 nm/RIU; the fitted data ($\Delta\lambda_{fit}$) corresponding to each RI are used to calculate the R^2 coefficient as 0.9946, which is a high value. The use of R^2 provides a data-independent metric on the quality of the fit; values over 0.95 are an acceptable estimate, while $R^2 > 0.99$ provides a very good result that shows negligible calibration errors.

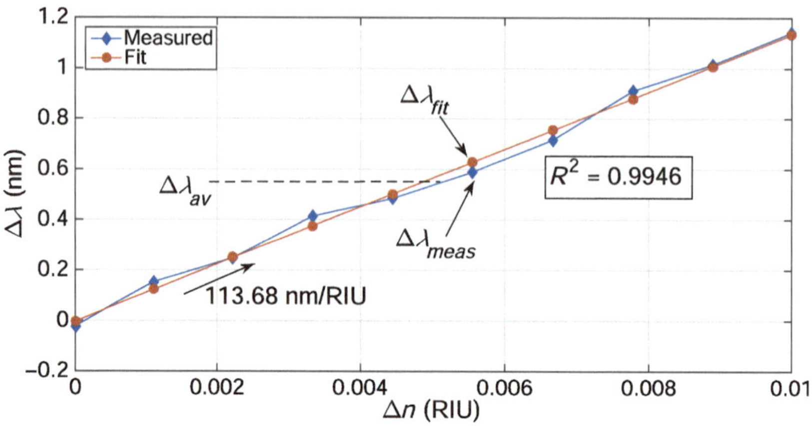

Figure 8.6 Sketch of the linear fitting, sensitivity estimation, and R^2 calculation for a generic optical fiber biosensor, given the measured wavelength shift $\Delta\lambda$ as a function of the RI change Δn.

The calibration of the sensor response to the different analyte concentrations is largely dependent upon the type of analyte, and how the sensor has been functionalized to its specific detection. For example, sensors can respond to the analyte concentration in a linear way, or in a logarithmic way, or in different other forms. For this reason, more than a specific protocol, we can outline a family of characterizations that define the main performance criteria.

The analysis of the wavelength shift with respect to the analyte change is providing an estimate of the LoD of the biosensor, which is the key metric to assess the capability to detect at low levels of concentration (Chiavaioli et al., 2017). The LoD defines, in experimental conditions, the minimum of concentration of analyte that the biosensor can detect without ambiguity. There are three main methods to evaluate the LoD from a characterization curve:

1. Evaluate the LoD from the RI characterization curve, after determining the uncertainty of the sensor. First, the minimum wavelength shift that can be detected and the sensitivity of the sensor need to be estimated (the sensitivity as shown in Fig. 8.6, while the accuracy of the detector is usually given on the datasheet of the instrument or can be determined experimentally). This process allows estimating the smallest RI change that the sensor can detect. Then, we can convert the RI change into the analyte concentration change, by estimating the maximum surface density concentration. This method is quite common for SPR sensors, as well as for emerging applications where a characterization with many data points is impractical.
2. Evaluate the LoD as the *blank sample*, obtained by measuring at zero-level concentration (and therefore in reference condition), and adding three times the standard deviation of the characterization curve. This method requires a thorough calibration of the analyte-dependent behavior in many data points; the function is then fitted according to the trend of the curve (e.g., a linear function or a log-dependent curve). Then, the standard

deviation of the fit is estimated, and the LoD is derived from this measurement. This method is recommended by IUPAC (International Union of Pure and Applied Chemistry) and is typically recommended for optical labeled biosensors, which can operate at very low concentration; its adaptation to fiber-optic biosensors is mainly limited by the availability of data points at low concentration, where the sensor has a marginal response.

3. The final approach, recommended from ACS (American Chemical Society), is derived from some of the chemical and gas sensors, and is based on the standard deviation of the measured wavelength shift only at low concentrations. The process involves repeated (7–10) measurements of the blank samples, and other repeated measurements at a concentration of one to five times the guessed value of LoD. Then, the response of the sensor is characterized, under the statistical point of view, with the *t*-Student's function and this allows a purely statistical evaluation of the LoD. This method is reliable, but more sensitive to the types of analyte (e.g., proteins) that tends to have a logarithmic response to the concentration.

The sensorgram reports the working conditions of a biosensor, reporting the wavelength shift in a continuous recording while exposing the sensor to different working conditions; an example of sensorgram is shown in Fig. 8.7. The sensor is first tested during the surface immobilization procedure, measuring the wavelength shift with respect to the initial conditions. Then, the surface

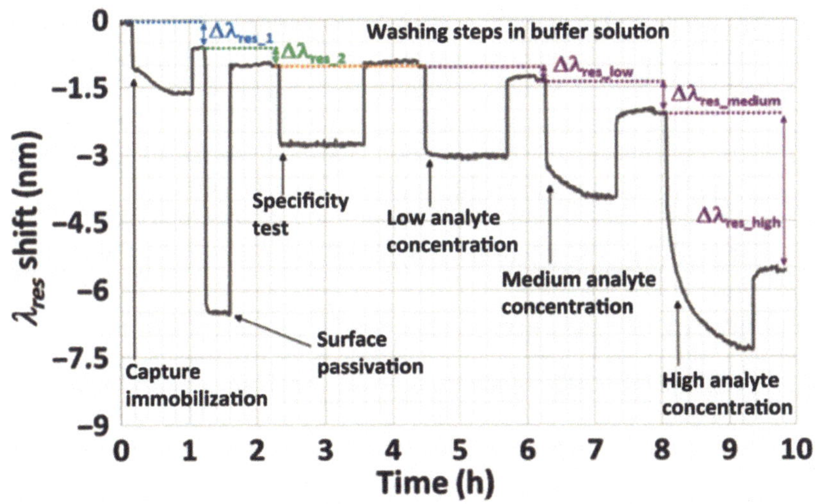

Figure 8.7 Example of sensorgram chart of a fiber optic biosensor. The chart reports the continuously recorded wavelength shift for a biosensor exposed in different working conditions. *Blue* = capture immobilization; *green* = surface passivation; *purple* = analyte interaction. Source: *From Chiavaioli, F., Gouveia, C. A., Jorge, P. A., & Baldini, F. (2017). Towards a uniform metrological assessment of grating-based optical fiber sensors: From refractometers to biosensors.* Biosensors, *7(2), 23.*

passivation is recorded, followed by a specificity test that assesses the response of the sensor to controls. Finally, the sensor is tested for the interaction with the analyte, from low to high concentration. This also allows recording the speed of detection, as the response is not instantaneous but progresses over time. The sensorgram allows a detailed visualization of the response (either toward positive or negative values of wavelength shift) when the sensor is exposed to analyte, controls, and through the surface passivation.

The other two key parameters of interest in biosensing are the *selectivity* or specificity, and the *regeneration* or reusability. The selectivity measures the capability of the sensor to selectively detect only to the analyte of interest, and not respond to other analytes. While the sensitivity is an optical parameters, which measures the capability of the sensor to respond to the surrounding changes, the selectivity is a biochemical figure of merit, because it defines the quality of the surface functionalization to chemically bind to the analyte and reject other analytes. Two main methods are used to test the selectivity of a biosensor in working conditions: the first approach is to introduce a negative control, by introducing a solution that contains other analytes, while the second method is to spike the analyte with a complex solution that contains other analytes. Whichever way, this test allows verifying the influence of other analytes on the detection: a good biosensor will have a response to other analytes showing a negligible wavelength change, or even an opposite trend, and in this case the cross-sensitivity can be considered negligible compared with the LoD. Conversely, a significant response to one of the control analyte shows an unwanted affinity that diminishes the selectivity of the biosensor. Appropriate selectivity tests are done using control analytes that have a known surface affinity with respect to the analyte under consideration, and at relatively high concentration to evaluate the amount of response under significant changes of concentrations. The regeneration measures the capability of the biosensor to be regenerated, or reused, for multiple cycles of detection, as opposite to work for a single measurement. This is important in some applications, where the sensor detects in cycles and therefore the quality of repeated detections is tested.

8.4 Conclusions

In conclusion, this section presented the interrogation hardware, software, and test protocols for optical fiber biosensors. The methods for interrogation, with reference to commercial instruments and their suitability for specific interrogation, have been discussed together with the software on board of interrogator. Although often underestimated, it is important to recall that the performance of a biosensor does not depend only on the working principle, or the quality of the functionalization, but have a strong dependence on the quality of the interrogation hardware. For example, sensors with poor sensitivity can still work with a low LoD thanks to high-resolution interrogators that can resolve wavelength shift levels of the order of the picometer. Similarly, software also has a very important role in the definition of the biosensor performance: a simple change of spectral feature detection might radically change the LoD of the system.

In current biosensors, the software and hardware are very well integrated; peak tracking methods are often programmed on board of the interrogator software, or the original software can be reprogrammed for a specific type of detection. To date, few spectrometers or interrogators already have biosensing-ready software, as typical routines are designed for rapid and accurate spectral detection, leaving the user with the task of programming the detection method. Nevertheless, unified methods for spectral detection start to appear, and they are usually compatible with graphical programming languages such as LabVIEW, or computational languages such as MatLab that are also well interfaced with LabVIEW.

On the other hand, the methods for calibrating and testing biosensors are more standardized, as the key metrics have been identified and are also allowing scientists to compare different detection methods (not limited only to fiber optic sensors). Hence, future efforts might be addressed to standardize interrogation methods and software programs for detection, to build a datasheet-type characterization of each biosensor in simulated working conditions.

References

Ayupova, T., Shaimerdenova, M., Korganbayev, S., Sypabekova, M., Bekmurzayeva, A., Blanc, W., ... Tosi, D. (2019). Fiber optic refractive index distributed multi-sensors by scattering-level multiplexing with MgO nanoparticle-doped fibers. *IEEE Sensors Journal, 20*(5), 2504–2510.

Chen, Y., Liu, J., Yang, Z., Wilkinson, J. S., & Zhou, X. (2019). Optical biosensors based on refractometric sensing schemes: A review. *Biosensors and Bioelectronics, 144*, 111693.

Chiavaioli, F., Gouveia, C. A., Jorge, P. A., & Baldini, F. (2017). Towards a uniform metrological assessment of grating-based optical fiber sensors: From refractometers to biosensors. *Biosensors., 7*(2), 23.

de Boor, Carl (1978). *A practical guide to splines*. New York: Springer-Verlag.

Fallauto, C., Liu, Y., Perrone, G., & Vallan, A. (2013). Compensated surface plasmon resonance sensor for long-term monitoring applications. *IEEE Transactions on Instrumentation and Measurement, 63*(5), 1287–1292.

Froggatt, M., & Moore, J. (1998). High-spatial-resolution distributed strain measurement in optical fiber with Rayleigh scatter. *Applied Optics, 37*(10), 1735–1740.

Haber, T. C.Micron Optics Inc. (2017). Method for enabling system operation based on a spectral fingerprint. *United States Patent 9,851,249.*

Lagarias, J. C., Reeds, J. A., Wright, M. H., & Wright, P. E. (1998). Convergence properties of the Nelder-Mead simplex method in low dimensions. *SIAM Journal of Optimization, 9*(1), 112–147.

Lamberti, A., Vanlanduit, S., De Pauw, B., & Berghmans, F. (2014). A novel fast phase correlation algorithm for peak wavelength detection of fiber Bragg grating sensors. *Optics Express, 22*(6), 7099–7112.

Loyez, M., Lobry, M., Wattiez, R., & Caucheteur, C. (2019). Optical fiber gratings immunoassays. *Sensors.*, *19*(11), 2595.

Loyez, M., Ribaut, C., Caucheteur, C., & Wattiez, R. (2019). Functionalized gold electroless-plated optical fiber gratings for reliable surface biosensing. *Sensors and Actuators B: Chemical*, *280*, 54–61.

Marin, Y. E., Nannipieri, T., Oton, C. J., & Di Pasquale, F. (2018). Current status and future trends of photonic-integrated FBG interrogators. *Journal of Lightwave Technology*, *36*(4), 946–953.

Poh, A. H., Adikan, F. R., & Moghavvemi, M. (2020). The past, present, and prospective on UV–VIS–NIR skin photonics and spectroscopy—A wavelength guide. *Medical and Biological Engineering and Computing*, *58*, 1159–1175.

Shaimerdenova, M., Bekmurzayeva, A., Sypabekova, M., & Tosi, D. (2017). Interrogation of coarsely sampled tilted fiber Bragg grating (TFBG) sensors with KLT. *Optics Express*, *25*(26), 33487–33496.

Socorro-Leránoz, A. B., Santano, D., Del Villar, I., & Matias, I. R. (2019). Trends in the design of wavelength-based optical fibre biosensors (2008–2018). *Biosensors and Bioelectronics: X*, *1*, 100015.

Sypabekova, M., Aitkulov, A., Blanc, W., & Tosi, D. (2020). Reflector-less nanoparticles doped optical fiber biosensor for the detection of proteins: Case thrombin. *Biosensors and Bioelectronics*, *165*, 112365.

Sypabekova, M., Korganbayev, S., González-Vila, Á., Caucheteur, C., Shaimerdenova, M., Ayupova, T., ... Tosi, D. (2019). Functionalized etched tilted fiber Bragg grating aptasensor for label-free protein detection. *Biosensors and Bioelectronics*, *146*, 111765.

Tosi, D. (2017). Review and analysis of peak tracking techniques for fiber Bragg grating sensors. *Sensors.*, *17*(10), 2368.

Yamaguchi, T., Ishihara, K., & Shinoda, Y. (2019). Field-programmable gate array-based multichannel measurement system for interrogating fiber Bragg grating sensors. *IEEE Sensors Journal*, *19*(15), 6163–6172.

II

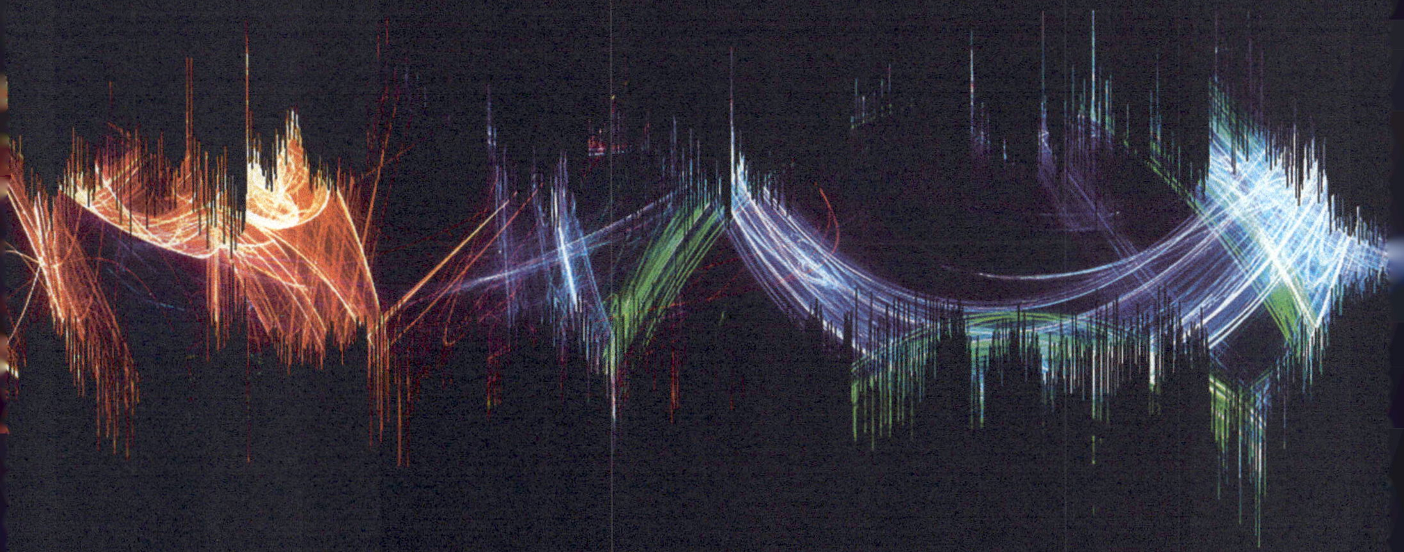

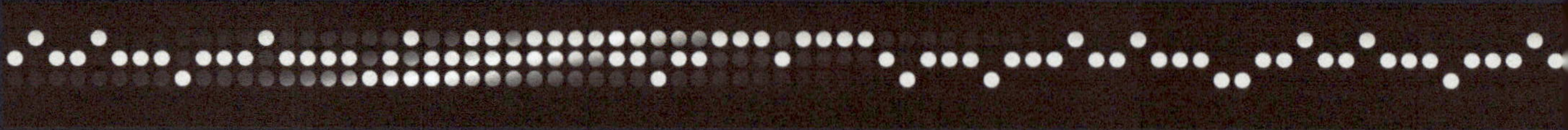

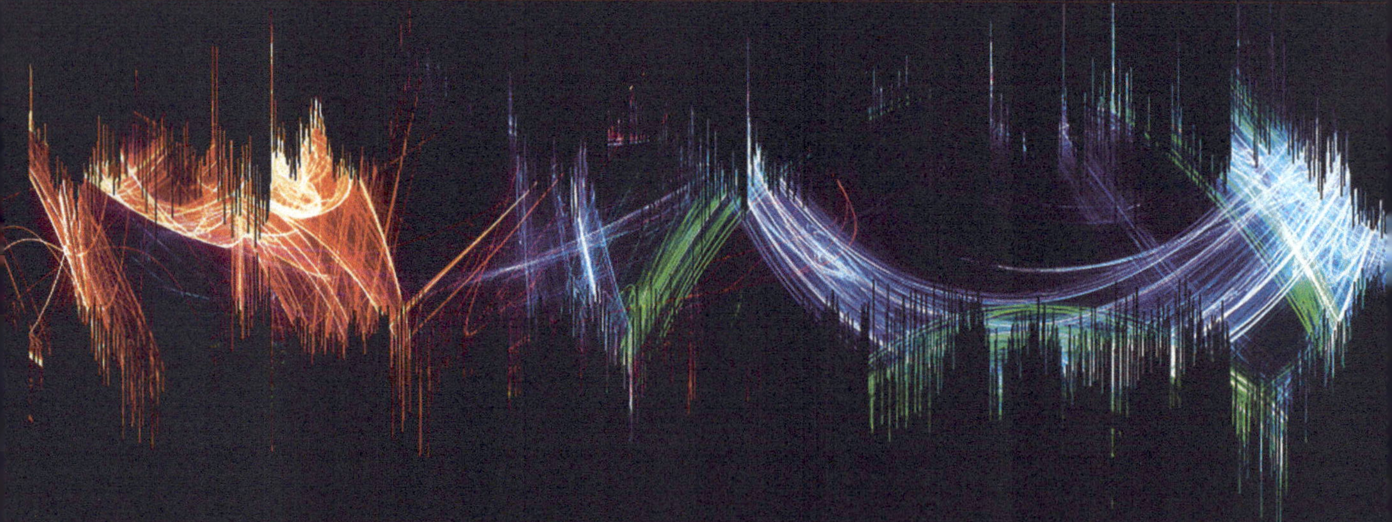

9

Bioreceptors on fiber surface

Bioreceptors are the molecular species that are responsible for the biochemical recognition mechanism. Bioreceptor is considered as the key player for determining the specificity of the biosensor. The selective biological interaction between the bioreceptor and the analyte is then detected and converted into a measurable and quantifiable signal. There are different types of bioreceptors available and they can be generally classified into four different major categories: (1) antibody/antigen, (2) enzymes, (3) nucleic acids [deoxyribonucleic acid (DNA), ribonucleic acid (RNA)], (4) cells and cellular structures (Vo-Dinh & Cullum, 2000).

9.1 Antibody

Antibodies are protective proteins released into the bloodstream and tissue, which are produced by the cells of the immune system called B lymphocytes (B cells). They are also called immunoglobulins (Ig) and their primary function within the living organism is to neutralize and eliminate the infectious agents and toxins produced by the infectious antigen. Antibodies are extremely specific to the foreign molecule and they have a Y-shaped structure consisting of four polypeptide chains (Fig. 9.1A), two long (also called heavy chain) and two short (also called light chain) chains. The four polypeptide chains of the antibody are held together by disulfide (S–S) bond. Two identical short chains and long chains have a molecular mass of 22 and 53 kDa, respectively, with an overall approximate molecular mass of 150 kDa and dimensions $14 \times 10 \times 4$ nm (Crivianu-Gaita & Thompson, 2015; Lu, Smyth, & O'Kennedy, 1996). Both long and short chains contain constant and variable regions. The constant region (indicated as **c**) or Fc region of the antibody is involved in activation of biological effect associated with immune response for infection elimination. Two or several Y-shaped antibody can be grouped together to form multiple antibodies. There are five classes of antibodies that are classified based on their constant regions: IgM, IgG, IgE, IgD, and IgA (Fig. 9.1B). The variable region (indicated as **v**, also called antigen-binding site) or Fab region varies greatly and can be specific to infectious agents, proteins, DNA, RNA, and polysaccharides.

Optical Fiber Biosensors.
DOI: https://doi.org/10.1016/B978-0-12-819467-6.00002-0

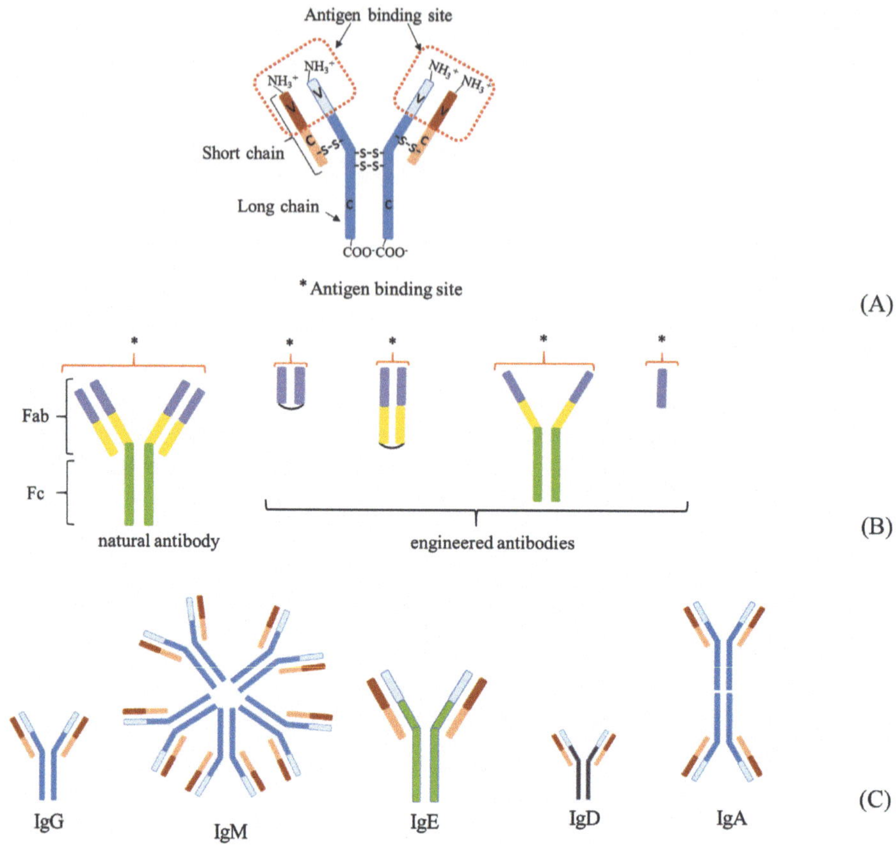

Figure 9.1
(A) Antibody structure. Antibody contains two identical long chains and short chains. Long and short chains are connected by flexible and strong disulfide bridges. (B) Classes of antibodies. (C) Schematic representation of natural antibody and engineered antibodies.

For biosensor applications, this variable region is used for the sensitive and specific detection and capture of the target molecule. In a living body, the genetic variation and combination can produce different types of variable regions almost to all kinds of foreign molecules. Those antibodies can be extracted, purified, and used as bioreceptors in the biosensing system. Antibodies can also be engineered and produced to other types of antigens not present within human body. Moreover, with the help of molecular engineering the overall antibody size can be decreased and stability can be increased by synthesizing the fragments of antibodies such as antigen-binding fragment or even single-chain fragment (Trilling, Beekwilder, & Zuilhof, 2013). Such manipulations with the antibody usually do not alter the antigen-binding specificity. The interaction between the antigen-binding site and the antigen is similar to lock and key systems where a part of the antigen is called epitope that perfectly fits its antigen-binding site thereby promoting only the specific detection. For these characteristics antibodies are used as bioreceptors on fiber surfaces for the specific target detection and in some literature such biosensors are also called immunosensors. The interaction between the antibody and the antigen in most cases is irreversible meaning that antibody-based biosensors are more suitable for single-use studies. Antibodies or fragments of antibodies have been used for the detection of antigens in different quantitative assays such as enzyme-linked immunosorbent assay (ELISA), surface plasmon resonance (SPR), electrochemical biosensors, piezoelectric biosensors, and optical biosensors.

The biosensor's sensitivity is dependent on how the antibody is immobilized on the fiber surface. The perfect antibody immobilization strongly relies on optimized surface density, maintenance of native conformation, and orientation without changing its binding activity and specificity. It is important to maintain the antigen-binding site available for successful antigen binding. The immobilization of the antibody and further detection of the antigen is usually maintained in physiological conditions that are required for antibody functionality. Antibodies have several reactive groups ready to interact with the fiber surface, therefore they can orient themselves in different ways (Fig. 9.2).

The attachment of the antibody on the fiber surface can be based on two types of attachment modes noncovalent and covalent. Noncovalent attachment of the antibodies is based on physical absorption and hence it does not have a control over the specific orientation of the antibodies. However the orientation in this case can be slightly manipulated by changing the pH of the reaction solutions or by electrochemically immobilizing the antibodies on the surface with the help of voltage application (Um et al., 2011; Zhao et al., 2012). Nevertheless, the noncovalent attachment of antibodies is considered as weak, relatively unstable with poor analytical performance (Trilling et al., 2013). Alternatively, the antibodies can be tightly attached to the surface via linker proteins (Fig. 9.3A). Such linker proteins have a natural affinity to the fc portion of the antibody (Huy et al., 2011; Shen, Cai, Wang, & Lu, 2011; Vashist, Dixit, MacCraith, & O'Kennedy, 2011). This type of interaction enables the antibody to be oriented in a tail-on mode and hence promoting the availability of the antigen-binding site for the interaction.

Optical fibers are usually made of glass (SiO_2), glass with polymer (PMMA, PVC), or polymer only. The surface of the optical fibers is hydrophobic making them difficult to interact with the hydrophilic antibodies. Therefore the surface

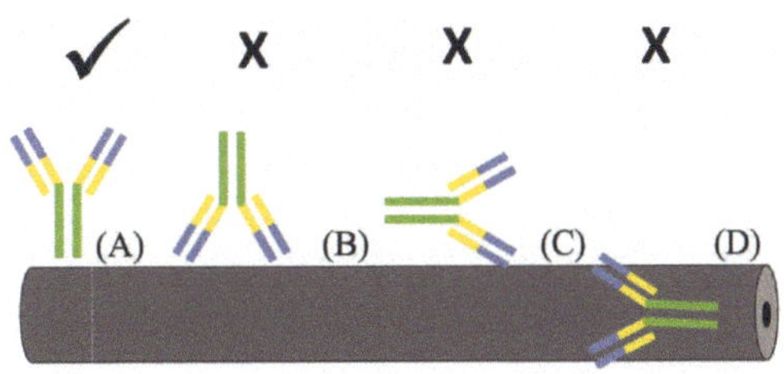

Figure 9.2
The orientation of the antibodies on the fiber surface (A) tail-on; (B) head-on; (C) side-on; (D) flat-on.

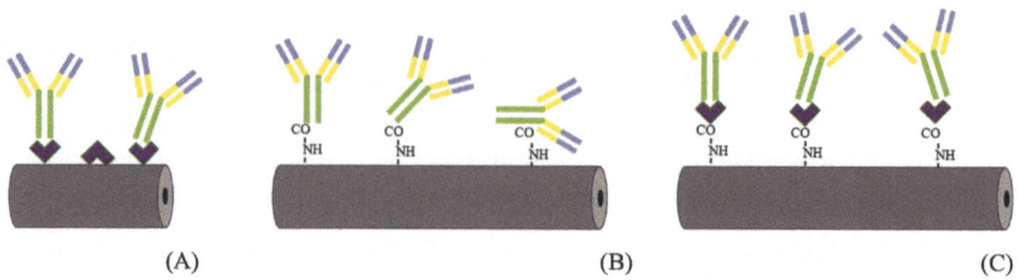

Figure 9.3 Types of antibody and fiber surface interaction (A) via linker proteins, (B) covalent bond, (C) combination of covalent bond and linker proteins.

of the fiber undergoes several types of treatment. The functionalization of the surface with specific groups can be done either directly on the fiber surface or with the help of functionalized self-assembled monolayers. The direct attachment of the functional groups on the fiber starts from cleaning with a detergent in the form of ethanol or isopropanol to remove any of the bound particles. Then the fiber is dried under the stream of gas (N_2) for preparation for further functionalization steps. Treatment with gasses such as CO_2 or N_2/H_2 is used to introduce functional groups such as carboxyl or amine groups for further covalent binding with the antibody (Pâslaru et al., 2014). Cleaning the fiber surface with solutions such as piranha (H_2SO_4:H_2O_2; 1:3) can introduce hydroxyl functional groups, which then used to functionalize the antibodies on the surface.

Covalent bond is a stable chemical bond where shared atoms are being held together between the surface and the antibody. An input energy is required to break the bond since the bond is relatively strong. Therefore the covalent immobilization of the antibody on the fiber surface ensures the stability and high sensitivity due to the tail on orientation.

The building block of an antibody is amino acid. All amino acids share the same chemical groups NH_3^+ and COO^- and are connected using these groups and eventually forming covalent amide bond. Some amino acids have side chains that contain functional groups and are available for the attachment on the surface. Amino acids such as lysine with NH_3^+ side chain and aspartate and glutamate with COO^- side chains are examples of such amino acids. In a folded antibody, the available surface exposed functional chemical groups take part in making a covalent bonding with the pretreated fiber surface (Fig. 9.3B). For more oriented immobilization of the antibodies on the surface, the combination of linker proteins and covalent attachment can be used (Fig. 9.3C). The disulfide bond between the chains can also be reduced and used for the antibody immobilization. Alternatively, the antibody can be engineered to contain synthetic amino acids that can be used for the surface immobilization, it can be fragmented into binding region, or it can be labeled with fluorescent molecules.

The common method of detecting antigen using antibodies in clinic is ELISA. ELISA involves multiple incubations and wash steps as well as the use of the tagged secondary antibodies. The level of the antigen in such method is determined by a colorimetric assay and acquired using the optical plate reader. In addition to multistep incubations, the assay does not allow the detection of the antigen in real time. To device a biosensor that could detect the analyte in real-time, efficient, fast, and on-site researchers developed many sensing platforms that could potentially replace ELISA taking into account not only the sensitivity and the response time but also the size and simplicity of the sensor. Due to the size and advantage in terms of the application and immunity to external electromagnetic field, optical fiber–based biosensors draw considerable attention in biosensing field.

Table 9.1 shows the collection of such biosensors using FBG, LPG, TFBG, and other types of fibers. The steps of antibody immobilization and the type of antibody vary in optical fiber–based biosensors. One such biosensor was developed using the LPG fiber and a special coating film based on three layers of polymer poly(allylamine hydrochloride) and gold-coated silica nanoparticles (Liu et al., 2018) (Fig. 9.4B). Polymer in this case was used to form and imbed the layers of silica nanoparticles on the surface of the optical fiber. The silica nanoparticles increased the surface-to-volume ratio and hence the sensitivity of the device. Then the surface of the silica nanoparticles was coated with Au in order to generate localized SPR. Gold-coated nanoparticles were then treated with the coadsorbent in the form of 11-MUA (11-Mercaptoundecanoic acid), followed by the EDC/NHS activation and consequent antibody immobilization and blocking with bovine serum albumin (BSA) (Fig. 9.4C). The sensor was used to immobilize the IgM antibody for the detection of human IgM, the earliest antibody that appears after the infection. IgM can be detected in blood and lymph fluid and plays an important role in diagnosis of diseases such as dengue virus infection and atherosclerosis. The low level of IgM (<20 mg/dL) during the infection is an implicative factor of an immune disorder. The current IgM diagnosis is mainly based on a traditional ELISA assay, which requires multiple incubation, whereas optical fiber–based IgM detection provides low cost, highly specific, and ability to be used in point of care diagnostics. The optical fiber–based biosensor setup consisted of halogen light source, CCD spectrometer, and computer for processing the data (Fig. 9.4A). IgM with concentrations from 15.6 μg/mL to 1 mg/mL was tested and acquired limit of detection (LOD) was 15 pg/mm^2 in a buffer solution. The detection range was useful in diagnosing diseases associated with low levels of IgM.

The other work used standard FBG fiber for the detection of the C-reactive protein (CRP) (Sridevi, Vasu, Asokan, & Sood, 2015). CRP is a biomarker involved in inflammatory process. The elevated level of CRP in human body was also found in certain types of cancer (Allin, Bojesen, & Nordestgaard, 2009). The standard FBG itself is insensitive to the surrounding refractive index (RI) change,

Table 9.1 Methods for fiber optic biosensing based on antibody receptors, and their surface chemistry.

Analyte (substrate)	Receptor (antibody)	Detection limit	Surface chemistry (sensing film)	Fiber type	References
CRP	CRP antibody (C-reactive protein)	0.01 mg/L	Graphene oxide formation, EDC/NHS activation, antibody conjugation	Standard FBG, etched	Sridevi et al. (2015)
Aquaporin 2	Aquaporin 2 antibody	1.5 ng/mL	Au coating, 11-Mercaptoundecanoic acid formation, EDC/NHS activation and antibody conjugation	TFBG, tilt angle 20 degrees	Han et al. (2017)
Transferrin	Transferrin antibody	10^{-6} g/mL	Au coating, 6-Mercaptohexanoic acid formation, EDC/NHS activation and antibody conjugation	TFBG, tilt angle 6 degrees	Voisin et al. (2014)
CK17	Cytokeratin 17 antibody	$\leq 10^{-12}$ g/mL	Au coating, Mercaptopoly(ethylene glycol) carboxylic acid formation, EDC/NHS activation and antibody conjugation, blocking with BSA	TFBG, tilt angle 7 degrees	Caucheteur, Loyez, González-Vila, and Wattiez (2018), Loyez et al. (2018, 2019), Ribaut et al. (2017)
		$\sim 10^{-9}$ g/ml	Silanization, cross-linking antibody via glutaraldehyde, blocking with BSA		
Escherichia coli bacteria	*E. coli* antibody		Silanization, cross-linking antibody via glutaraldehyde, blocking with BSA	FBG	Srinivasan, Umesh, Murali, Asokan, and Siva Gorthi (2017)
Epithelial cells	Epidermal growth factor receptor (EGFR) antibody	3×10^6 cells /mL	Au coating, conjugation of antibody via Dojindo's carboxylic acid	TFBG, tilt angle 5–8 degrees	Malachovská et al. (2015)
Newcastle disease virus (NDV)	NDV antibody	0.42 pM	Au coating, silanization, Au nanospheres conjugation, staphylococcal protein attachment via cystamine, NDV antibody attachment	TFBG, tilt angle 81 degrees	Luo et al. (2018)
Antihuman IgM	IgM antibody	22 pg/mm^2	Poly(allylamine hydrochloride)/gold-coated silica nanoparticles, 11-Mercaptoundecanoic acid (11-MUA) formation, EDC/NHS activation and antibody conjugation, blocking with BSA	LPG, periodicity 110 μm	Liu et al. (2018)
Antihuman IgG	IgG antibody	2 μg/mL	Silanization, cross-linking antibody via glutaraldehyde	LPG	DeLisa et al. (2000)
Antihuman IgG	IgG antibody	0.04 μg/mL	Graphene oxide/silver coated polymer formation, EDC/NHS activation, antibody conjugation	PCS (polymer cladding silica), core diameter 600 μm	Wang and Wang (2018)
Antihuman IgG	IgG antibody	2 μg/mL	Silanization, polydopamine-modified gold film formation, antibody conjugation	Multimode optical fiber, core diameter 400 μm	Shi et al. (2015)

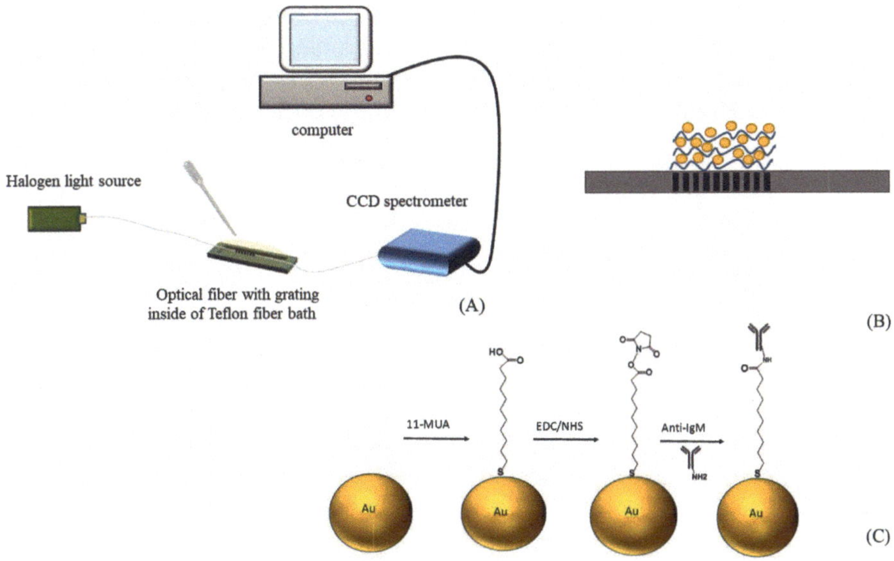

Figure 9.4 (A) LPG sensor setup. (B) Schematic diagram of the layer-by-layer modification of LPG. (C) The modification of LPG for the detection of IgM. Source: *Adapted from Liu, L.L., Marques, L., Correia, R., Morgan, S.P., Lee, S.W., Tighe, P., . . ., Korposh, S. (2018). Highly sensitive label-free antibody detection using a long period fibre grating sensor.* Sensors Actuators B: Chemical, *https://doi.org/10.1016/j.snb.2018.05.109.*

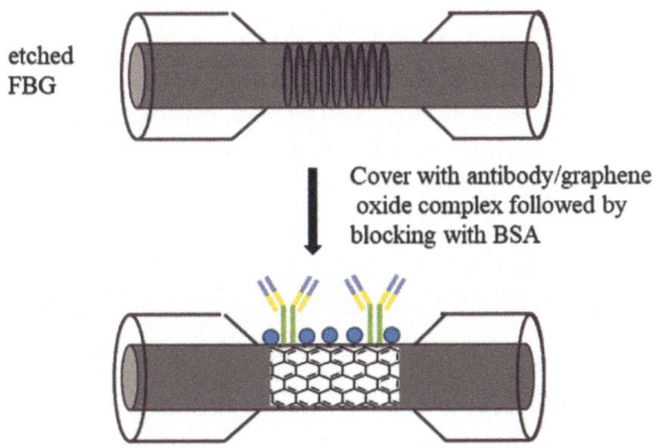

Figure 9.5 The schematic representation of the functionalized surface of the etched FBG for the detection of CRP using anti-CRP antibodies.

therefore to make it sensitive to the surrounding RI the part of the fiber is usually etched (Bekmurzayeva et al., 2018). Prior to immobilization the CRP antibody was primarily allowed to interact with the graphene oxide to form a complex (Fig. 9.5). The complex was then used to cover the surface of the fiber and used for the following detection of the CRP after blocking with BSA. The lowest detectable concentration was 0.01 mg/L. The sensor was tested for the specificity for CRP in contrast to other molecules such as glucose, urea, and creatinine and showed that CRP–graphene oxide complex–coated eFBG sensors had a high specificity to CRP even in the presence of the above molecules.

Large number of optical fiber biosensors exploit the SPR phenomenon, which require the deposition of thin metal layer over the sensitive area surface. This is due to the fact that SPR increases the sensitivity of the most optical fiber sensors to surrounding RI changes. For instance, gold-coated TFBG functionalized with transferrin antibody for label free biosensing was developed by Voisin, Pilate, Damman, Mégret, and Caucheteur (2014). Transferrin is a blood plasma protein that binds to iron molecules and thus controls the level of iron. Transferrin has a clinical significance in diagnosing the iron-deficient anemia. The TFBG fiber was fist coated with thin layer of Au and then covered with mercaptohexanoic acid to allow the formation of a self-assembled monolayer. The surface was then activated with EDC/NHS complex and conjugated with antibody (Fig. 9.6). The transmitted amplitude spectra were recorded with optical vector analyzer through external linear polarizer. The real-time monitoring of each functionalization step ensured the effectiveness of the surface coverage. The limit of the detection of the device was in the range between 10^{-7} and 10^{-6} g/mL and the binding process was repeatable as well as the surface was used several times after the regeneration cycles.

Due to the advancement in surface chemistry, the antibody immobilization on optical fiber surface can be also achieved without the thin metal layer. The antibody immobilization strategy on the surface of the bare glass optical fibers affects the overall sensitivity of the device. Loyez, Albert, Caucheteur, and Wattiez (2018) studied the difference between covalent antibody immobilization, physical adsorption, and antibody immobilization via linker proteins for the detection of cytokeratin 17 protein (CK17) using the anti-CK17 antibody (Fig. 9.7). CK17 is a biomarker and elevated level is associated with lung cancer. The study used TFBG optical fiber with tilt angle being at 7 degrees. In all

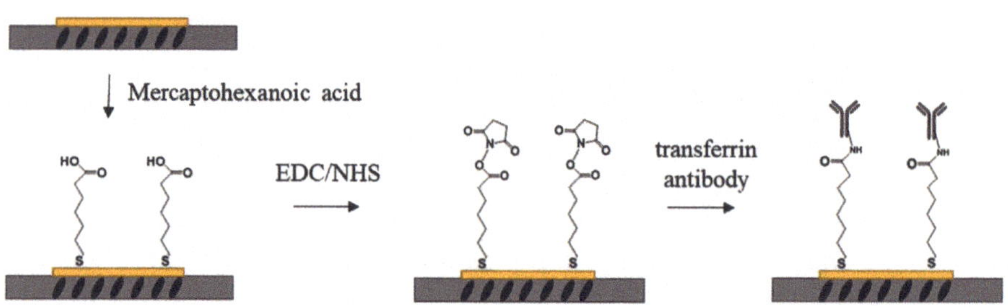

Figure 9.6 The schematic representation of the functionalized surface of Au-coated TFBG for the detection of transferrin using anti-Transferrin antibodies.

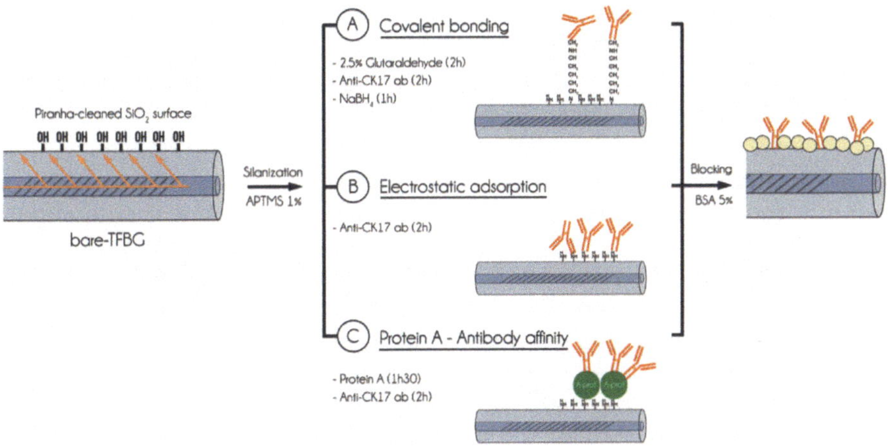

Figure 9.7 Illustration of the main steps of the three functionalization processes used for the immobilization of antibodies onto silica optical fiber gratings. The first method considered is a covalent binding of anti-CK17 antibodies (A) while electrostatic adsorption (B) and the use of Protein A intermediate are also represented (C). Source: *Adapted from Loyez, M., Albert, J., Caucheteur, C., & Wattiez, R. (2018). Cytokeratins biosensing using tilted fiber gratings.* Biosensors, 8, *74.*

three cases the surface of the optical fiber was silanized, a common method for the functionalization of the glass optical fibers and after each respective antibody immobilization strategy the surface was blocked with BSA to eliminate the nonspecific binding. The binding efficiently was tested by incubating the optical fiber with increasing CK17 protein concentrations from 10^{-12} g/mL up to 10^{-6} g/mL and measuring the consequent amplitude and wavelength shift. According to the results, covalent bonding of antibodies showed a detection limit of $\sim 10^{-9}$ g/mL, immobilization method based on linker showed unstable signal and the results were difficult to reproduce. Interestingly, the most reliable functionalization method as compared to the other two methods studied was the electrostatic adsorption exhibiting a LOD of 14 pM. Overall the study showed that the sensitivity range and LOD for the thin metal–coated optical fibers are better than those of bare fibers. However, bare gratings could be used in applications where the low LOD is not an essential point as opposed to the overall detection.

To conclude, antibodies are natural bioreceptors, which can be used to capture a target molecule on special detection platforms and hence serve as a key element in biosensor development. The immobilization of the antibody and orientation on the surface of the optical fiber is important for the better sensitivity and specificity of the sensor. The surface chemistry as well as the fiber type also plays an important role in biosensor sensitivity characteristics. Antibodies have a limited shelf life and they are sensitive to temperature variations. However they can be engineered on purpose to make them stable and small and hence suitable for the biosensor development.

9.2 Enzymes

Enzymes are catalytic proteins that speed up a reaction without being consumed by the reaction. They regulate chemical reactions occurring within living organisms. They are heavily involved in cell metabolism and hence play a crucial role. In the absence of enzymes, chemical reactions in the metabolic pathways would take such a long time. Every chemical reaction between biomolecules involves bond breaking and bond formation. The investment of energy (e.g., heat) is required to contort the molecules involved in the reaction process. An enzyme catalyzes the reaction by lowering this energy (activation energy) and enabling the molecules to interact even at moderate temperatures. Enzymes are extremely selective to the reactions they catalyze and they determine the order and timing for any chemical reaction taking place within the cell. The molecule to which enzyme binds is called substrate and together they form enzyme–substrate complex. The specificity of the enzyme enables it to recognize its substrate even among closely related to substrate compounds. The catalytic properties of the enzyme usually convert substrate into the product and this is usually carried only at specific region called an active site (Fig. 9.8). Like in antibodies, the building block of most enzymes is amino acid, except for enzyme made from RNAs. Only few amino acids are involved in interaction with the substrate and the rest of the amino acids determine the overall shape and configuration of the active site. The shape of the active site and the shape of the substrate need to be fit and compatible so to induce the specific reaction. Within this fitted configuration, those few amino acids that make up the active site catalyze the conversion of the substrate into the product. After the reaction, the product leaves the active site and making it available for another set of reaction with the substrate. The rate of the reaction is extremely fast. For instance, one enzyme can catalyze up to a thousand molecule per second by functioning over and over again in a series of cycles.

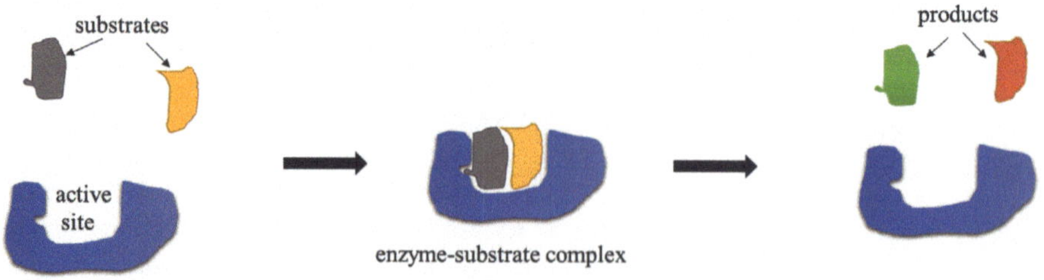

Figure 9.8 The schematic of the catalytic activity of an enzyme.

There are enzymes that catalyze reaction in both directions, that is, forward and reverse reaction. Those enzymes mostly try to reach the balance of substrate and product concentration thereby reaching the equilibrium.

The structure and activity of enzymes like many other proteins are dependent on conditions of the surrounding environment such as pH, temperature, and other chemicals. The optimal condition is considered where the active site of the enzyme maintains active confirmation and optimal catalytic activity. With an increasing temperature the rate of an enzymatic reaction increases also, however, up to a certain point. Most human enzymes have optimal activity at temperatures between 35°C and 40°C. There are also bacterial enzymes that work well at 70°C and above. Most of the enzymes work well at pH 6–8 but not all. For instance enzymes that are present in human digestive system function well in acidic environments where the pH level is 2.

To function at full extent many of the enzymes require addition of small organic molecules called cofactors or coenzymes. These can be metal atoms such as iron or copper. Some chemicals on the contrary can selectively inhibit the catalytic activity of an enzyme and they are called inhibitors. If the inhibitor binds the active site and competes with the substrate, it is called a competitive inhibitor. If the inhibitor does not compete for the same active site but binds to another part of the enzyme, it is called noncompetitive inhibitor. Noncompetitive inhibitors causes the change in enzyme shape and hence stops the binding of the substrate to the active site of an enzyme (Fig. 9.9). Table 9.2 lists different types of optical fiber–based biosensor where an enzyme was used as a bioreceptor.

The highly selective properties of the enzyme for a specific analyte have been used to develop enzyme-based fiber optic biosensors (Monk & Walt, 2004). One of the mostly studied biosensors for the detection of glucose levels is based on the enzyme named glucose oxidase (GO). GO catalyzes the conversion reaction of the substrate glucose into the product gluconalactone or gluconic acid and hydrogen peroxide. The detection of glucose levels is important for the prevention and treatment of serious diseases such as diabetes. The immobilization of the GO on the fiber surface could be based on approaches such as

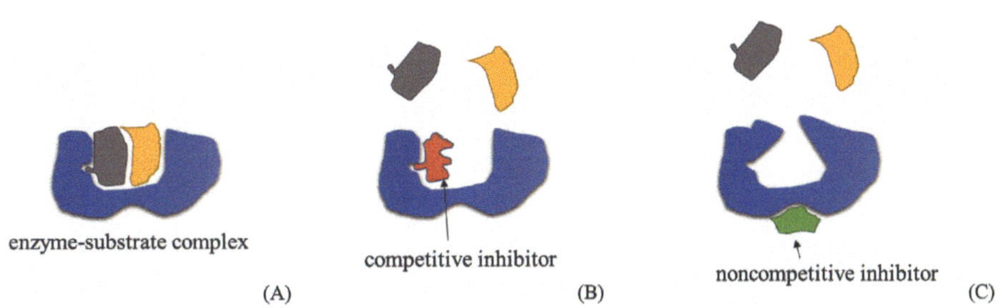

Figure 9.9
The schematic of the enzyme inhibition (A), by competitive (B) and noncompetitive (C) inhibitors.

Table 9.2 Methods for fiber optic biosensing based on enzyme receptors, and their surface chemistry.

Analyte (substrate)	Receptor (enzyme)	Detection limit	Surface chemistry (sensing film)	Fiber type	Sensitivity	Detection range	References
Glucose	Glucose oxidase	0.1–3 mg/mL	Salinization with APTES	LPG, standard SMF periodicity 550 μm		10–300 mg/dL	Deep et al. (2012)
		0.013–0.02 mg/mL	Salinization with APTES	TFBG, standard SMF, tilt angle 78 degrees	1.514 nm/mg/mL	0–5 mg/mL	Luo et al. (2015)
		1 nM	Multilayer poly (ethylenimine) (PEI)/poly (acrylic acid) (PAA)	LPG, $d = 80$ μm SMF, periodicity 390 μm		2–10 μM	Yin et al. (2016)
			Graphene oxide cross-linking via EDC/NHS	TFBG, hydrogen-loaded standard SMF, tilt angle 82 degrees	0.24 nm/mM	0–8 mM	Jiang et al. (2018)
		10 nM	Polyaniline cross-linking via Gluteraldehyde	Multimode optical fiber of core/cladding 425/320 μm		10 nM–100 mM	Pahurkar et al. (2015)
			Silica gel matrix	0.5 m long Y-bundle 120 silica fibers in a circular arrangement	89.06 ± 13.67 mV/mM^{-1}	0–60 mM	Portaccio et al. (2009)
			Metal organic framework	LPG standard SMF, periodicity 400 μm	0.5 nm/mM	1–8 mM	Zhu et al. (2019)
		0.142 mg/mL	SiO_2 nanoparticles and polyacrylamide gel	Multimode optical fiber $d = 600$ μm	0.14 nm/(mg/dL)	0–80 mg/dL	Yuan et al. (2017)
			Salinization with APTES	LPG, SMF thin cladding boron–germanium-doped fiber $d = 80$ μm, periodicity 300 μm	4298.20 nm/RIU	0.1–3.2 mg/mL	Badmos et al. (2017)
		25.79 nM,6.43 μM	Quantum dots/cellulose acetate complex sensitive film	Quartz optical fiber $d = 600$ μm		10–100 nmol/L, 10–200 μmol/L	Yu et al. (2019)
Triacylglyceride	Lipase	17.71 mg/dL	Salinization with APTES	LPG, Boron–Germanium codoped fiber, periodicity 581 μm	0.5 nm/mM	2–6 mg/mL	Baliyan, Sital, Tiwari, Gupta, and Sharma (2016)
D sorbitol	Sorbitol dehydrogenase	0.020 nM	Tantalum pentaoxide nanoflowers on silver-coated fiber	Multimode plastic optical fiber, core $d = 600$ μm	3.6 ng/mL	0.1–1.1 μg/mL	Kant et al. (2017)
Acetylcholine	Acetylcholine transferase	38 nM			8.709 nm/μM	0–10 μM	Kant and Gupta (2018)
Acetylcholine	Acetylcholine transferase	23 nM	Salinization with APTES	SMF $d = 125$ μm, tapered waist 10 μm		0.12–31 μM	Arjmand, Aray, Saghafifar, and Alijanianzadeh (2020)
Methyl-parathion	Acetylcholine transferase	0.24 nM	Salinization with APTES	SMF $d = 125$ μm, tapered fiber		10^{10} M to 5×10^5	Arjmand, Saghafifar, Alijanianzadeh, and Soltanolkotabi (2017)
Ethanol	alcohol dehydrogenase (ADH) enzyme and its coenzyme nicotinamide adenine dinucleotide (NAD)	15.34 μM	Hydrogel (polyacrylamide)	Multimode plastic optical fiber, core $d = 600$ μm		0.1–10 mM	Semwal et al. (2016)

physical absorption, cross-linking, and covalent bonding as well as integration of nanoparticles, composite membranes, and other technologies.

A glucose biosensor was developed using the LPG where the GO was absorbed on the poly(ethylenimine) (PEI) and poly(acrylic acid) (PAA) multilayer film. The film in this case was used to detect and enhance the signal whereas the GO was used to detect the glucose level. The conversion of the glucose into the gluconic acid by the GO resulted in the change in pH in the local microenvironment. This change then initiated the swelling of the PEI/PAA multilayer and the swelling degree was dependent on the glucose concentration. The proposed device showed LOD of 1 nM. The overall setup was integrated in a microfluidic chip, which enabled fast and low-sample glucose analysis (Yin, Huang, Gao, Zhang, & Ye, 2016) (Fig. 9.10).

In another example, the GO was immobilized on a graphene oxide–coated TFBG fiber. Graphene oxide contains many oxygen containing groups and hence it was used to covalently link the GO onto the fiber surface. In particular the carboxyl COO^- group of graphene oxide was used to covalently connect with the amino NH_2^+ groups of GO via EDC/NHS surface chemistry. Once the glucose was added on the sensor surface, GO-specific catalytic reaction took place, which was observed as a resonant wavelength shift. The catalytic reaction from GO to gluconic acid and hydrogen peroxide promoted the RI change in local environment. The device could detect low concentrations of glucose in

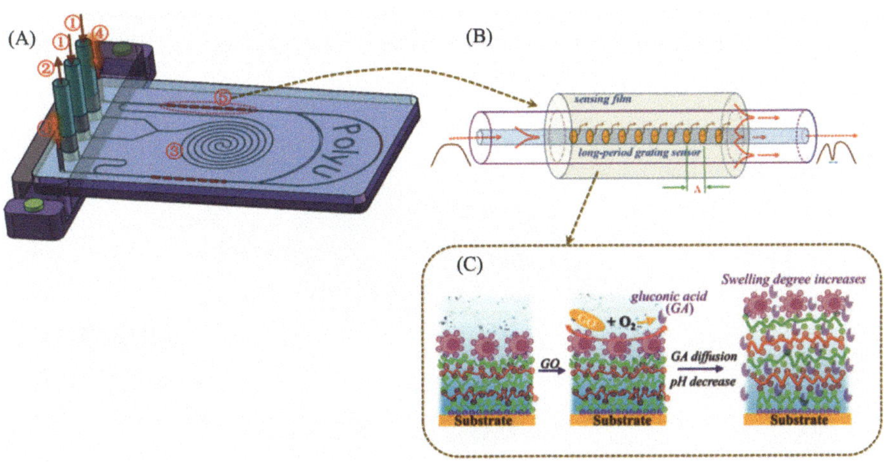

Figure 9.10 (A) Schematic design of the optical fiber biosensor–integrated microfluidic chip: 1 are two inlets, 2 is outlet, 3 is a spiral mixture, 4 are optical fibers, and 5 is the embedded LPG sensor. (B) The mode coupling and optical resonance in the LPG biosensor. (C) Working mechanism of the multilayer film for glucose sensing and signal enhancement. Source: *Reprinted/Adapted with permission from © The Optical Society. Ming-jie Yin, Bobo Huang, Shaorui Gao, A. Ping Zhang, and Xuesong Ye, "Optical fiber LPG biosensor integrated microfluidic chip for ultrasensitive glucose detection," Biomed. Opt. Express 7, 2067-2077 (2016).*

the range of 0–8 mM with a response coefficient of ~0.24 nm/mM (Jiang et al., 2018) (Fig. 9.11).

The work where the polyaniline was used as the matrix for the GO attachment on the multimode optical fiber of core/cladding dimensions 425/320 μm showed increased device stability where it could deliver consistent results for up to 36 days. This is important aspect as it could contribute to the continuous glucose level monitoring. The polyaniline is a porous material and it provided a supportive base for the GO immobilization by cross-linking via glutaraldehyde. According to the results the sensor exhibited LOD at 10 nM and showed stability and reproducibility (Pahurkar, Tamgadge, Gambhire, & Muley, 2015).

The other porous material that was used to immobilize the GO on the fiber surface was based on metal organic frameworks (MOFs). MOFs are made of metal ions that are linked to form a porous substrate for trapping and attaching enzymes. In this interesting work, the protein encapsulation inside the pores showed a good efficiency and increased activity and stability under harsh conditions. Enzymes are tend to be sensitive to both temperature and pH and this mode of immobilization showed a great stability even after placing the sensor in boiling water. The MOF-encapsulated GO was placed on the surface of the LPG fiber and the change in glucose level resulted in the wavelength shifts, which are linearly correlated with glucose concentrations in the range of 1–8 mM (Zhu et al., 2019) (Fig. 9.12).

Fiber glucose biosensor based on fluorescent carbon quantum dots (CQDs)-GO/cellulose acetate (CA) complex sensitive film was fabricated and used for the detection of glucose real time over a period of time by measuring the

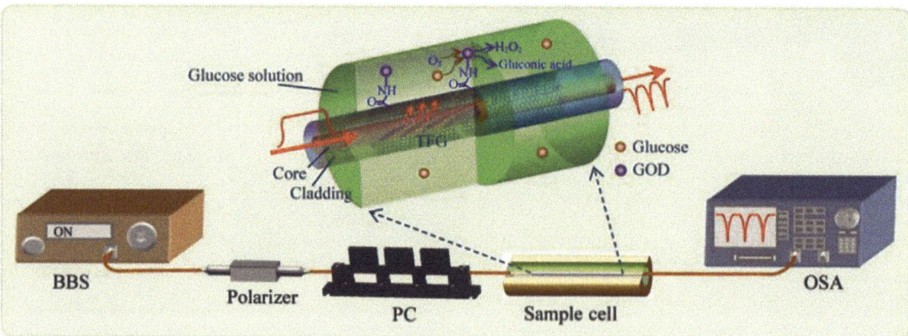

Figure 9.11 Experimental setup for surrounding medium and glucose detection. The upward inset shows the schematically dissection diagram of GOD-GO-modified TFG. *BBS*, Broadband source; *PC*, polarization controller; *OSA*, optical spectral analyzer. Source: *Reprinted from Jiang, B., Zhou, K., Wang, C., Sun, Q., Yin, G., Tai, Z., . . ., Zhang, L. (2018). Label-free glucose biosensor based on enzymatic graphene oxide-functionalized tilted fiber grating.* Sensors Actuators B: Chemical, *254, 1033–1039. https://doi.org/10.1016/j.snb.2017.07.109.*

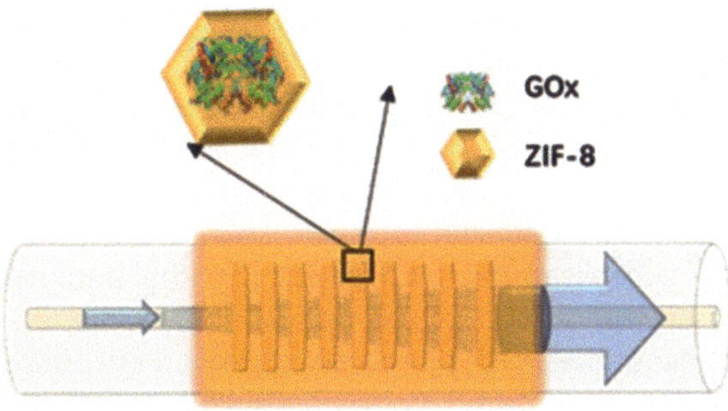

Figure 9.12 Schematic diagram of MOF coated LPG. Source: *Reprinted from Zhu, G., Zhang, M., Lu, L., Lou, X., Dong, M., & Zhu, L. (2019). Metal-organic framework/enzyme coated optical fibers as waveguide-based biosensors.* Sensors Actuators B: Chemical, 288, *12–19. https://doi.org/10.1016/j.snb.2019.02.083.*

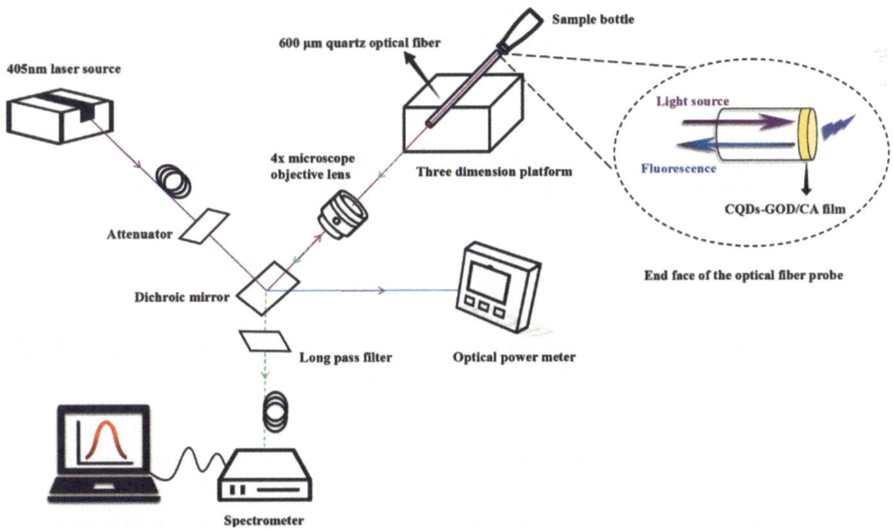

Figure 9.13 The schematic diagram of the optical fiber sensor platform based on CQDs-GO/CA precursor. Source: *Reprinted from Yu, S., Ding, L., Lin, H., Wu, W., & Huang, J. (2019). A novel optical fiber glucose biosensor based on carbon quantum dots-glucose oxidase/cellulose acetate complex sensitive film.* Biosensors & Bioelectronics, 146. *https://doi.org/10.1016/j.bios.2019.111760.*

fluorescence intensity (Yu, Ding, Lin, Wu, & Huang, 2019). The CQDs-GO complex was prepared by the chemical cross-linking method where the GO was immobilized on the COD's surface via the EDC/NHS coupling chemistry. Then the prepared CQDs-GO/CA precursor casting solution was deposited on the tip of the 600 μm quartz optical fiber. The proposed biosensor showed change in fluorescence intensity linear with the change in glucose concentration at nanomolar level (Fig. 9.13).

The optical fiber biosensor for the detection of sorbitol with the sorbitol dehydrogenase enzyme (SDH) entrapped on tantalum pentaoxide nanoflowers shows another example of how enzymes could be placed and used as a sensing device. SDH is an enzyme, which catalyzes the conversion reaction of D sorbitol into the fructose. The identification of the D sorbitol is important since the level of the molecule gets disrupted in patients with diabetes and causes complementary complications such as neuropathy and microvascular damage. The study used multimode plastic optical fiber with core diameter of 600 μm. The use of nanoflower in biosensor development draw attention due to their enzyme entrapment and stabilizing ability. Nanoflowers exhibit higher surface-to-volume ratio as compared to nanoparticles and hence promote the efficient catalytic activity of the entrapped enzyme. The application of both metal later (silver) and nanoflowers resulted in increased SPR signal generation. The sensitivity and the LOD for such biosensor was 3.6 ng/mL (Kant, Tabassum, & Gupta, 2017). The same principle of operation was also applied for the entrapment of the acetylcholinesterase enzyme for the detection of the neurotransmitter acetylcholine (Kant & Gupta, 2018).

There is also a possibility of using hydrogels as a matrix for the enzyme entrapment and further detection on the surface of the optical fiber (Semwal, Shrivastav, Verma, & Gupta, 2016). Hydrogels are 3D cross-linked polymer networks able to enlarge by absorbing large amount of water or other fluids. Enzymes alongside with their coenzymes can be trapped in such hydrogels and used for biosensing purposes. Hydrogels such as polyacrylamide were used to entrap alcohol dehydrogenase (ADH) enzyme and its coenzyme nicotinamide adenine dinucleotide (NAD) for the detection of ethanol. Such configuration increased the rate of the catalytic reaction of the enzyme and hence detection and conversion of the substrate into to product (Fig. 9.14).

To conclude, the use of an enzyme as receptor results in the detection of the either enzyme substrate or a product of the reaction between the enzyme and substrate. Different enzyme immobilization strategies can be exploited to deliver the sensitive detection. The main strategy is based on enzyme entrapment on the surface of the optical fiber via either direct immobilization, the use of nanoparticles, cross-linking or via gel matrices. The sensitivity of the enzyme-based biosensors could be also improved by addition of coenzymes and different types of optical fibers. Most of the enzymes require a certain temperature conditions in order to operate at full capacity, therefore, maintaining of such conditions is also important during signal recording.

9.3 Oligonucleotides

Oligonucleotides are short single- or double-stranded DNA or RNA molecules. The building block of oligonucleotides is nucleic acid. There are five nucleic

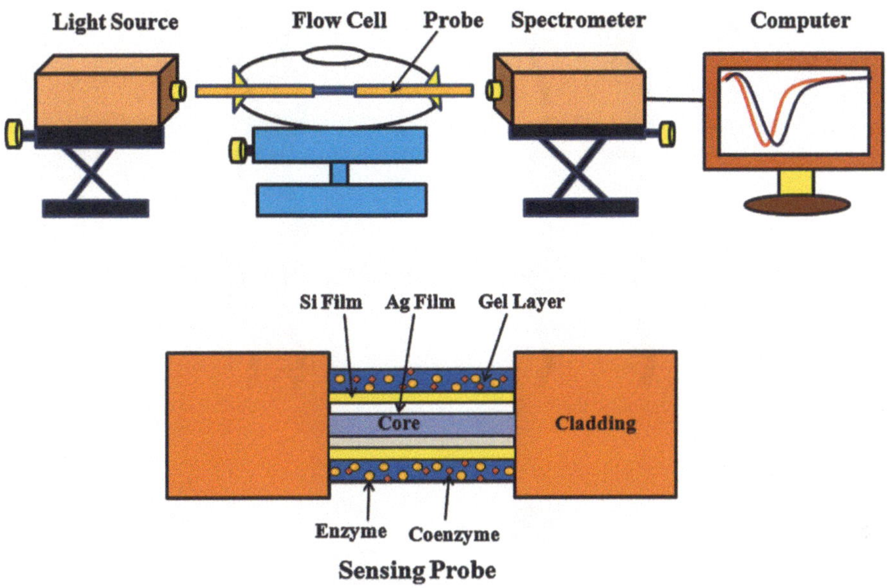

Figure 9.14 Schematic diagram of the experimental setup and hydrogel entrapment of the enzyme and coenzyme on unclad optical fiber. Source: *Reprinted from Semwal, V., Shrivastav, A.M., Verma, R., & Gupta, B.D. (2016). Surface plasmon resonance based fiber optic ethanol sensor using layers of silver/silicon/hydrogel entrapped with ADH/NAD.* Sensors Actuators B: Chemical, 230, *485–492. https://doi.org/10.1016/j.snb.2016.02.084.*

acids [Adenine (A), Thymine (T), Guanine (G), Cytosine (C), and Uracil (U)] in total and each nucleotide acid pairs with another complementary nucleic acid (A:T; G:C; A:U) to form a hydrogen bond. Each nucleic acid is consisted of three components: a 5-carbon sugar, a phosphate group, and a nitrogenous base. If the sugar is made of compound ribose, the oligonucleotide is called RNA; if the sugar is derived from ribose as deoxyribose, the oligonucleotide is called DNA. Each nucleotide binds its complementary pair via Watson-Crick base paring (Fig. 9.15) to form a spiral-shaped two oligonucleotide strands.

Oligonucleotides are generally used in biology, biochemistry, molecular diagnostics, genetics, and molecular biology experiments. The main function of oligonucleotides is to hybridize to its own complimentary strand thereby promoting only the specific interaction. Oligonucleotides could be used for gene expression manipulation, therapeutic application, detection (forensic sciences, biosensing field), and treatment. In optical fiber biosensing field, oligonucleotides have been used as a receptor for capturing complementary strand or a protein. The ends of the nucleotide could be modified as such as to enable them to attach on the surface of the optical fibers. For instance, such modifications include adding amino (NH_2) or thiol groups (SH) to one of the extremities of the nucleotide. In addition, linkers could be attached to the

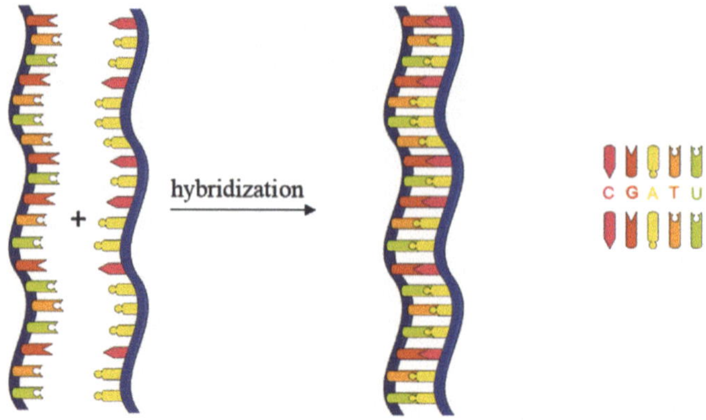

Figure 9.15
The schematic representation of the oligonucleotides and nucleic acids.

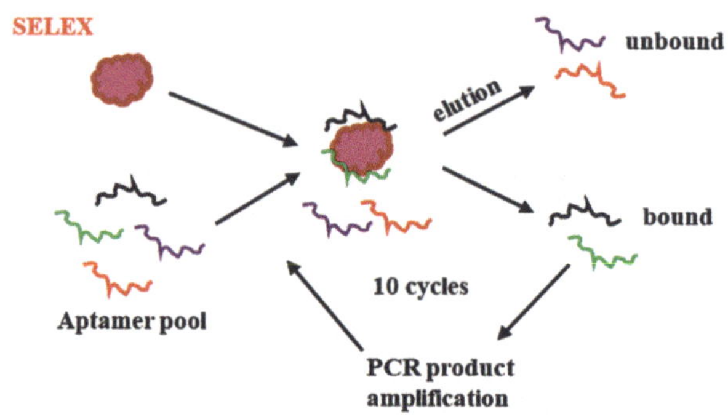

Figure 9.16
The schematic representation of SELEX-systematic evolution of ligands by exponential enrichment.

oligonucleotides for extending them from the surface and probes/fluorescent molecules could be attached for the labeled detection. The most commonly used oligonucleotide as a receptor in biosensing field is aptamer. Aptamer is a short single- or double-stranded oligonucleotide (15–80 nucleotides). Unlike antibodies and enzymes, aptamers are relatively cheap, extremely stable and functional under broad range of conditions defined by the user based upon the intended end (Sypabekova, Jolly, Estrela, & Kanayeva, 2019). Aptamers are selected by a process called systematic evolution of ligands by exponential enrichment (SELEX) (Fig. 9.16), where oligonucleotide library consisting of randomly generated sequences of fixed length allowed to incubate with the target molecule. The bound sequences were then eluted and amplified before the next round of cycle. Overall, 6–20 cycles are needed in order to select only the specific aptamers with distinct sequences for the target molecule.

The specific sequences are then used as receptors for the detection of the target molecule in optical fiber–based biosensors. The target molecule type for an aptamer varies from ions, proteins, viruses, and cells. Aptamers are tend to form a stable 3D structure, which allow them to bind to the target molecule (Fig. 9.17). Table 9.3

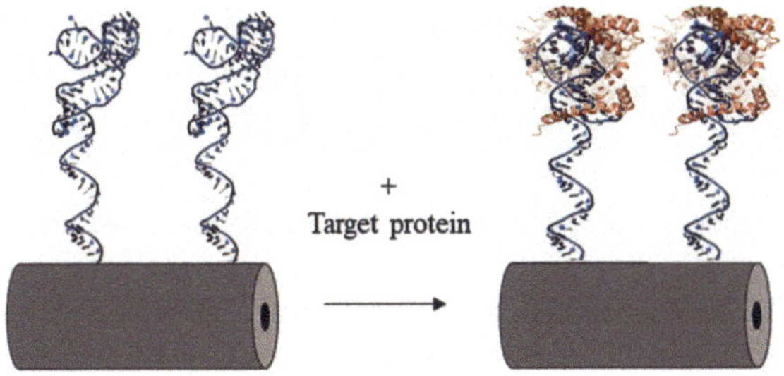

Figure 9.17 Structural modeling of aptamers and the protein. Schematic representation of the target binding on optical fiber surface. Source: *Modified and adapted from Joseph, D.F., Nakamoto, J.A., Garcia Ruiz, O.A., Peñaranda, K., Sanchez-Castro, A.E., Castillo, P.S., & Milón, P. (2019). DNA aptamers for the recognition of HMGB1 from Plasmodium falciparum.* PLoS One. *https://doi.org/10.1371/journal.pone.0211756 and modified.*

Table 9.3 Methods for fiber optic biosensing based on oligonucleotide receptors, and their surface chemistry.

Analyte	Receptor (oligonucleotide)	Detection limit	Surface chemistry (sensing film)	Fiber type	References
ssDNA	PNA probe (peptide nucleic acid)	0.01 μm	Silanization, DMF (*N,N*-dimethylformamide) conjugation and attachment of the probe	TFBG (double) tilt angle 3.2 degrees	Candiani et al. (2012)
	Leptospira bacteria DNA	0.1 fM	Silanization with APTES, cross-linking DNA via glutaraldehyde	SMF, tapered, wait $d = 12$ μm	Zainuddin et al. (2018)
	20 bp dnaK gene of *E. coli*	0.7 μg/mL	Silanization with APTES, cross-linking DNA via glutaraldehyde	FBG, etched ($d = 5$ μm)	Chryssis et al. (2005)
Thrombin	Aptamer-NH_2	0.075–0.110 nM	Silanization with APTES and cross-linking aptamers via glutaraldehyde, blocking with BSA	TFBG, etched	Sypabekova, Korganbayev et al. (2019)
	Aptamer-SH	22.6 nM	Aptamer conjugation via S-S bond	TFBG, excitation of SPR (50 nm Au) tilt angle 10 degrees	Shevchenko et al. (2011)
	1 Aptamer-SH2 Aptamer-SH	1 nM	Aptamer conjugation via S-S bond	TFBG, excitation of SPR, LSPR (50 nm Au, 13 nm AuNP's) tilt angle 20 degrees	Lao et al. (2019)
HER-2 (human epidermal growth factor receptor-2)	Aptamer-SH	10^{-12} g/mL	Aptamer conjugation via S-S bond and blocking with MCH	TFBG, tilt angle 7 degrees	Lobry et al. (2020)
Dopamine	Aptamer	10^{-13} M	Graphene film deposition, aptamer immobilization via $\pi-\pi$ interaction	TFBG, excitation of SPR (2–3 nm Cr, 32 nm Au) tilt angle 20 degrees	Hu et al. (2018)
Circulating breast cancer cell	Aptamer-SH (mammaglobin-A)	49 cells/mL	Aptamer conjugation via S-S bond and blocking with MCH	TFBG, excitation of SPR, LSPR (50 nm Au, 10 nm AuNPs) tilt angle 8 degrees	Loyez et al. (2020)
Immunoglobulin E	Biotinylated-aptamers	2 nM	Hydroxyl/carboxyl mercapto-PEG formation, EDC activation, streptavidin immobilization	Multimode fiber $d = 400$ m	Pollet et al. (2009)

briefly summarizes the use of oligonucleotides in the form of single-stranded DNA and aptamers in the development of optical fiber–based biosensors.

Zainuddin et al. (2018) used SMF-tapered fiber for the functionalization of short single-stranded DNA. The sensor was developed for the detection of the complementary DNA strand of the bacterium *Leptospira* a causative agent of Leptospirosis disease. The DNA receptor was immobilized on the fiber surface after the silanization process. The setup consisted of tapered optical fiber region positioned within the microchannel groove of connected at one end to optical spectrum analyzer and at another to light source (Fig. 9.18). DNA binding with functionalized tapered optical fiber with probe DNA changed the effective RI of the surface, which resulted in shift of transmission spectra. The biosensor was able to detect the low concentrations of complementary DNA strand at 0.1 fM. The specificity test with control DNA sequence also showed that the signal was indeed generated from the specific binding the complementary strand.

Similar study used the single-stranded DNA aptamers for the detection of thrombin protein but using etched TFBG fibers (Sypabekova, Korganbayev et al., 2019). The thrombin molecule and its aptamer interaction are well established and had been used in the development of different types of biosensors. The surface chemistry based on silanization of the surface of the optical fiber followed by the immobilization of amine terminated aptamer (Fig. 9.19). The unreacted surface was blocked using the BSA to limit the nonspecific binding. The binding of the thrombin protein initiated the wavelength shift, which enabled to detect protein at low concentrations. The theoretical LOD according the study was 7.5 pM and the biosensor was able to distinguish different RI changes at the interface of the sensor surface and the buffer.

Another study developed a sandwich assay for the detection of thrombin using gold-coated TFBG fiber (Lao et al., 2019). In this study two different thiolated (SH) thrombin aptamers were used, one aptamer had a sequence of 15 nucleotides and the other had 29 nucleotides. Both aptamers bind well to the thrombin molecule and possibly without competing for the same binding site, thereby allowing to use both aptamers in one detection assay. Firstly, 29 nucleotide long aptamer was attached to the gold-coated TFBG fiber via thiol bond. Gold provides a good

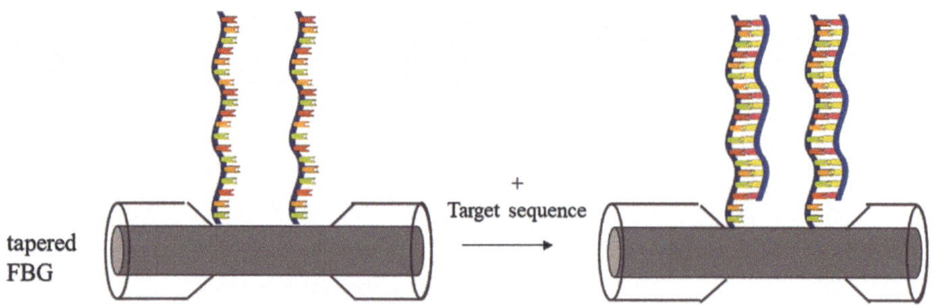

Figure 9.18
DNA hybridization detection on the fiber-tapered optical fiber.

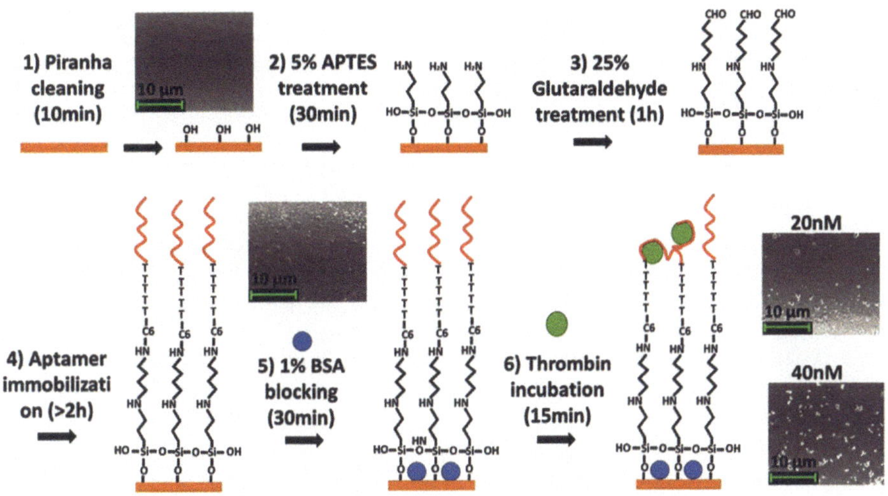

Figure 9.19 Schematic overview of the functionalization of the etched TFBG with thrombin aptamer and thrombin detection. SEM images for clean, aptamer-immobilized fiber surface, and after thrombin detection (20 and 40 nM). Source: *Reprinted from Sypabekova, M., Korganbayev, S., González-Vila, Á., Caucheteur, C., Shaimerdenova, M., Ayupova, T., . . ., Tosi, D. (2019). Functionalized etched tilted fiber Bragg grating aptasensor for label-free protein detection.* Biosensors & Bioelectronics, *146, 111765. https://doi.org/10.1016/j.bios.2019.111765 with permission from Elsevier.*

platform for the formation of stable thiol bond therefore it has been extensively used in many biosensors. In addition gold aids the generation of the SPR signal required for the detection. Secondly, 15 nucleotide long aptamer was attached to 13 nm gold nanoparticles. Gold nanoparticles, in addition to SPR, generated localized SPR. The additional localized SPR signal overall increased the sensitivity of the device and demonstrated stable and reproducible response to thrombin concentration down to a LOD of 1 nM. The results showed that the application of additional aptamer-coated gold nanoparticles increased the sensitivity three order of magnitude as compared to other optical fiber–based thrombin biosensors. The experimental setup consisted of broadband light source connected to the sensing fiber through the polarizer and polarization controller. The transmission spectrum was monitored by optical spectrum analyzer.

Aptamers were also used for the detection of small molecules such as neurotransmitter dopamine using the TFBG fibers (Hu et al., 2018). Low level of dopamine has been associated with Parkinson's disease and other neurological disorders. Aptamers could be functionalized on the surface of the optical fibers covered with thin layer of gold and single layer of graphene. Graphene served as a platform for adsorbing single-stranded DNA aptamers specific to dopamine via $\pi-\pi$ stacking. In the presence of the dopamine the aptamer specific binding process initiates the macromolecular structure of the aptamer confirmation (Fig. 9.20). The conformational change of aptamers in the presence of dopamine molecule triggered the surface RI change and hence the signal detection.

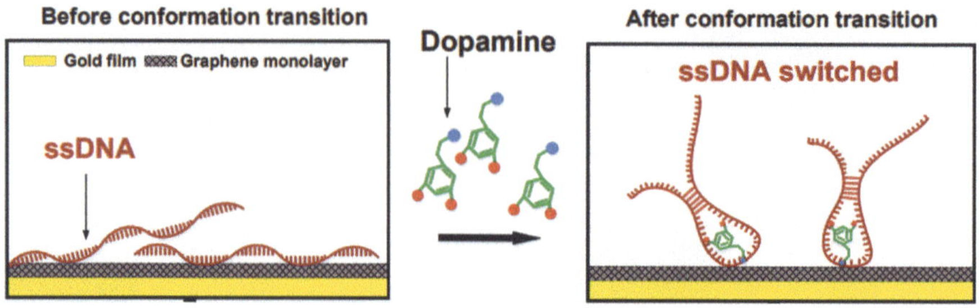

Figure 9.20 Schematic of the aptamer-based dopamine sensing mechanism: the conformation of the ssDNA aptamer is transformed by mall dopamine molecules. Source: *Reprinted from Hu, W., Huang, Y., Chen, C., Liu, Y., Guo, T., & Guan, B.-O. (2018). Highly sensitive detection of dopamine using a graphene functionalized plasmonic fiber-optic sensor with aptamer conformational amplification.* Sensors Actuators B: Chemical, 264, *440–447. Copyright (2020), with permission from Elsevier.*

The sensor exhibited a low LOD of 10^{-13} M. The sensor was tested in serum samples in order to check the reliability in real samples. However the sensitivity decreased possibly due to the complex molecular component of the serum.

To conclude, oligonucleotides serve as stable and specific receptors used in the development of the optical fiber–based biosensor. The simple chemistry based on DNA hybridization and further detection of complimentary strand using the optical fibers is feasible, which allow optical fiber–based detection in different fields including diagnostics and forensic sciences. Receptors such as aptamer sequences could be also immobilized on the optical fiber surface using different strategies and used for the detection of biomarkers, small molecules, and cells. Overall oligonucleotides are easy to modify, small, and could be synthesized chemically and hence used as cheap receptors that can bind to the target with high affinity.

9.4 Cells

Optical fiber–based biosensor was used for the detection of cellular growth and biofilm formation. In the case of the cellular growth, the surface of the optical fibers was covered with a surface molecules to which cells tend to attach. In the case of biofilm formation, optical fibers were inserted inside the incubator or a reactor where the organisms can grow well. In most cases optical fibers coated with thin metal layer were placed in a reactor where cells are grown and left until the cells attach and start growing directly on the surface of the fiber. The role of the thin metal layer was first to generate the SPR signal and second serve as a platform for cell and organism attachment. The evanescence field created as the result of SPR decays away from the surface to a distance of a few micrometers and hence sufficient for the detection of cells on the optical fiber surface. The cell growth and biofilm formation could be monitored in real time and without introducing any labeling technologies based on the same principle of detecting the surrounding RI change. As opposed to cell type both human cell line growth as well as bacterial biofilm formation could be monitored using the optical fibers. Since optical fibers are miniature and can fit into any environment, they are convenient to study the effect of the different stimuli such as chemicals and drugs on the cell proliferation, attachment, and detachment from the surface.

Shevchenko et al. (2014) used the single mode TFBG fiber for the detection of the cellular behavior of the NIH-3T3 fibroblast cells. A simple optical fiber in this case was inserted inside the cell culture equipment for the real-time and label free detection of the cellular behavior in response to the chemical stimuli such as trypsin, serum, and sodium azide. The fibroblast cells were attached on the surface of the optical fiber using a molecule fibronection, a cell adhesion protein. As the result of the stimuli, it was possible to monitor the cell detachment, uptake, and inhibition of cellular mechanism using the TFBG fiber exhibiting SPR phenomenon (Fig. 9.21).

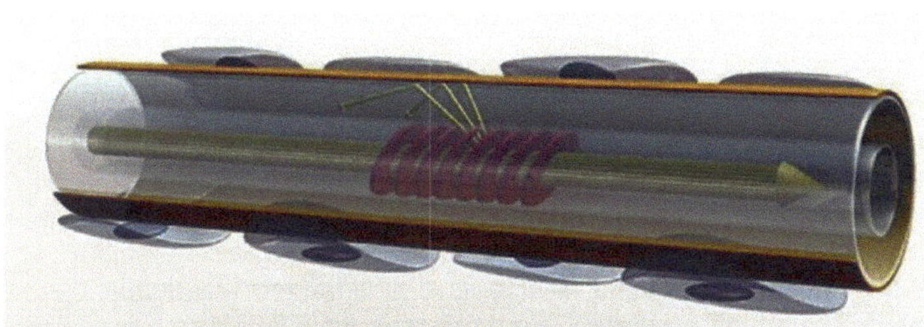

(A)

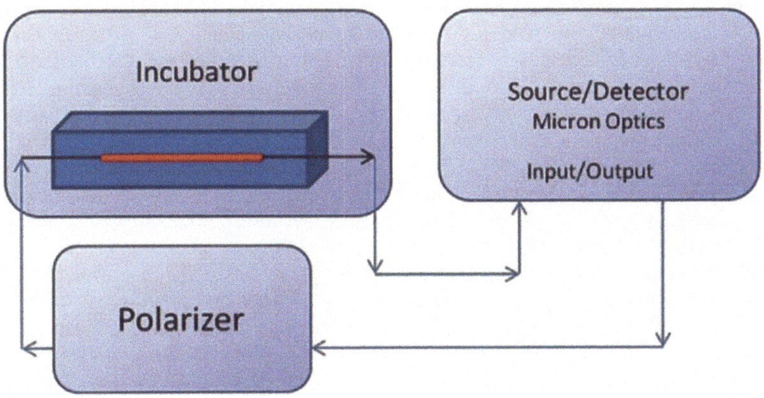

(B)

Figure 9.21 Optical fiber configuration. (A) 3D illustration of a fiber sensor with cells attached to the surface of the gold coating. Fringes in the core of the fiber indicate the tilted grating that redirects the light toward the surface of the fiber. (B) Schematic of the optical interrogation setup (all the *line arrows* represent single mode fiber connections). Source: *Reprinted from Shevchenko, Y., Camci-Unal, G., Cuttica, D.F., Dokmeci, M.R., Albert, J., & Khademhosseini, A. (2014). Surface plasmon resonance fiber sensor for real-time and label-free monitoring of cellular behavior. Biosensors & Bioelectronics, 56, 359–367. https://doi.org/10.1016/j.bios.2014.01.018. Copyright (2020), with permission from Elsevier.*

Table 9.4 Method for optical fiber cells sensors.

Analyte (surface colonization)	Detection limit	Surface chemistry (sensing film)	Fiber type	References
Pseudomonas aeruginosa	81 μg/cm	Silanization, polymer (ethylene glycol dicylcopentenyl ether acrylate (EGDPEA) and di (ethylene glycol) methyl ether methacrylate (DEGMA) monomers) coating	LPG, periodicity 109 μm	Kurmoo et al. (2020)
NIH-3T3 fibroblast cells		Fibronectin coating	TFBG, excitation of SPR (50 nm Au)	Shevchenko et al. (2014)

To conclude, optical fiber–based biosensors can used for the detection of not only small molecules in the form of proteins and oligonucleotides, but also larger macromolecules such as separate cells as well the cellular complexes. This is a good indicator of the fact that such biosensors are universal and are not limited to analyte type and most importantly size (Table 9.4).

References

Allin, K. H., Bojesen, S. E., & Nordestgaard, B. G. (2009). Baseline C-reactive protein is associated with incident cancer and survival in patients with cancer. *Journal of Clinical Oncology: Official Journal of the American Society of Clinical Oncology*. Available from https://doi.org/10.1200/JCO.2008.19.8440.

Arjmand, M., Aray, A., Saghafifar, H., & Alijanianzadeh, M. (2020). Quantitative analysis of methyl-parathion pesticide in presence of enzyme substrate using tapered fiber optic biosensor. *IEEE Sensors Journal*. Available from https://doi.org/10.1109/jsen.2020.2968895.

Arjmand, M., Saghafifar, H., Alijanianzadeh, M., & Soltanolkotabi, M. (2017). A sensitive tapered-fiber optic biosensor for the label-free detection of organophosphate pesticides. *Sensors Actuators B: Chemical*. Available from https://doi.org/10.1016/j.snb.2017.04.121.

Badmos, A. A., Sun, Q., Sun, Z., Zhang, J., Yan, Z., Lutsyk, P., ... Zhang, L. (2017). Enzyme-functionalized thin-cladding long-period fiber grating in transition mode at dispersion turning point for sugar-level and glucose detection. *Journal of Biomedical Optics*. Available from https://doi.org/10.1117/1.jbo.22.2.027003.

Baliyan, A., Sital, S., Tiwari, U., Gupta, R., & Sharma, E. K. (2016). Long period fiber grating based sensor for the detection of triacylglycerides. *Biosensors & Bioelectronics*. Available from https://doi.org/10.1016/j.bios.2015.12.089.

Bekmurzayeva, A., Dukenbayev, K., Shaimerdenova, M., Bekniyazov, I., Ayupova, T., Sypabekova, M., ... Tosi, D. (2018). Etched fiber bragg grating biosensor functionalized with aptamers for detection of thrombin. *Sensors*, *18*, 4298.

Candiani, A., Sozzi, M., Cucinotta, A., Selleri, S., Veneziano, R., Corradini, R., ... Pissadakis, S. (2012). Optical fiber ring cavity sensor for label-free DNA detection. *IEEE Journal of Selected Topics in Quantum Electronics*. Available from https://doi.org/10.1109/JSTQE.2011.2166110.

Caucheteur, C., Loyez, M., González-Vila, Á., & Wattiez, R. (2018). Evaluation of gold layer configuration for plasmonic fiber grating biosensors. *Optics Express*, *26*, 24154–24163.

Chryssis, A. N., Saini, S. S., Lee, S. M., Yi, H., Bentley, W. E., & Dagenais, M. (2005). Detecting hybridization of DNA by highly sensitive evanescent field etched core fiber Bragg grating sensors. *IEEE Journal of Selected Topics in Quantum Electronics*. Available from https://doi.org/10.1109/JSTQE.2005.857724.

Crivianu-Gaita, V., & Thompson, M. (2015). Immobilization of Fab′ fragments onto substrate surfaces: A survey of methods and applications. *Biosensors & Bioelectronics, 70*, 167–180.

Deep, A., Tiwari, U., Kumar, P., Mishra, V., Jain, S. C., Singh, N., ... Bharadwaj, L. M. (2012). Immobilization of enzyme on long period grating fibers for sensitive glucose detection. *Biosensors & Bioelectronics*. Available from https://doi.org/10.1016/j.bios.2011.12.051.

DeLisa, M. P., Zhang, Z., Shiloach, M., Pilevar, S., Davis, C. C., Sirkis, J. S., & Bentley, W. E. (2000). Evanescent wave long-period fiber bragg grating as an immobilized antibody biosensor. *Analytical Chemistry, 72*, 2895–2900. Available from https://doi.org/10.1021/ac9912395.

Han, L., Guo, T., Xie, C., Xu, P., Lao, J., Zhang, X., ... Guan, B. O. (2017). Specific detection of aquaporin-2 using plasmonic tilted fiber grating sensors. *Journal of Lightwave Technology*. Available from https://doi.org/10.1109/JLT.2016.2645233.

Hu, W., Huang, Y., Chen, C., Liu, Y., Guo, T., & Guan, B.-O. (2018). Highly sensitive detection of dopamine using a graphene functionalized plasmonic fiber-optic sensor with aptamer conformational amplification. *Sensors Actuators B: Chemical, 264*, 440–447.

Huy, T. Q., Hanh, N. T. H., Van Chung, P., Anh, D. D., Nga, P. T., & Tuan, M. A. (2011). Characterization of immobilization methods of antiviral antibodies in serum for electrochemical biosensors. *Applied Surface Science, 257*, 7090–7095. Available from https://doi.org/10.1016/j.apsusc.2011.03.051.

Jiang, B., Zhou, K., Wang, C., Sun, Q., Yin, G., Tai, Z., ... Zhang, L. (2018). Label-free glucose biosensor based on enzymatic graphene oxide-functionalized tilted fiber grating. *Sensors Actuators B: Chemical, 254*, 1033–1039. Available from https://doi.org/10.1016/j.snb.2017.07.109.

Joseph, D. F., Nakamoto, J. A., Garcia Ruiz, O. A., Peñaranda, K., Sanchez-Castro, A. E., Castillo, P. S., & Milón, P. (2019). DNA aptamers for the recognition of HMGB1 from *Plasmodium falciparum*. *PLoS One*. Available from https://doi.org/10.1371/journal.pone.0211756.

Kant, R., & Gupta, B. D. (2018). Fiber-optic SPR based acetylcholine biosensor using enzyme functionalized Ta_2O_5 nanoflakes for Alzheimer's disease diagnosis. *Journal of Lightwave Technology*. Available from https://doi.org/10.1109/JLT.2018.2856924.

Kant, R., Tabassum, R., & Gupta, B. D. (2017). A highly sensitive and distinctly selective D-sorbitol biosensor using SDH enzyme entrapped Ta_2O_5 nanoflowers assembly coupled with fiber optic SPR. *Sensors Actuators B: Chemical*. Available from https://doi.org/10.1016/j.snb.2016.09.178.

Kurmoo, Y., Hook, A. L., Harvey, D., Dubern, J. F., Williams, P., Morgan, S. P., ... Alexander, M. R. (2020). Real time monitoring of biofilm formation on coated medical devices for the reduction and interception of bacterial infections. *Biomaterials Science*. Available from https://doi.org/10.1039/c9bm00875f.

Lao, J., Han, L., Wu, Z., Zhang, X., Huang, Y., Tang, Y., & Guo, T. (2019). Gold nanoparticle-functionalized surface plasmon resonance optical fiber biosensor: In situ detection of thrombin with 1 nM detection limit. *Journal of Lightwave Technology, 37*, 2748–2755. Available from https://doi.org/10.1109/JLT.2018.2822827.

Liu, L. L., Marques, L., Correia, R., Morgan, S. P., Lee, S. W., Tighe, P., ... Korposh, S. (2018). Highly sensitive label-free antibody detection using a long period fibre grating sensor. *Sensors Actuators B: Chemical*. Available from https://doi.org/10.1016/j.snb.2018.05.109.

Lobry, M., Loyez, M., Hassan, E. M., Chah, K., DeRosa, M. C., Goormaghtigh, E., ... Caucheteur, C. (2020). Multimodal plasmonic optical fiber grating aptasensor. *Optics Express*. Available from https://doi.org/10.1364/oe.385747.

Loyez, M., Albert, J., Caucheteur, C., & Wattiez, R. (2018). Cytokeratins biosensing using tilted fiber gratings. *Biosensors, 8*, 74.

Loyez, M., Hassan, E. M., Lobry, M., Liu, F., Caucheteur, C., Wattiez, R., ... Albert, J. (2020). Rapid detection of circulating breast cancer cells using a multiresonant optical fiber aptasensor with plasmonic amplification. *ACS Sensors*, *5*, 454–463. Available from https://doi.org/10.1021/acssensors.9b02155.

Loyez, M., Larrieu, J.-C., Chevineau, S., Remmelink, M., Leduc, D., Bondue, B., ... Caucheteur, C. (2019). In situ cancer diagnosis through online plasmonics. *Biosensors & Bioelectronics*, *131*, 104–112.

Lu, B., Smyth, M. R., & O'Kennedy, R. (1996). Tutorial review. Oriented immobilization of antibodies and its applications in immunoassays and immunosensors. *Analyst*, *121*, 29R–32R.

Luo, B., Xu, Y., Wu, S., Zhao, M., Jiang, P., Shi, S., ... Liu, Y. (2018). A novel immunosensor based on excessively tilted fiber grating coated with gold nanospheres improves the detection limit of Newcastle disease virus. *Biosensors & Bioelectronics*, *100*, 169–175. Available from https://doi.org/10.1016/j.bios.2017.08.064.

Luo, B., Yan, Z., Sun, Z., Liu, Y., Zhao, M., & Zhang, L. (2015). Biosensor based on excessively tilted fiber grating in thin-cladding optical fiber for sensitive and selective detection of low glucose concentration. *Optics Express*. Available from https://doi.org/10.1364/oe.23.032429.

Malachovská, V., Ribaut, C., Voisin, V., Surin, M., Leclère, P., Wattiez, R., & Caucheteur, C. (2015). Fiber-optic SPR immunosensors tailored to target epithelial cells through membrane receptors. *Analytical Chemistry*. Available from https://doi.org/10.1021/acs.analchem.5b00159.

Monk, D. J., & Walt, D. R. (2004). Optical fiber-based biosensors. *Analytical and Bioanalytical Chemistry*. Available from https://doi.org/10.1007/s00216-004-2650-x.

Pahurkar, V. G., Tamgadge, Y. S., Gambhire, A. B., & Muley, G. G. (2015). Glucose oxidase immobilized PANI cladding modified fiber optic intrinsic biosensor for detection of glucose. *Sensors Actuators B: Chemical*. Available from https://doi.org/10.1016/j.snb.2014.12.125.

Pâslaru, E., Baican, M. C., Hitruc, E. G., Nistor, M. T., Poncin-Epaillard, F., & Vasile, C. (2014). Immunoglobulin G immobilization on PVDF surface. *Colloids Surfaces B Biointerfaces*, *115*, 139–149.

Pollet, J., Delport, F., Janssen, K. P. F., Jans, K., Maes, G., Pfeiffer, H., ... Lammertyn, J. (2009). Fiber optic SPR biosensing of DNA hybridization and DNA-protein interactions. *Biosensors & Bioelectronics*. Available from https://doi.org/10.1016/j.bios.2009.08.045.

Portaccio, M., Lepore, M., Della Ventura, B., Stoilova, O., Manolova, N., Rashkov, I., & Mita, D. G. (2009). Fiber-optic glucose biosensor based on glucose oxidase immobilised in a silica gel matrix. *Journal of Sol-Gel Science and Technology*. Available from https://doi.org/10.1007/s10971-009-1915-4.

Ribaut, C., Loyez, M., Larrieu, J.-C., Chevineau, S., Lambert, P., Remmelink, M., ... Caucheteur, C. (2017). Cancer biomarker sensing using packaged plasmonic optical fiber gratings: Towards in vivo diagnosis. *Biosensors & Bioelectronics*, *92*, 449–456.

Semwal, V., Shrivastav, A. M., Verma, R., & Gupta, B. D. (2016). Surface plasmon resonance based fiber optic ethanol sensor using layers of silver/silicon/hydrogel entrapped with ADH/NAD. *Sensors Actuators B: Chemical*, *230*, 485–492. Available from https://doi.org/10.1016/j.snb.2016.02.084.

Shen, G., Cai, C., Wang, K., & Lu, J. (2011). Improvement of antibody immobilization using hyperbranched polymer and protein A. *Analytical Biochemistry*, *409*, 22–27. Available from https://doi.org/10.1016/j.ab.2010.09.028.

Shevchenko, Y., Camci-Unal, G., Cuttica, D. F., Dokmeci, M. R., Albert, J., & Khademhosseini, A. (2014). Surface plasmon resonance fiber sensor for real-time and label-free monitoring of cellular behavior. *Biosensors & Bioelectronics*, *56*, 359–367. Available from https://doi.org/10.1016/j.bios.2014.01.018.

Shevchenko, Y., Francis, T. J., Blair, D. A. D., Walsh, R., DeRosa, M. C., & Albert, J. (2011). In situ biosensing with a surface plasmon resonance fiber grating aptasensor. *Analytical Chemistry*, *83*, 7027–7034.

Shi, S., Wang, L., Su, R., Liu, B., Huang, R., Qi, W., & He, Z. (2015). A polydopamine-modified optical fiber SPR biosensor using electroless-plated gold films for immunoassays. *Biosensors & Bioelectronics*. Available from https://doi.org/10.1016/j.bios.2015.06.080.

Sridevi, S., Vasu, K. S., Asokan, S., & Sood, A. K. (2015). Sensitive detection of C-reactive protein using optical fiber Bragg gratings. *Biosensors & Bioelectronics*. Available from https://doi.org/10.1016/j.bios.2014.10.033.

Srinivasan, R., Umesh, S., Murali, S., Asokan, S., & Siva Gorthi, S. (2017). Bare fiber Bragg grating immunosensor for real-time detection of Escherichia coli bacteria. *Journal of Biophotonics*. Available from https://doi.org/10.1002/jbio.201500208.

Sypabekova, M., Jolly, P., Estrela, P., & Kanayeva, D. (2019). Electrochemical aptasensor using optimized surface chemistry for the detection of *Mycobacterium tuberculosis* secreted protein MPT64 in human serum. *Biosensors & Bioelectronics*, 123. Available from https://doi.org/10.1016/j.bios.2018.07.053.

Sypabekova, M., Korganbayev, S., González-Vila, Á., Caucheteur, C., Shaimerdenova, M., Ayupova, T., ... Tosi, D. (2019). Functionalized etched tilted fiber Bragg grating aptasensor for label-free protein detection. *Biosensors & Bioelectronics, 146*. Available from https://doi.org/10.1016/j.bios.2019.111765.

Trilling, A. K., Beekwilder, J., & Zuilhof, H. (2013). Antibody orientation on biosensor surfaces: A minireview. *Analyst*. Available from https://doi.org/10.1039/c2an36787d.

Um, H. J., Kim, M., Lee, S. H., Min, J., Kim, H., Choi, Y. W., & Kim, Y. H. (2011). Electrochemically oriented immobilization of antibody on poly-(2-cyano-ethylpyrrole)-coated gold electrode using a cyclic voltammetry. *Talanta, 84*, 330–334. Available from https://doi.org/10.1016/j.talanta.2011.01.013.

Vashist, S. K., Dixit, C. K., MacCraith, B. D., & O'Kennedy, R. (2011). Effect of antibody immobilization strategies on the analytical performance of a surface plasmon resonance-based immunoassay. *Analyst*. Available from https://doi.org/10.1039/c1an15325k.

Vo-Dinh, T., & Cullum, B. (2000). Biosensors and biochips: Advances in biological and medical diagnostics. *Fresenius' Journal of Analytical Chemistry, 366*, 540–551. Available from https://doi.org/10.1007/s002160051549.

Voisin, V., Pilate, J., Damman, P., Mégret, P., & Caucheteur, C. (2014). Highly sensitive detection of molecular interactions with plasmonic optical fiber grating sensors. *Biosensors & Bioelectronics, 51*, 249–254. Available from https://doi.org/10.1016/j.bios.2013.07.030.

Wang, Q., & Wang, B.-T. (2018). Surface plasmon resonance biosensor based on graphene oxide/silver coated polymer cladding silica fiber. *Sensors Actuators B: Chemical, 275*, 332–338. Available from https://doi.org/10.1016/j.snb.2018.08.065.

Yin, M., Huang, B., Gao, S., Zhang, A. P., & Ye, X. (2016). Optical fiber LPG biosensor integrated microfluidic chip for ultrasensitive glucose detection. *Biomedical Optics Express, 7*, 2067–2077. Available from https://doi.org/10.1364/boe.7.002067.

Yu, S., Ding, L., Lin, H., Wu, W., & Huang, J. (2019). A novel optical fiber glucose biosensor based on carbon quantum dots-glucose oxidase/cellulose acetate complex sensitive film. *Biosensors & Bioelectronics*. Available from https://doi.org/10.1016/j.bios.2019.111760.

Yuan, Y., Yang, X., Gong, D., Liu, F., Hu, W., Cai, W., ... Yang, M. (2017). Investigation for terminal reflection optical fiber SPR glucose sensor and glucose sensitive membrane with immobilized GODs. *Optics Express*. Available from https://doi.org/10.1364/oe.25.003884.

Zainuddin, N. H., Chee, H. Y., Ahmad, M. Z., Mahdi, M. A., Abu Bakar, M. H., & Yaacob, M. H. (2018). Sensitive Leptospira DNA detection using tapered optical fiber sensor. *Journal of Biophotonics*. Available from https://doi.org/10.1002/jbio.201700363.

Zhao, X., Pan, F., Garcia-Gancedo, L., Flewitt, A. J., Ashley, G. M., Luo, J., & Lu, J. R. (2012). Interfacial recognition of human prostate-specific antigen by immobilized monoclonal antibody: Effects of solution conditions and surface chemistry. *Journal of the Royal Society, Interface/the Royal Society, 9*, 2457–2467. Available from https://doi.org/10.1098/rsif.2012.0148.

Zhu, G., Zhang, M., Lu, L., Lou, X., Dong, M., & Zhu, L. (2019). Metal-organic framework/enzyme coated optical fibers as waveguide-based biosensors. *Sensors Actuators B: Chemical, 288*, 12–19. Available from https://doi.org/10.1016/j.snb.2019.02.083.

10

Fiber surface modifications for biosensing

10.1 Introduction

To fabricate an optical fiber biosensor, it is necessary to attach a ligand (bioreceptor) on the glass surface, which will bind the analyte of interest. Compared to polymers, proteins (including antibodies) cannot bind the surface of optical fiber directly (Debs, Ebendorff-Heidepriem, Quinton, & Monro, 2009). Plasmonic optical fiber biosensors are first coated with gold (or other metal) layer before further functionalization with ligands. Silanization is a common technique [especially for cladding-etched Fiber Bragg Grating (FBG) sensors] in various types of optical biosensors as the first adlayer. Different polymers are also used as the first layer on optical fiber for the fabrication of biosensors. These three methods are discussed in this chapter (Fig. 10.1).

10.2 Pretreatment of optical fiber

Before applying a suitable functional coating, the protective coating of optical fiber needs to be removed and fiber surface has to be cleaned with an appropriate solvent. One of the first steps of fiber functionalization is its pretreatment to remove contaminants and increase hydroxyl groups on the surface. A variety of solutions such as Piranha solution (H_2SO_4:H_2O_2), alkaline- or acid-based solutions are used both with and without heating the solution or sonicating as shown in Table 10.1. The effect of surface pretreatment on the subsequent functionalization has not been extensively studied; and the choice of the solution might be dictated by the nature of the fiber nature (glass or plastic), availability of the solutions, and availability of the equipment (ultrasonicator, oven for heating during or after pretreatment, or incandescent lamp). Glass fiber cannot be treated with hydrofluoric acid since it will be etched; while plastic fibers are cleaned with base Piranha solution instead of Piranha with sulfuric acid.

Polishing is another method commonly used for surface pretreatment for polymer fibers rather than glass optical fibers. Polymer-clad silica multimode optical

Optical Fiber Biosensors.
DOI: https://doi.org/10.1016/B978-0-12-819467-6.00010-X

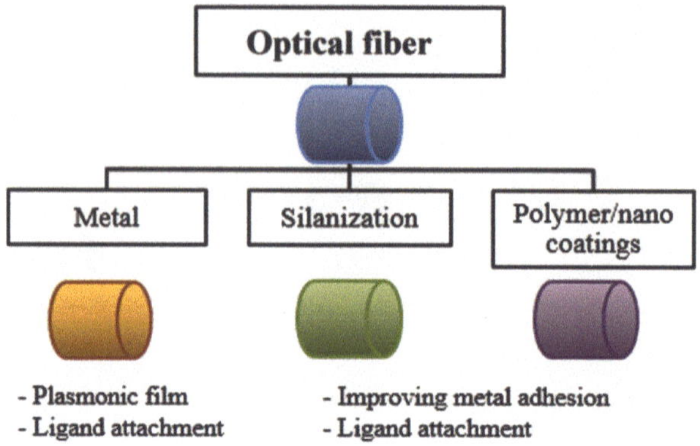

Figure 10.1 First layer in functionalization of optical fiber biosensors and their applications.

fiber was polished with polishing films (roughness 5, 3, 1, and 0.3 μm sequentially) (Cao, Tu, Sun, & Grattan, 2013). A plastic optical fiber [core—poly (methyl methacrylate) resin; cladding—fluorinated polymer] was polished to maximize the light coupling before being U-shaped and gold-coated (Arcas, Dutra, Allil, & Werneck, 2018). Fine polishing papers (roughness 1200 and 3 μm) were used to furnish and polish the ends of the plastic optical fiber after it was connected to connectors to improve its light-gathering ability (Botewad, Pahurkar, & Muley, 2018).

10.3 Coating of optical fiber surface (general consideration)

Several coating techniques including drop casting, dip coating, optical deposition, electrospinning/electrospraying, and layer-by-layer deposition are known. These methods have their own advantages and disadvantages as shown in Table 10.2. Among these techniques, drop casting and dip coating are the simplest ones, whereas optical deposition allows monitoring the process of coating, but its mechanism is not fully understood. During electrospinning/ electrospraying the material of interest is first electrically charged by applying large potential difference between the needle of the syringe (serves as an electrode) and the grounded surface. Depending on the distance between electrodes, applied voltage and the concentration of the solution, two types of materials are formed on the surface: nanofibers (electrospinning) or nanoparticles (electrospraying). Layer-by-layer deposition can include one or more above-mentioned techniques and often results in an ultra-thin film containing nanostructured materials (Tan, Ibsen, & Tjin, 2019). A range of coatings, including dopamine, carbon nanotubes, graphene, metallic, or ceramic nanoparticles, were fabricated on optical fiber surface using these methods. These sensors were used to detect humidity, hydrogen, ethanol, isopropanol, *p*-xylene, and acetone (Gonzalez-Sierra

Table 10.1 Surface pretreatment of optical fiber for further functionalization.

Pretreatment conditions	After pretreatment	Optical fiber type	Purpose of pretreatment (as shown in the corresponding Ref.)	Further application of surface	Ref.
H_2O:H_2O_2:NH_4OH (5:1:1)	Washing with DI water	EFBG	Hydrophilic surface	Immobilization of antibody–graphene complex	Sridevi, Vasu, Asokan, and Sood (2015)
NaOH (0.2 N) at 40°C for 3.5 h NaOH for 30 min	Rinsing with DI water 10 min	EFBG	Hydrophilic surface	Few hydroxyl groups Coating with single-walled carbon nanotubes or graphene oxide	Sridevi, Vasu, Jayaraman, Asokan, and Sood (2014)
Piranha 30 min	– Exhaustive rinsing with DI water – Heated in a hot air oven at 112°C for 60 min	SMF-TCSMF-SMF	Oxidizing the surface	Silanization, crosslinker, antibody	Zheng, Lang, Shen, and Shen (2018)
– NaOH (4–5 M) for 15 min and sonicated for 2–3 min – Thorough rinsing in DI water – Base Piranha at 70°C–80°C for 15 min	– Exhaustive rinsing with DI water – Heating in a hot air oven at 112°C for 1 h	Plastic cladded silica optical fiber LSPR	Removing any organic contamination	Silanization, gold nanoparticles, silicon nitride film	Chauhan, Punjabi, Sharma, and Mukherji (2016)
Piranha solution (sulfuric acid 70%) for 30 min	- Thoroughly rinsing with DI water- 100°C for 1 h	Polymer-clad silica MM fiber LSPR		Silanization, gold nanoparticles, gold nanorods	Cao et al. (2013)
– HNO_3 solution (5% v/v) ~2 h at 40°C – Washed thoroughly with DI water and ethanol intermittently – Piranha 1 h	Drying under an incandescent lamp (40 W; 240 V; ~24 h; ~40°C)	Dual peak LPG	– Removing all contaminations; – Activating the hydroxyl groups	Immobilization of enzyme	Badmos et al. (2017)
– HNO_3 (5%; v/v) for 2 h at 40°C – Thoroughly washed in water and ethanol – Piranha 1 h	Drying in a convection oven for 16 h at 80 C	TFBG	– Removing contamination – Activating hydroxyl groups	Silanization, gold nanoparticles, antibodies	Luo et al. (2018)
– HNO_3 (5%) at 90°C for 2 h – Rinse with ethanol and DI water	Drying	LPG	– Cleaning – Activating hydroxyl groups	Silanization	Baliyan, Sital, Tiwari, Gupta, and Sharma (2016)

(*Continued*)

Table 10.1 Continued

Pretreatment conditions	After pretreatment	Optical fiber type	Purpose of pretreatment (as shown in the corresponding Ref.)	Further application of surface	Ref.
– Sulfuric acid 1 h					
– Ethanol (99%)/HCl (conc.) (1:1; v/v) (to wash after etching) – Piranha 30 min	– Quickly rinsing with DD water – Dry	EFBG	– Enhancing the exposure of hydroxyl groups	Silanization	Wang, Pang, Zhang, and Wang (2009)

Base Piranha - ammonium hydroxide H_2O_2 (30%); 3:1 v/v; *DI*, deionized; *NA*, not available in the source; Piranha: H_2SO_4 (conc.): H_2O_2 (30%); 3:1 v/v; *LPG*, Long Period Grating; *LSPR*, Localized Surface Plasmon Resonance; *SMF*, single-mode optical fiber; *SPR*, Surface Plasmon Resonance; *TCSMF*, long thin core single-mode fiber; *TFBG*, Tilted Fiber Bragg Grating.

Table 10.2 Different methods used for coating optical fiber surface (mostly based on optical fiber for metal ion detection).

Method	Procedure	Advantage	Disadvantage	Examples
Drop casting	1. Solution containing particles or nanosheets dropped on the surface 2. Drying (heating/evaporation)	The simplest	• Only for very small nanoparticles/ nanosheets • Not strong adhesion	• Palladium • Carbon nanotube
Dip coating	1. Immersion (controlled lowering of the fiber into solution for a fixed time) 2. Deposition (controlled pulling of the fiber) 3. Curing (removal of excess material, drying/heating)	Can deposit monolayer	Time-consuming	• Microgel • Dopamine • Nanoparticles • PMMA
Optical deposition	Coating at interface of fiber guided light and the coating solution	• Controlling specific amount of coating • Can be monitored (back reflection of light; a circulator and power meter)	• Usually at fiber end only • Mechanism not fully understood	• Graphene • Carbon nanotube
Electrospin/ electrospraying	Electrically charged particles: • as the liquid jet to form nanofibers (electrospinning) • as a dispersed spray of nanoparticles (electrospraying)	Can be used for composite nanostructured materials	Special equipment required	• Nanofibers • Nanoparticles • Polyacytelene • Polypyrrole • Carbon nanotube
Layer-by-layer deposition	1. Fiber treated to gain charged surface 2. Treating with opposing charged material by a suitable coating method (any of the five methods can be used; first coating layer) 3. Rinse to remove excess/dry 4. Treating with opposing charged material by a suitable coating method (any of the five methods can be used; second coating layer) Until desired number of layers is achieved	Ultra-thin film containing nanostructured material	Time-consuming	• Polyelectrolytes • Metallic or ceramic nanoparticles • Carbon nanotubes Semiconductor quantum dots • Chromophores • Fluorophores

PMMA, Polymeric polymethylmethacrylate.

Source: Prepared based on Gonzalez-Sierra et al. (2017); Li, Liu et al. (2020); Rivero et al. (2019); Shabaneh et al. (2015); Su et al. (2020); Tan et al. (2019); Urrutia et al. (2013).

et al., 2017; Li, Liu et al., 2020; Rivero, Goicoechea, Arregui, & Layer-by-Layer, 2019; Shabaneh et al., 2015; Su, Dai, & Gan, 2020; Tan et al., 2019; Urrutia, Goicoechea, Rivero, Matias, & Arregui, 2013).

10.4 Coating of optical fiber surface with metal layer

For biosensing, optical fiber surface is coated with metal layers for the following reasons:

- plasmonic layer for the production of Surface plasmon resonance (SPR);
- adhesion layer for attaching ligands directly (with thiol groups);
- adhesion layer for attaching intermediate layer (for further coupling with ligands).

The most widely used plasmonic materials on optical fiber are gold and silver or their combination (Khalil et al., 2018). Different combinations of these metals or alternative materials to gold as a plasmonic material are being investigated. Combining Ag and Au with ZnO layer (Ag/Au/ZnO) has better performance capabilities for SPR-based sensors compared to Ag/ZnO, Au/ZnO, Au/Ag/ZnO (Tabassum & Gupta, 2015). Another study used titanium nitride (TiN) which was successfully used on photonic crystal fiber (PCF) to detect Refractive Index (RI) range of 1.32–1.34 (Khalil et al., 2018).

Conventional techniques used to coat optical fiber sensors with plasmonic materials include electroless deposition, electroplating (electrolysis plating), and sputtering (Albert, Lepinay, Caucheteur, & DeRosa, 2013); the last being the most widely used and results in high-quality gold surfaces (Albert et al., 2013). Electroless deposition and sputtering will be discussed in this section.

In electroless deposition, as the name suggests, electrical potential is not used and the method is based on the reduction of metallic ions from solution to optical fiber surface. As shown in Fig. 10.2, before electroless deposition optical fiber surface is first hydroxylated, pretreated with intermediate layer (silanization or dopamine polymerization), and coated with gold nanoparticles (GNP). Fiber, functionalized in this manner, is ready for electroless deposition itself. For this, it is immersed in an aqueous plating solution, which has two main components: complex metal ions solution and reducing agent. GNP on the surface become bigger and form more or less continuous films because of the reducing agent (Albert et al., 2013).

Forming noncontinuous self-assembled monolayers (SAMs) of GNP without electroless deposition is another approach of modifying the optical fiber surface for plasmonic metal layer. GNP used for optical fiber include different-shaped particles including gold nanospheres (GNS), gold nanorods (GNR), gold nanocages (GNC). Although there are examples of direct coating fibers (both silica and plastic) with

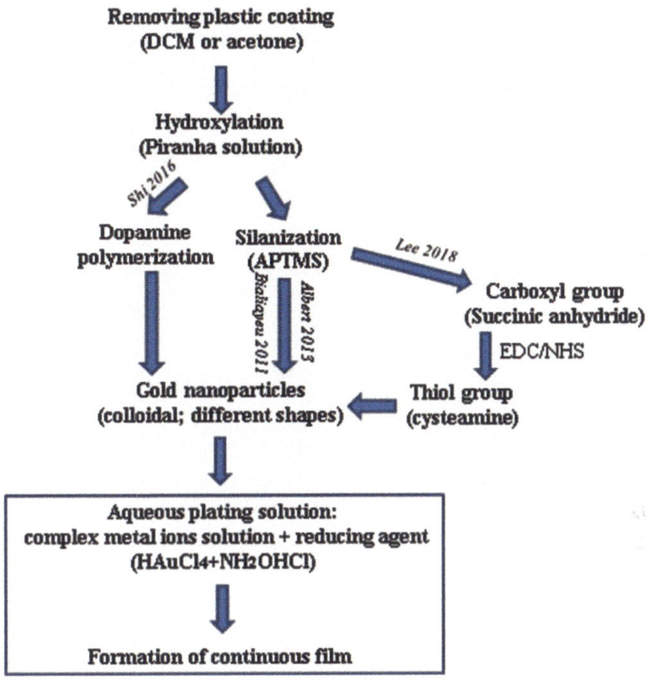

Figure 10.2 Electroless deposition of metal layer on optical fiber surface after coating it with gold nanoparticles. Surface preparation and actual electroless deposition (in box) are shown. Source: *Based on Albert et al. (2013), Bialiayeu, Caucheteur, Ahamad, Ianoul, and Albert (2011), Lee, Park, Byun, Kim, and Kim (2018), Shi et al. (2016).*

GNP (Li, Li et al., 2020; Tyagi et al., 2018), very often, the surface has to be pretreated with an intermediate layer as discussed in Section 10.6.1.

Sputtering is a more traditional way among the three discussed methods and results in high-quality plasmonic layer on the fiber (Caucheteur, Guo, & Albert, 2015; Shi et al., 2016). Main challenges of forming gold film on optical fiber by sputtering and ways to solve them are shown in Fig. 10.3. Two main issues must be solved to get a high-quality gold layer: (1) improving film adhesion and (2) uniform gold thickness (Hu et al., 2018). Gold or other metal adhesion on optical fiber surface can be improved by a thin layer of other metals such as Cr [2–3 nm (Hu et al., 2018); ~5 nm (Kaushik, Tiwari, Pal, & Sinha, 2019)] or silanization (see Section 10.6.1). A thermal treatment after gold adhesion is another method for improving the adhesion of gold on optical fiber. Thermal treatment conditions include 20 minutes (Malachovska et al., 2015) or 2 hours at ~200°C (Lobry et al., 2019).

The small cylindrical shape of optical fiber makes a traditional flat-plane sputtering method not suitable without modification (Hu et al., 2018). Often optical fiber requires rotation along the axis to ensure uniform plasmonic material coating as was done in several works (Albert et al., 2013; Hu et al., 2018). Rotating the fiber inside the chamber while sputtering (if available in the instrument) might be a better option. Rotation speed of 9 rpm (7 rotation cycles) (Kaushik

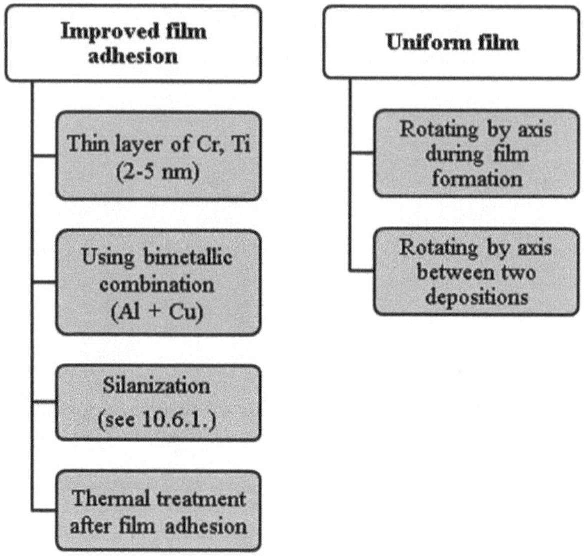

Figure 10.3 Main challenges of forming gold (or other plasmonic) film on optical fiber by sputtering and ways to solve them.

et al., 2019) or 100 rpm (Arghir, Spasic, Verlinden, Delport, & Lammertyn, 2015) was used. The optimal gold layer thickness was found to be 50 nm, while others report 32 nm (Hu et al., 2018) or 35 nm (Lobry et al., 2019). Electroplating and sputtering are considered standard methods that can be used to coat multiple samples simultaneously resulting in reproducible sensors (Guo, 2017). Interestingly, nonuniformity resulted from rotation (during sputtering) did not change SPR generation (Albert et al., 2013).

Performance of sensors can be affected by the gold coating method used. Loyez, Lobry, Wattiez, and Caucheteur (2019) compared four different configurations of Tilted Fiber Bragg Grating (TFBG) biosensors [bare, sputter coated, electroless deposited, and hybrid (sputtering then electroless deposition)] for biomarker detection in complex medium. Biosensor with sputtered gold coating resulted in the highest sensitivity and best SNR in complex conditions.

Silver is also a widely used metal in plasmonic optical fiber biosensors. Electroless deposition of silver on optical fiber is illustrated in Fig. 10.4. Electroless plating of silver by silver mirror reaction or Tollen's reaction is done by the precipitation of metallic silver on optical fiber surface from the solution of ammoniacal silver nitrate with a reducing agent (Klantsataya, Francois, Ebendorff-Heidepriem, Hoffmann, & Monro, 2015). After cleaning the fiber, the surface can be sensitized with $SnCl_2$ in 0.1 M HCl as described in Klantsataya et al. (2015). When the fiber is rinsed with water, the sudden increase in pH leads to the precipitation of soluble tin ions on the fiber surface. Tin ions are thought to provide nucleation site for silver layer to be formed

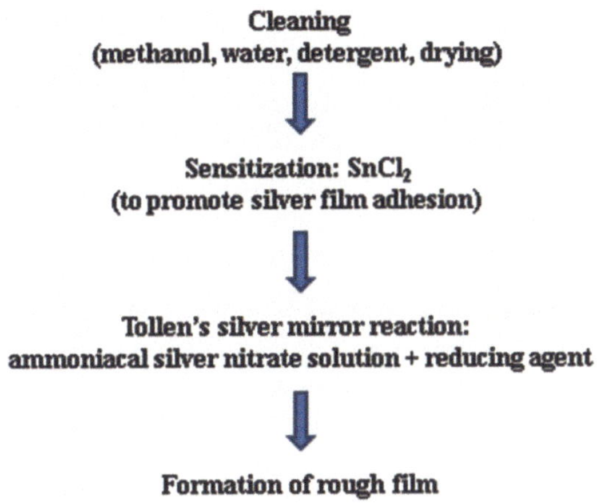

Figure 10.4 Electroless deposition of silver on optical fiber surface. Source: *Based on Klantsataya E., Francois A., Ebendorff-Heidepriem H., Hoffmann P., Monro T. M. (2015). Surface plasmon scattering in exposed core optical fiber for enhanced resolution refractive index sensing.* Sensors, *15 (10):25090–25102.*

$$CH_2OH(CHOH)_4COH + 2Ag(NH_a)_2^+ + 2OH^- \rightarrow 2Ag + CH_2OH(CHOH)_4COOH + 4NH_a + H_2O \quad (1)$$

$$2AgNO_a + 2KOH \rightarrow Ag_2O + 2KNO_a + H_2O \quad (2)$$

$$Ag_2O + 4NH_a + 2KNO_a + H_2O \rightarrow 2Ag(NH_a)_2NO_a + 2KOH \quad (3)$$

Figure 10.5 Silver mirror reaction or Tollens' reaction used to deposit silver on optical fiber surface. Source: *Reprinted with permission from Boehm J., Francois A., Ebendorff-Heidepriem H., Monro T. M. (2011). Chemical deposition of silver for the fabrication of surface plasmon microstructured optical fibre sensors.* Plasmonics, *6(1):133–136. (Order license ID1096268-1; RightsLink).*

during electroless deposition (Klantsataya et al., 2015). Tollen's reaction consists of reduction of silver ammonium complexes to form silver nanoparticles [Fig. 10.5; Debs et al. (2009)] when reducing agent (e.g., glucose) is added (Boehm, Francois, Ebendorff-Heidepriem, & Monro, 2011).

Tollen's reaction is an easy and inexpensive method for producing reflective surface on optical fiber surface. A tip covered with thick silver layer having high reflectance (90%–95%) can be obtained if it is immersed into Tollen's reaction. Silver oxidation can be prevented by coating it with epoxy resin (Esteban, Diaz-Herrera, Navarrete, & Gonzalez-Cano, 2006). Produced surface is significantly rough: *ca.* 5.5 nm for a 60 nm thick film (Boehm et al., 2011).

Electroless deposition by Tollen's reaction was optimized to reach the same performance as in the radiofrequency sputtering method (Boehm et al., 2011).

Fibers (based on metal organic frameworks) were compared in terms of resonance signal and response to solutions with different RI.

Electroless silver plating can be done in a selective manner where some regions are not coated for practical reasons. By irradiating only the tip of tapered optical fiber, the catalyst (Pd(II)-based activation colloidal solution) does not bind it and silver is not coated on that region when the whole fiber is immersed into electroless silver plating solution (Tao et al., 2016).

To build a reflection mirror, the tip of optical fiber must be coated with a completely reflecting layer of metal. This can be done either by using a special silver glue (Ribaut et al., 2017) or by coating with silver using the Tollen's reaction (Lee et al., 2018; Quero et al., 2016).

10.5 Ligands on gold-coated optical fiber

To fabricate a biosensor, optical fiber surface coated with metal (in case of plasmonic biosensors) is subsequently modified to selectively bind analyte of interest. Gold-coated optical fiber can be further modified in a number of ways to attach ligands as shown in Fig. 10.6 and Table 10.3.

The main two methods include physical immobilization or covalent immobilization. Physical adsorption is known to be a fast and easy method resulting in good coverage of the surface; however, the method is less reproducible and produces instable coating with a possible change to the structure of ligands. Covalently linked molecules are usually more stable, are more reproducible, and have more coverage. There are two types of covalent linking: one-step and two-step receptor immobilization (Albert et al., 2013). In one-step method,

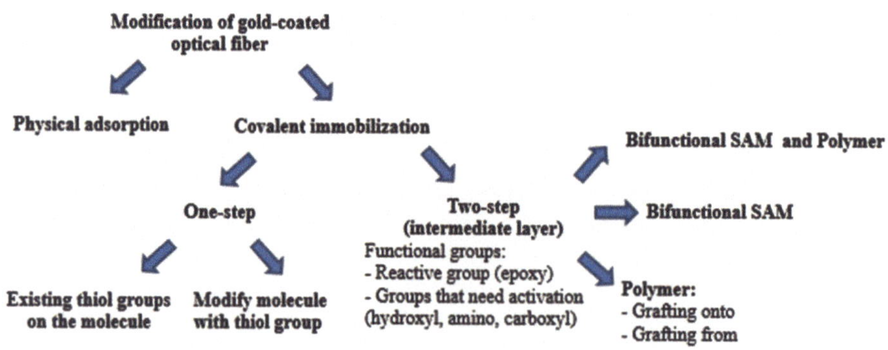

Figure 10.6 Surface modification of gold-coated optical fiber for biosensing purpose. Source: *Based on Albert J., Lepinay S., Caucheteur C., DeRosa M. C. (2013). High resolution grating-assisted surface plasmon resonance fiber optic aptasensor.* Methods (San Diego, Calif.)*;63(3):239–254.*

Table 10.3 Functionalization of optical fibers coated with gold/silver with ligands for fabrication of biosensors.

Surface	Intermediate layer	Functional groups of intermediate layer molecule	Cross-linkers	Ligand	Refs.
Gold (sputtered)	–	–	–	Biotinylated thiols	Voisin et al. (2014)
Gold (sputtered)	–	–	–	Thiolated aptamer	Shevchenko et al. (2011)
GNR	–	–	TCEP	Thiolated aptamer*	Lee et al. (2018)
MPTMSGNP	Cysteamine	Thiol, amine 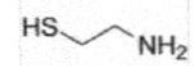	–	Protein (antibody)*	Luo et al. (2018)
Gold (sputtered)	MHA	Thiol, carboxyl 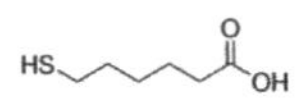	EDC/NHS	Protein (antibody)	Voisin et al. (2014)
Gold (sputtered)	S2-PEG6-COOH	Two thiol, carboxyl 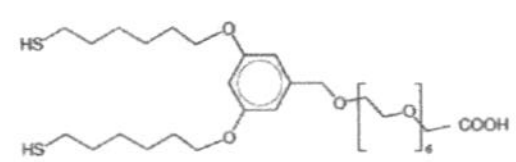	EDC/NHS	Protein (antibody)	Ribaut et al. (2017)
GNP	MAA	Thiol, carboxyl 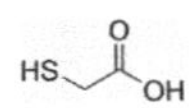	–	Protein (antibody)	Tyagi et al. (2018)
PAH/SiO_2 APTES GNP	MUA	Thiol, carboxyl 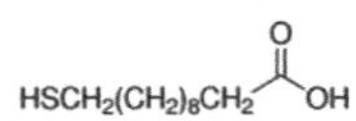	EDC NHS	Biotin	Liu, Marques et al. (2018)
APTMSGNS			EDC/Sulfo-NHS	Protein (antibody)	Cao et al. (2013)
MPTMS CTAB GNR					Cao et al. (2013)
Gold (sputter)			EDC/NHS	Protein (antibody)	Lin et al. (2007)
Gold (sputter)					Han et al. (2017)
APTMS Silver NP					Chen, Shi et al. (2015)

Ligand is activated (not surface).

GNR, Gold nanorods; *MUA*, 11-mercaptoundecanoic acid; *S_2-PEG6-COOH*, dithiolalkanearomatic PEG6-COOH; *MAA*, mercaptoacetic acid; Biotinylated alkylthiol(mercaptoundecyl-hexaethyleneoxybiotin amide); *MHA*, 6-mercaptohexanoicacid; *NP*, nanoparticles; *TCEP*, Tris(2-carboxyethyl)phosphine hydrochloride.

molecules to be coated are first thiolated as was the case when biotinylated thiols were covered on a gold-coated FBG (Voisin, Pilate, Damman, Megret, & Caucheteur, 2014). In other one-step approaches, an existing thiol-reacting group is utilized. Cysteine residues on protein are one of the native thiols, which can be utilized for SAM formation. Unfortunately, protein structure can be disrupted and its binding with the analyte can be affected (Albert et al., 2013). Examples of both one-step and two-step approaches are shown in Table 10.3.

Oligonucleotides modified with thiol groups can be directly coated on the gold surface of optical fibers. Thiolation of oligonucleotides is an established process. Thiolated aptamers in high concentrations (10–20 μM) can be directly immobilized on gold-coated fiber surface usually in buffers containing salts [$MgCl_2$ and NaCl (Shevchenko et al., 2011)]. Thiol groups on oligonucleotides are activated before incubating with the gold surface by cleaving disulfide bonds. For this, they are usually treated with tris(2-carboxyethyl)phosphine hydrochloride [5 mM for 30 minutes (Lee et al., 2018)]. Attaching thiolated (and activated) aptamer on gold nanorods on the optical fiber surface was done by incubating them for 5 minutes [10 mM acetate buffer (pH 5.6)]. More than one oligonucleotides can be bound on the surface as was done with two aptamers in a 1:4 molar ratio for detection of toxin using Localized Surface Plasmon Resonance (LSPR) sensor (Lee et al., 2018). This approach might have improved selectivity of the sensor. Moreover, attaching different thiolated ligands could also be used for multiplexing of the senor to detect several analytes.

The two-step approach includes the use of intermediate layers, bifunctional SAMs, and/or polymers which are able to react both with the surface and the ligand (Albert et al., 2013). 11-Mercaptoundecanoic acid (MUA) is one of the most commonly used intermediate layers on gold-coated optical fibers (Fig. 10.7). Carboxyl groups on MUA can also be activated by incubating the surface with *N*-(3-dimethylaminopropyl)-*N′*-ethylcarbodiimide hydrochloride (EDC) and/or *N*-hydroxysulfosuccinimide (Sulfo-NHS) before incubation with antibodies (Cao et al., 2013; Han et al., 2017; Tyagi et al., 2018). EDC/NHS pair is a commonly used cross-linking pair. EDC is a carbodiimide, a cross-linker, which activates carboxyl groups on the molecules to form *o*-acylisourea active ester which is however unstable. NHS (*N*-hydroxysuccinimide) and sulfo-NHS are often added into the reaction to improve its efficiency or create dry-stable (amine-reactive) intermediates. Sulfo-NHS is different from NHS only in having sulfonate ($-SO_3$) group on the *N*-hydroxysuccinimide ring and being more hydrophilic in nature.

Together with MUA, commercially available reagents (with proprietary content) for carboxylic SAMs which are designed to minimize a nonspecific protein adsorption on the surface can also be used in a two-step approach for antibody immobilization (Malachovska et al., 2015).

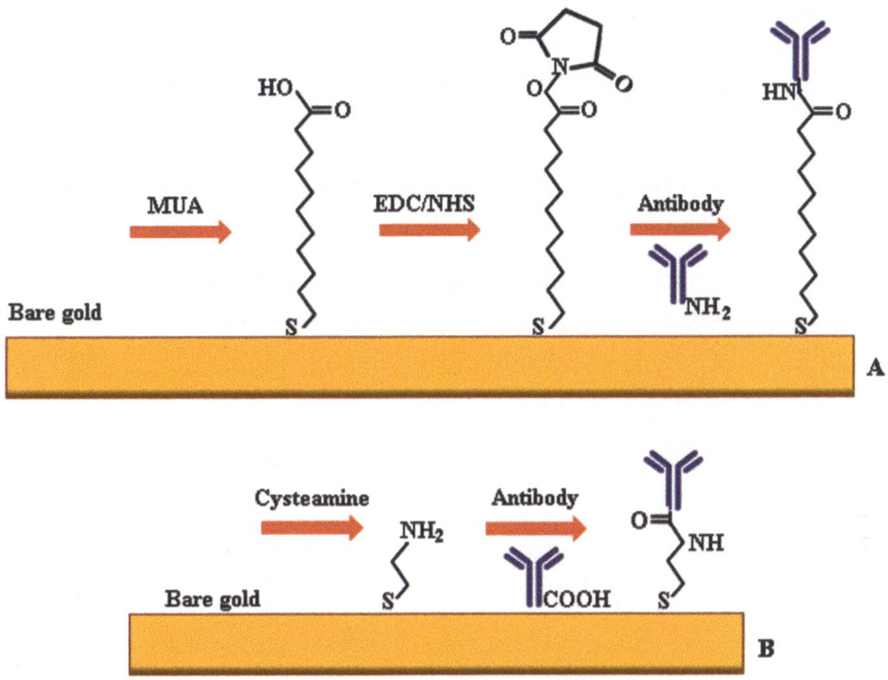

Figure 10.7 Functionalization of gold-coated optical fiber with antibodies after cross-linking with MUA (A) and cysteamine (B). *MUA*, 11-Mercaptoundecanoic acid.

Despite thiolated oligonucleotides forming compact layers on gold, there are multiple contacts between each strand and the surface including adsorption due to amine moieties. This leads to interference of hybridization (in case of DNA sensor) and binding of the target (in case of aptamer sensor). Using a small molecule called 6-mercapto-1-hexanol can solve this issue by disrupting the contacts between DNA and the surface, and forces DNA to attach on the surface mostly by their thiol groups. As a result, DNA ligands are less constrained on the surface and are more accessible to analytes (Steel, Levicky, Herne, & Tarlov, 2000).

Gold can also be treated with mercaptohexanoic acid or MHA (2 mM for 12 hours) for the formation of SAMs (Voisin et al., 2014). After MHA the surface can be activated with EDC/NHS antibodies (30 μg/mL in 10 mM acetate buffer, pH 5) for 30 minutes (Voisin et al., 2014).

Biotinylated thiols (mercaptoundecyl-hexaethyleneoxy biotin amide) can be used as a bifunctional SAM, which are reactive with both gold surface and streptavidin (Voisin et al., 2014). Biotin can then be used to bind streptavidin or entities bound with streptavidin. Streptavidin has high affinity toward biotin making it in one of the strongest noncovalent interactions (Liu, Marques et al., 2018). Biotinylated surface can also be coated with neutravidin which has four sites for biotin and therefore can be used for binding other biotinylated molecules in a sandwich manner (Sciacca, Francois, Hoffmann, & Monro, 2013).

Cysteamine (Fig. 10.7) can be used to render gold-coated optical fiber with amine groups as this was done for immobilization of protein A (Luo et al., 2018) or biotin (Liu, Marques et al., 2018). Thiol groups of cysteamine bind gold with strong ion-exchange interaction (Arcas et al., 2018) and form Au–S bond (Luo et al., 2018). Then, carboxyl groups on the proteins or other molecules can be activated by EDC/NHS (Luo et al., 2018) or NHS (Liu, Marques et al., 2018) for covalent attachment on the aminated surface.

10.6 Silanization of optical fiber surface

Due to its nature, optical fiber has chemically active surface hydroxyl groups which can be used in silanization. Silane-coupling agents (SCAs) are silicon-based materials that have a general formula of $R'(CH_2)_nSi(OR)_3$, where R′ is an organofunctional group and R is a hydrolyzable alkoxy group (Liu et al., 2013). During hydrolysis, alkoxy groups are converted into silanol groups (SiOH) when silanes are mixed with water/ethanol solution. During the next step of condensation, they form hydrogen bonds with surface hydroxide groups, while the excess of silanol groups form siloxane network (Si–O–Si). This network is chemically stable and shows resistance to corrosion (Liu, Cao, Yu, & Chen, 2015; Wang et al., 2009).

Silanization of optical fiber biosensors has the following main functions in optical fiber biosensor fabrication:

- improvement of metal adhesion (mainly gold);
- adhesion layer (having different functional groups) for attaching ligands directly;
- adhesion layer for attaching intermediate layer (for further coupling with ligands).

10.6.1 Silanization as an adhesion promoter

Intermediate thin layer of metals (Ti, Cr, Al) between optical fiber and gold significantly improves adhesion of gold; however, this requires specialized equipment and the film can interfere with signal response of SPR sensor by partially absorbing propagating light during excitation (Arghir et al., 2015). Using SCA as an intermediate layer between optical fiber and gold can be an alternative to metal films. SCAs also have been used as a protective layer and for improving adhesion of

Table 10.4 Conditions of coating optical fiber surface with nanoparticles.

Fiber	Intermediate layer	GNP type	Conditions of GNP coating	Ref.
Polymer-clad silica MM	APTMS	GNS Diameter 60 nm	6 h	Cao et al. (2013)
Polymer-clad silica MM	MPTMS	GNR (CTAB coated) Aspect ratio 4.1	6 h	Cao et al. (2013)
LPFG	No	GNS (MUA coated for attaching antibody)	*NA*	Tyagi et al. (2018)
Exc. TFBG	MPTMS	GNS (diameter 80 nm)	12 h at RT	Luo et al. (2018)
LPFG	Three layers of silica nanoparticles and PAH; APTES	GNP (diameter 2–5 nm)	1 h	Liu, Marques et al. (2018)
TFBG	APTMS GA Cysteamine	GNC (edge length 30 nm) GNS (diameter 30 nm) Both coated with MUA	2 h (GNC) 1 h (GNS)	Lepinay, Staff, Ianoul, and Albert (2014)
Silica-based MM	MPTMS	Silver NP	Dipping 160 °C for 5 h	Cao, Zhao, and Qin (2019)

APTMS, (3-Aminopropyl) trimethoxysilane; *CTAB*, cetrimonium bromide; *Exc. TFBG*, excessively tilted FBG; *GA*, glutaraldehyde; *GNC*, gold nanocubes; *GNS*, gold nanosphere; *MM*, multimode; *MPTMS*, (3-mercaptopropyl) trimethoxysilane; *MUA*, mercaptoacetic acid; *NA*, not available in the paper; *PAH*, poly(allylamine hydrochloride).

polymer coatings (Debs et al., 2009). GNP have low poor adhesion toward optical fiber and are therefore used as colloids and SCAs are used as linkers (Bonyar, Wimmer, & Csarnovics, 2014). These linkers are used not only to attach GNP but also to reduce nonspecific binding (Liu, Marques et al., 2018). GNP due to their negative charge attach on positively charged groups of SCA by electrostatic force. Table 10.4 shows conditions of coating optical fiber surface with GNP.

Most commonly used SCAs for gold adhesion improvement are (3-mercaptopropyl) trimethoxysilane (MPTMS), (3-Aminopropyl) trimethoxysilane (APTMS), and 3-aminopropyltriethoxysilane (APTES). APTES has been first used for glass modification back in 1969 (Adiguzel & Kulah, 2014). For improvement of gold adhesion it has been used in several studies including Houngkamhang et al. (2018). APTMS-silanized optical fiber surface was treated with GNS for SAM formation (Cao et al., 2013; Chauhan et al., 2016). GNC and GNS were also coated on the fiber surface after it was silanized (APTMS) and treated with glutaraldehyde and cysteamine (Lepinay et al., 2014).

Types of SCA differ in their ability to attach to gold. Thus APTMS has a weaker interaction with gold (weak electrostatic NH_2—Au interaction), whereas MPTMS forms stronger bonds (covalent S—Au bonds) (Fig. 10.8; Arghir et al., 2015).

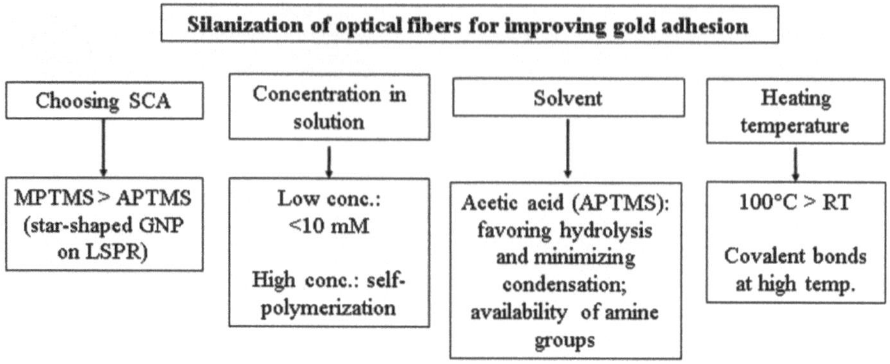

Figure 10.8 Silanization of optical fibers for improving gold adhesion. Source: *Based on Arghir et al. (2015), Chauhan et al. (2016), Zhang et al. (2012).*

Moreover, when star-shaped GNP were coated on two different silane layers on tapered optical fibers, a more sensitive LSPR sensors were obtained when MPTMS was used and not APTMS. This was observed by a bigger decrease of transmission spectra for thiolated SCA than aminated one (Zhang et al., 2012). In another study, using MPTMS as a promoter for gold adhesion in SPR sensor resulted in a robust and stable sensor as illustrated in different testing conditions (mechanical, chemical, and thermal treatments) (Arghir et al., 2015). For the formation of covalent bonds between GNP and the surface, fiber can be coated MPTMS to bind GNR coated with positively charged cetrimonium bromide (Cao et al., 2013).

Silanization was also utilized for adhesion of graphene to produce highly sensitive LPFG for detection of hemoglobin (Liu, Xu et al., 2018). Graphene oxide (GO) attaches to amine groups of APTES by its epoxy groups. Fiber surfaces silanized with different SCA [APTES, APTMS, glycidyloxypropyl-trimethoxysilane (GOPS)] were also successfully used for attaching polymer layers (Cao et al., 2013; Gao et al., 2016; Sciacca et al., 2013) used as intermediate layers for ligand attachment as discussed below.

10.6.2 Silanization for ligand attachment

Another important application of SCA in optical fibers is providing the surface with functional groups for binding of ligands to provide specific binding in biosensing. Ligand (or bioprobe) adds specificity to optical fiber since only analytes of interest should be able to bind the surface. After silanization, either groups on the surface or on the bioreceptor need to be activated using cross-linkers. For example, one terminal of glutaraldehyde (GA) forms amino bond with APTES and the second terminal is available for immobilizing amine-terminated oligonucleotide (for DNA hybridization or aptamers against various molecules) (Saini et al., 2007; Tang et al., 2016; Yildirim et al., 2014). Silanized optical fiber surfaces were used as platforms for ligand attachment in a number of ways shown in Table 10.5.

Table 10.5 Functionalization of silanized optical fibers for fabrication of biosensors.

Surface	Crosslinker	Ligand	Ref.
APTES	–	Protein (antibody)	Zheng et al. (2018)
APTES	–	Protein (antibody)	Baliyan et al. (2016)
APTES	–	Protein (enzyme)	Badmos et al. (2017)
APTES	–	Protein	Cao et al. (2017)
APTES	–	Protein (enzyme)	Baliyan et al. (2016)
APTES	EDC	Phosphorylated DNA oligo* (with 1-methylimidazole)	Delgado-Pinar et al. (2017)
GOPS	EDC/NHS	Antibody fragment (reduced with cysteine)	Tedeschi, Domenici, Ahluwalia, Baldini, and Mencaglia (2003)
APTES	GA	Aminated DNA oligo	Saini et al. (2007)
APTES	GA	Aminated DNA oligo	Yildirim et al. (2014)
APTES	GA	Aminated DNA oligo	Tang et al. (2016)
APTES	GA	Aminated DNA oligo	Chryssis et al. (2005)
APTS	SulfoSMCC	Antibody fragment (reduced with cysteine)	Delgado-Pinar et al. (2017)
APTES	EDC/NHS	Phosphorylated DNA oligo	Chen, Liu et al. (2015)
MPTMS	GMBS	Protein (antibody)	Long et al. (2010)
APTES	SA DIC/NHS	PNA	Bertucci et al. (2015)
APTES	GA	Aminated DNA oligo?	Dagenais et al. (2005)
APTES	GA EDC/NHS	Dethiobiotin**	Wang, Xiang, Zhou, Liu, and Shi (2015)
APTES	GA	Protein (antibody)	Sun, Ran, and Wang (2017)
APTES	SulfoSMCC	Thiolated protein (antibody)	Tedeschi et al. (2003)
APTES	GA	Protein (antibody)	Zheng et al. (2018)
APTES	GA	Protein	Mustapa, Abu Bakar, Kamil, Syahir, and Mahdi (2018)
APTES	SA DIC/NHS	PNA	Bertucci et al. (2015)
APTES	EDC	Phosphorylated DNA oligo	Delgado-Pinar et al. (2017)

APTS, (3-(2-aminoethylamino)propyl-trimethoxysilane); *SA*, succinic anhydride; * glass surface but not optical fiber; *APTES*, (3-aminopropyl) triethoxysilane; *APTMS*, (3-(2-aminoethylamino)propyl-trimethoxysilane); *DIC*, *N,N'*-Diisopropylcarbodiimide; *GA*, gluteraldehyde; *GOPS*, glycidyloxypropyl-trimethoxysilane; *MPTMS*, (3-mercaptopropyl)trimethoxysilane; *PNA*, peptide nucleic acid; *SA*, succinic anhydride. ** Ligand is activated (not surface).

One of the silanization molecules widely used for silanization of optical fibers is APTES. Chen et al. functionalized optical fiber with a covalently immobilized phosphorylated oligonucleotides via EDC-mediated reaction after silanization with APTES. Phosphate group on oligonucleaotide is activated by EDC in the presence of imidazole to conjugate to primary amines. This optical fiber was then used to detect hybridization of DNA (Chen, Liu et al., 2015). In another study, antibodies were immobilized on fiber after silanizing it with MPTMS, a SCA with a thiol group at the end (Long et al., 2010).

Although conditions such as low concentration of SCA, high heat treatment temperature, and type of SCA shown in Fig. 10.7 also apply for ligand attachment, protocols used for silanization of optical fiber vary enormously in terms of the conditions applied. Concentration of SCA in solutions ranges from 0.2% (Stanford, Dagenais, Park, & DeShong, 2008) to as high as 10% (Chen, Liu et al., 2015; Tedeschi et al., 2003); the solvents where they are dissolved include acetone, ethanol, propanol, toluene, or water . Heat treatment temperature ranges from 60°C (Tedeschi et al., 2003) up to 200°C (Tang et al., 2016).

Silanization can result in a surface with a variety of functional groups depending on the SCA type. Aminated surfaces are generated when surface is silanized with APTES, APTS, APTMS, while MPTMS gives thiolated surface, and treatment with GOPS results in epoxy group-functionalized surface. The type of SCA does not only dictate the downstream reaction (type of crosslinker or functional group on the ligand molecule) but it can also affect the performance of the biosensor as this was demonstrated by silanizing the surface with APTMS or MPTMS (Cao et al., 2013) as seen in Fig. 10.9.

Different functionalization methods after silanizing the surface with APTMS (random noncovalent where proteins were immobilized directly on APTMS;

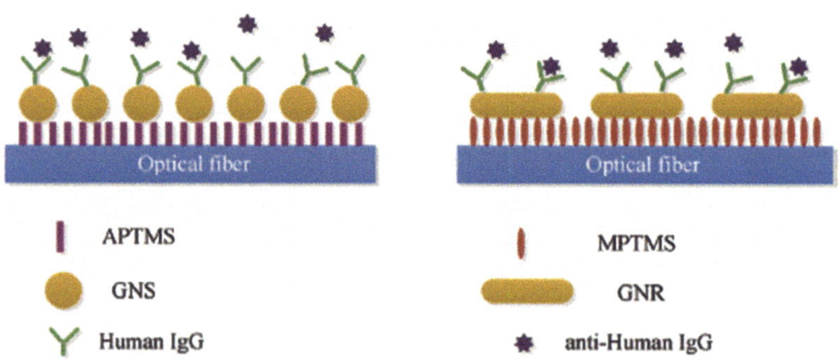

Figure 10.9 Schematics of biosensing approaches using GNS- (left) and GNR- (right) based LSPR sensors. *APTMS*, (3-(2-aminoethylamino)propyl-trimethoxysilane); *IgG*, immunoglobulin G; *GNS*, gold nanospheres; *GNR*, gold nanorods; *LSPR*, Localized Surface Plasmon Resonance; *MPTMS*, (3-mercaptopropyl) trimethoxysilane. Source: *Reprinted with permission from Cao et al. (2013) (License Number 5003480878168 RightsLink).*

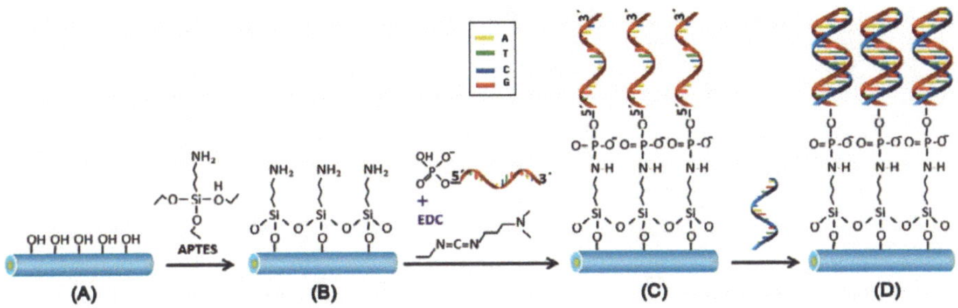

Figure 10.10 Schematic diagram of biofunctionalization of optical fiber biosensor: (A) cleaned glass fiber surface; (B) silanization of glass fiber surface by APTES; (C) covalent immobilization of 5′-phosphorylated oligonucleotides via EDC-mediated reaction; (D) hybridization with the complementary oligonucleotides. Source: *Modified from Chen X., Liu C., Hughes M., Nagel D., Hine A., Zhang L. (2015). EDC-mediated oligonucleotide immobilization on a long period grafting optical biosensor.* Journal of Biosensors and Bioelectronics;*6(2). Open-access article distributed under the terms of the Creative Commons Attribution License.*

covalent—via EDC; and oriented covalent—through protein A before EDC-mediated binding) were compared (Fig. 10.10) (Loyez, Albert, Caucheteur, & Wattiez, 2018). Interestingly, among the three methods, electrostatic immobilization of antibodies was found to have better performance in terms of limit of detection. Another study showed that GOPS can be used in alkaline and neutral conditions for immobilization of dextran and thiol groups of antibody fragments respectively (Tedeschi et al., 2003).

10.7 Other coatings on optical fiber (polymer and nanocoatings)

Apart from gold/silver as plasmonic material and silanization for ligand attachment, other types of materials are under investigation for fabricating optical fiber biosensors. Alternative coatings in two-step ligand attachment include modification with polydopamine, graphene oxide, poly(allylamine hydrochloride) (PAH) (Table 10.6). Graphene as studied as an alternative plasmonic material or for improvement of plasmonic layer performance in several studies. Graphene is a novel 2D nanomaterial consisting of carbon atoms tightly packed into honeycomb structure (Liu, Xu et al., 2018). Graphene synthesized by thermal chemical vapor deposition method was applied to the core of plastic optical fiber producing SPR biosensor (Kim et al., 2013). Tong et al. (2018) proposed using graphene on D-shaped PCF biosensor before plasmonic layer (silver). Graphene was chosen due to its good transmittance and high surface area ratio for improving sensitivity of the proposed sensor. In another study, enzyme-based (cholesterol oxidase) biosensor utilized graphene oxide over silver-coated unclad fiber for increasing the number of immobilized enzymes (Semwal & Gupta, 2018). GO (oxidized derivative of graphene) has a large

Table 10.6 Functionalization of optical fibers for fabrication of biosensors (polymer/nanocoatings).

Polymer/ nanomaterial	Key properties	Surface pretreatment	Ligand	Linker/ activation	Ref
Dextran	• Polymeric network of hydrogel • Carboxyl functional group	Silanized surface (GOPS)	Antibodies	EDC/NHS	Tedeschi et al. (2003)
GO	• Hydrophilic • Hydroxyl, epoxy, carboxyl functional groups	Silanized surface (APTES)	Protein (enzyme)	EDC/NHS	Liu, Xu et al. (2018)
		Hydroxylated (NaOH)	PETIM (multivalent dendrimer)	–	Sridevi et al. (2014)
PAA	• Carboxyl functional group	Silanized surface (APTMS)	Protein	EDC/NHS	Cao et al. (2013)
PAH	• Amine functional group	Silver film (Tollen's reaction)	Biotin	EDC/NHS	Sciacca et al. (2013)
		Silver film (Tollen's reaction)	Protein (antibody)	EDC/NHS	Sciacca et al. (2013)
		–	Protein (antibody)	EDC/NHS	He, Tian, Zhu, Lavlinskaia, and Du (2011)
Biotin SAM	• Can bind to streptavidin/ neutravidin	Silanized surface (APTMS)	ssDNA (biotinylated)	Streptavidin	Arghir et al. (2015)
Carboxyl SAM	• Carboxyl functional group	Silanized surface (APTMS)	Protein (antibody)	SulfoEDC/ NHS	Arghir et al. (2015)
PLL	• Amine functional group	–	ssDNA	–	Gao et al. (2016)
PAGE	• Entrapment of ligand (enzyme) in its active form	Silver and silicon coating	Substrate	–	Kant, Tabassum, and Gupta (2016)
PDA		Silanized surface (APTMS) Gold coated	Protein (antibody)	–	Shi et al. (2015)
PDA					Shi et al. (2016)
PANI	• Amine functional group	–	Protein (enzyme)	GA	Botewad et al. (2018)

GO, graphene oxide; *PAGE*, polyacrylamide gel; *PAH*, poly(allylamine hydrochloride); *PANI*, polyaniline; *PETIM*, mannose-functionalized poly (propyl ether imine) dendrimers; *PAA*, polyacrylic acid; *PDA*, polydopamine; *PLL*, poly-L-lysine.

surface area that can be used to attach biomolecules (Li, Li et al., 2020). It has such chemical groups on its surface as hydroxyl, epoxy, carboxyl (Liu, Xu et al., 2018). It has also been used to improve the performance of D-shaped PCF when deposited between fiber and metal layer (Tong et al., 2018). EFBG after pretreatment to increase surface hydroxyl groups was incubated with GO to form a stable coating ready for further ligand attachment (Sridevi et al., 2014). Another approach is to form a GO–antibody complex first by activating GO with EDC, NHS, and then incubating with antibodies. Then using this complex to functionalize optical fiber sensor as it was demonstrated by Sridevi et al. (2015) for building biosensor for detection of inflammation biomarker based on EFBG.

Polydopamine is a polymer formed when dopamine is self-polymerized from dopamine (monomer) in a basic condition when Tris (tris(hydroxymethyl) aminomethane) is added. The continuous film which is formed has such functional groups as quinone and catechol. They can be utilized to covalently attach molecules with amine- or thiol groups (Lobry et al., 2019). Lectin protein was immobilized on polydopamine film formed on gold-coated FBG surface for glucose sensing. In another study, two layers of polydopamine are formed on TFBG sensor: one to enhance electroless deposition of GNP for producing SPR and the second one for fast immobilization of antibodies (Shi et al., 2016). Polydopamine surface was incubated with antibody solution to form stable layer by Schiff base and/or Michael addition reaction.

New materials for coating optical fiber for biosensing include nanocomposite zinc oxide (ZnO) and molybdenum disulfide (MoS_2), ZnO/MoS_2. MoS_2 nanosheet on gold-coated optical fiber gives more binding sites for antibodies and alleviates the need in cross-linkers. Characteristics of each material and the effect of using their combination allowed obtaining sensitive and specific platform (Kaushik et al., 2019). Lossy mode resonance sensor coated with ZnO/MoS_2 was used as a platform to attach molecularly imprinted polymers (MIP) designed for a toxic phenolic molecule (Usha and Gupta, 2018). MIP have high selective ability since they are formed using an analyte of interest as a template.

Other polymers which were coated on optical fiber are PAH and polymethylmethacrylate. PAH contains amine group, whereas polymethylmethacrylate provides carboxyl groups. After coating the surface with silver, biotin was immobilized using its carboxyl group using EDC/NHS on PAH (Sciacca et al., 2013). Polymethylmethacrylate was coated on side polished fiber after SnO_2 thin film for covalent immobilization of antibodies via activating its carboxyl groups with EDC/NHS (Chiavaioli et al., 2018).

Commercially available bifunctional SAM formation reagents (having two functionalities: one to attach on surface and another to bind a ligand) are also available. For instance biotin and carboxyl group formation SAM reagents were utilized to attach biotinylated ssDNA (after binding streptavidin) and antibodies (after activation of carboxyl groups) on SPR-based optical fiber biosensors (Arghir et al., 2015). These reagents can form highly organized thin layer of molecules by chemisorption. Dextran is also a promising polymer, which is widely used in commercial chips in bulky SPR instruments since it is hydrophilic and has carboxyl functional groups.

One study compared three ways of attaching bovine serum albumin (BSA) protein on TFBG surface (Maguis et al., 2008). In the first case of "ionic bondings only method" self-assembled layer of alternating polyethylene imine and dextran sulfate sodium are formed, to which negatively charged bioreceptor (BSA) (by putting into buffer with appropriate pH) is absorbed. Second method included the same layer but used strong interaction between extravidin and biotin by electrostatically attaching extravidin on the surface and then attaching biotinylated BSA. The third way of immobilization combined covalent attachment of polyacrylic acid layer onto silanized surface with an avidin–biotin linkage. Improved biological activity of bioreceptor and lower limit of detection of analyte (anti-BSA) was obtained for the second and third methods.

Polyacrylamide gel, which is routinely used in biological laboratories in gel electrophoresis, can also be used as supporting environment for the ligand. Enzymes were entrapped in the polymer and then immobilized on silver/silicon-coated fiber surface (Kant et al., 2016).

10.8 Attaching bacterial cells as ligands

Attaching complex ligands such as bacterial cells require preliminary growth of bacteria of interest. Bacteria were grown on gold-coated TFBG surface under optimal temperature for their growth under rotation and CrO_4. For some applications, bacterial strains with special characteristics are firstly isolated; for instance, by growing them in a media with metal ions (Cu^{2+}, Pb^{2+}, and CrO_4) to isolate metal-resistant ones. Then they were enriched in a medium without metal ions. Bacteria were then incubated with gold-coated TFBG with substance of interest (e.g., CrO_4) to ensure the purity of bacteria with special characteristics under certain temperature and rotation optimal for their growth and attachment (Cai et al., 2020). In other cases, bacteria of interest are grown and their suspension is mixed with sterile-filtered low viscosity alginate solution. Then the sensitive part of the optical fiber (e.g., cladding-etched part) is briefly dipped into this solution and then dipped into calcium chloride to form calcium alginate matrix with entrapped bacteria (Eltzov, Pavluchkov, Burstin, & Marks, 2011; Ivask et al., 2007).

10.9 Reducing nonspecific binding

Surface modification of optical fiber does not usually end with the attachment of ligand specific to the analyte of interest. Since the real samples are made of complex mixtures of proteins and other molecules, it is important to reduce their nonspecific binding on the surface. Due to physisorption, molecules can adsorb to the surface leading to high background signals interfering with the signal from analytes (Lichtenberg, Ling, & Kim, 2019). Hence blocking the surface after the bioreceptor is attached is an important step to reduce nonspecific binding. Blocking nonspecific binding results in improved stability of the signal when detecting analyte of interest as was demonstrated in the detection of cytokeratin protein TFBG-based biosensor (Loyez et al., 2018). Different approaches used for reducing nonspecific binding on optical fiber biosensors are shown in Fig. 10.11 and Table 10.7.

Most commonly used blocking protein in biosensor fabrication is BSA and it was widely used for optical fiber biosensors too. BSA is a widely used and readily available blocking agent (Wang et al., 2017). BSA was used to block the sensor surface after silanization, after activating functional groups (Table 10.7). However, using BSA has certain drawbacks; it can form nonuniform layer, have lot-to-lot variability and sometimes can be cross-reactive (Lichtenberg et al., 2019). A number of solutions with a proprietary composition for blocking are commercially and were successfully used such as "the Blocking Solution" (Candor).

Another approach to reduce nonspecific binding is deactivation (blocking residual reacting sites or quenching) of active groups on optical fibers by incubating with small molecules such as ethanolamine or sodium borohydride. Ethanolamine was used to deactivate carboxyl groups activated with EDC/NHS after attaching ligands in several studies. Despite using only ethanolamine for blocking unreacted groups, the surface was tested in diluted human serum for specific detection of antibodies (Zeni et al., 2020).

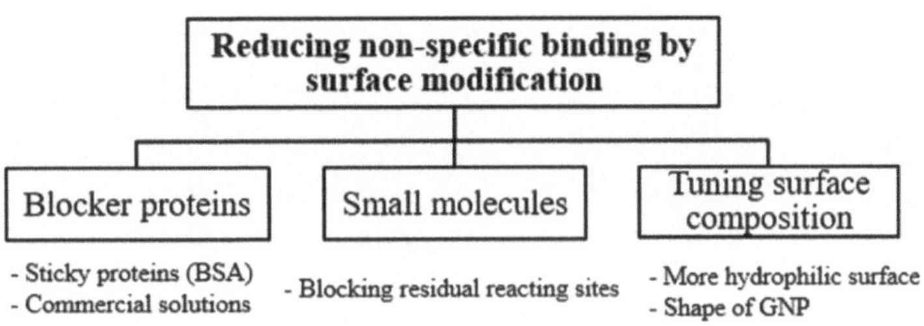

Figure 10.11 Reducing nonspecific binding on optical fiber by surface modification.

Table 10.7 Different blocking agents used to reduce nonspecific binding on optical fiber surface.

Blocking agent	Purpose	Blocking conditions	Ref.
Ethanolamine	Deactivate ester group	50 mM	Bertucci et al. (2015)
	SulfoEDC/NHS/antibody Deactivate carboxyl groups	50 mM	Arghir et al. (2015)
	SulfoEDC/NHS/antibody Deactivate carboxyl groups	1 M for 30 min	Zeni et al. (2020)
	MUA/EDC/NHS/antibody Deactivate carboxyl groups	1 M	Kaushik et al. (2019)
$NaBH_4$	Deactivate aldehyde group of GA ($CHO => CH_2OH$)	0.1 M	Le, Jimenez, Chainet, and Stambouli (2015)
BSA	Block unoccupied area on sensor by GO–antibody complex	0.01 mg/mL for 15 min	Sridevi et al. (2015)
	Block activated carboxyl groups (before ligand immobilization)	3% for 30 min	Zhou et al. (2018)
	Block activated carboxyl groups (unoccupied by ligand)	2 mg/mL for 1 h	Cao et al. (2013)
	Block amine groups (unoccupied by ligand)	5% for 1.5 h	Loyez et al. (2018)
	Block redundant NHS carbonate ester group	2% BSA (containing 0.01% tween 20)	Tyagi et al. (2018)
	Minimize nonspecific protein adsorption Cover potentially uncoated areas of sensor surface	1% for 1 h at 37°C	Quero et al. (2016)
	"Block unreacted cysteamine amine functional groups"	10 mM	Arcas et al. (2018)
HSA	Prevent nonspecific binding on surface not occupied by ligand	0.25 mg/mL	He et al. (2011)
Blocking Solution (Candor)	Unreacted binding sites	45 min	Sciacca et al. (2013)
Blocking buffer solution (B)	minimize the nonspecific binding of analyte to the surface		Nguyen et al. (2015)

GA, Glutaraldehyde.

Reducing nonspecific binding can also be done by reducing hydrophobicity of the surface by exploring the effect of shapes of GNP coating the fiber surface. It is well known that proteins stick nonspecifically to hydrophobic surface. Lepinay et al. (2014) in their TFBG biosensor used two shapes of nanoparticles and found that GNC lowered the hydrophobicity of the surface more than GNS due to more MUA binding on its surface.

References

Adiguzel, Y., & Kulah, H. (2014). Studies on visual detection and surface modification testing of glass microfiber filter paper based biosensor. *Biosensors & Bioelectronics, 54*, 27–34.

Albert, J., Lepinay, S., Caucheteur, C., & DeRosa, M. C. (2013). High resolution grating-assisted surface plasmon resonance fiber optic aptasensor. *Methods (San Diego, Calif.), 63*(3), 239–254.

Arcas, A. D., Dutra, F. D., Allil, R., & Werneck, M. M. (2018). Surface plasmon resonance and bending loss-based U-shaped plastic optical fiber biosensors. *Sensors., 18*(2).

Arghir, I., Spasic, D., Verlinden, B. E., Delport, F., & Lammertyn, J. (2015). Improved surface plasmon resonance biosensing using silanized optical fibers. *Sensors and Actuators B-Chemical, 216*, 518–526.

Badmos, A. A., Sun, Q. Z., Sun, Z. Y., Zhang, J. X., Yan, Z. J., Lutsyk, P., et al. (2017). Enzyme-functionalized thin-cladding long-period fiber grating in transition mode at dispersion turning point for sugar-level and glucose detection. *Journal of Biomedical Optics, 22*, 2.

Baliyan, A., Sital, S., Tiwari, U., Gupta, R., & Sharma, E. K. (2016). Long period fiber grating based sensor for the detection of triacylglycerides. *Biosensors & Bioelectronics, 79*, 693–700.

Bertucci, A., Manicardi, A., Candiani, A., Giannetti, S., Cucinotta, A., Spoto, G., et al. (2015). Detection of unamplified genomic DNA by a PNA-based microstructured optical fiber (MOF) Bragg-grating optofluidic system. *Biosensors & Bioelectronics, 63*, 248–254.

Bialiayeu, A., Caucheteur, C., Ahamad, N., Ianoul, A., & Albert, J. (2011). Self-optimized metal coatings for fiber plasmonics by electroless deposition. *Optics Express, 19*(20), 18742–18753.

Boehm, J., Francois, A., Ebendorff-Heidepriem, H., & Monro, T. M. (2011). Chemical deposition of silver for the fabrication of surface plasmon microstructured optical fibre sensors. *Plasmonics., 6*(1), 133–136.

Bonyar A., Wimmer B., & Csarnovics I. (2014). Development of a localised surface plasmon resonance sensor based on gold nanoparticles. In *Proceedings of the 2014 37th international spring seminar on electronics technology* (Isse) - Advances in Electronic System Integration.:371–376.

Botewad, S. N., Pahurkar, V. G., & Muley, G. G. (2018). Fabrication and evaluation of evanescent wave absorption based polyaniline-cladding modified fiber optic urea biosensor. *Optical Fiber Technology, 40*, 8–12.

Cai, S. S., Pan, H. X., Gonzalez-Vila, A., Guo, T., Gillan, D. C., Wattiez, R., et al. (2020). Selective detection of cadmium ions using plasmonic optical fiber gratings functionalized with bacteria. *Optics Express, 28*(13), 19740–19749.

Cao, J., Tu, M. H., Sun, T., & Grattan, K. T. V. (2013). Wavelength-based localized surface plasmon resonance optical fiber biosensor. *Sensors and Actuators B-Chemical, 181*, 611–619.

Cao, J., Zhao, D., & Qin, Y. Y. (2019). Novel strategy for fabrication of sensing layer on thiol-functionalized fiber-optic tapers and their application as SERS probes. *Talanta, 194*, 895–902.

Cao, Y., Wang, X. D., Guo, T., Ran, Y., Feng, X. H., Guan, B. O., et al. (2017). High-resolution and temperature-compensational HER2 antigen detection based on microwave photonic interrogation. *Sensors and Actuators B-Chemical, 245*, 583–589.

Caucheteur, C., Guo, T., & Albert, J. (2015). Review of plasmonic fiber optic biochemical sensors: Improving the limit of detection. *Analytical and Bioanalytical Chemistry, 407*(14), 3883–3897.

Chauhan, S. K., Punjabi, N., Sharma, D. K., & Mukherji, S. (2016). A silicon nitride coated LSPR based fiber-optic probe for possible continuous monitoring of sucrose content in fruit juices. *Sensors and Actuators B-Chemical, 222*, 1240–1250.

Chen, J. P., Shi, S., Su, R. X., Qi, W., Huang, R. L., Wang, M. F., et al. (2015). Optimization and application of reflective LSPR optical fiber biosensors based on silver nanoparticles. *Sensors., 15*(6), 12205–12217.

Chen, X., Liu, C., Hughes, M., Nagel, D., Hine, A., & Zhang, L. (2015). EDC-mediated oligonucleotide immobilization on a long period grafting optical biosensor. *Journal of Biosensors and Bioelectronics, 6*(2).

Chiavaioli, F., Zubiate, P., Del Villar, I., Zamarreno, C. R., Giannetti, A., Tombelli, S., et al. (2018). Femtomolar detection by nanocoated fiber label-free biosensors. *ACS Sensors., 3*(5), 936–943.

Chryssis, A. N., Saini, S. S., Lee, S. M., Yi, H. M., Bentley, W. E., & Dagenais, M. (2005). Detecting hybridization of DNA by highly sensitive evanescent field etched core fiber bragg grating sensors. *IEEE Journal of Selected Topics in Quantum Electronics, 11*(4), 864–872.

Dagenais M., Chryssis A. N., Yi H., Lee S. M., Saini S. S., & Bentley W. E., editors (2005). Optical bio-sensors based on etched fiber Bragg gratings. In *Conference on optoelectronic integrated circuits VII*; 2005 Jan 25–27; San Jose, CA. BELLINGHAM: Spie-Int Soc Optical Engineering.

Debs, J. E., Ebendorff-Heidepriem, H., Quinton, J. S., & Monro, T. M. (2009). A fundamental study into the surface functionalization of soft glass microstructured optical fibers via silane coupling agents. *Journal of Lightwave Technology, 27*(5–8), 576–582.

Delgado-Pinar, M., Shi, Q., Poveda-Wong, L., Delgado-Pinar, E., Xu, B. J., Zhao, J. L., et al. (2017). Oligonucleotide-hybridization fiber-optic biosensor using a narrow bandwidth long period grating. *IEEE Sensors Journal, 17*(17), 5503–5509.

Eltzov, E., Pavluchkov, V., Burstin, M., & Marks, R. S. (2011). Creation of a fiber optic based biosensor for air toxicity monitoring. *Sensors and Actuators B-Chemical, 155*(2), 859–867.

Esteban, O., Diaz-Herrera, N., Navarrete, M. C., & Gonzalez-Cano, A. (2006). Surface plasmon resonance sensors based on uniform-waist tapered fibers in a reflective configuration. *Applied Optics, 45*(28), 7294–7298.

Gao, R., Lu, D. F., Cheng, J., Jiang, Y., Jiang, L., Xu, J. D., et al. (2016). Fiber optofluidic biosensor for the label-free detection of DNA hybridization and methylation based on an in-line tunable mode coupler. *Biosensors & Bioelectronics, 86*, 321–329.

Gonzalez-Sierra, N. E., Gomez-Pavon, L. D., Perez-Sanchez, G. F., Luis-Ramos, A., Zaca-Moran, P., Munoz-Pacheco, J. M., et al. (2017). Tapered optical fiber functionalized with palladium nanoparticles by drop casting and laser radiation for H-2 and volatile organic compounds sensing purposes. *Sensors., 17*(9).

Guo, T. (2017). Fiber grating-assisted surface plasmon resonance for biochemical and electrochemical sensing. *Journal of Lightwave Technology, 35*(16), 3323–3333.

Han, L. Z., Guo, T. A., Xie, C., Xu, P., Lao, J. J., Zhang, X. J., et al. (2017). Specific detection of aquaporin-2 using plasmonic tilted fiber grating sensors. *Journal of Lightwave Technology, 35*(16), 3360–3365.

He, Z. H., Tian, F., Zhu, Y. N. A., Lavlinskaia, N., & Du, H. (2011). Long-period gratings in photonic crystal fiber as an optofluidic label-free biosensor. *Biosensors & Bioelectronics, 26*(12), 4774–4778.

Houngkamhang, N., Charoensuwan, S., Sonthipakdee, O., Nawattanapaiboon, K., Somboonkaew, A., & Amara, R. (2018). Gold-nanoparticle-based fiber optic sensor for sensing the refractive index of environmental solutions. *Chiang Mai Journal of Science, 45*(5), 2168–2177.

Hu, W. J., Huang, Y. Y., Chen, C. Y., Liu, Y. K., Guo, T. A., & Guan, B. O. (2018). Highly sensitive detection of dopamine using a graphene functionalized plasmonic fiber-optic sensor with aptamer conformational amplification. *Sensors and Actuators B-Chemical, 264*, 440–447.

Ivask, A., Green, T., Polyak, B., Mor, A., Kahru, A., Virta, M., et al. (2007). Fibre-optic bacterial biosensors and their application for the analysis of bioavailable Hg and As in soils and sediments from Aznalcollar mining area in Spain. *Biosensors & Bioelectronics*, *22*(7), 1396–1402.

Kant, R., Tabassum, R., & Gupta, B. D. (2016). Fiber optic SPR-based uric acid biosensor using uricase entrapped polyacrylamide gel. *IEEE Photonics Technology Letters*, *28*(19), 2050–2053.

Kaushik, S., Tiwari, U. K., Pal, S. S., & Sinha, R. K. (2019). Rapid detection of Escherichia coli using fiber optic surface plasmon resonance immunosensor based on biofunctionalized Molybdenum disulfide (MoS2) nanosheets. *Biosensors & Bioelectronics*, *126*, 501–509.

Khalil, A. E., El-Saeed, A. H., Ibrahim, M. A., Hashish, M. E., Abdelmonem, M. R., Hameed, M. F. O., et al. (2018). Highly sensitive photonic crystal fiber biosensor based on titanium nitride. *Optical and Quantum Electronics*, *50*(3).

Kim, J. A., Hwang, T., Dugasani, S. R., Amin, R., Kulkarni, A., Park, S. H., et al. (2013). Graphene based fiber optic surface plasmon resonance for bio-chemical sensor applications. *Sensors and Actuators B-Chemical*, *187*, 426–433.

Klantsataya, E., Francois, A., Ebendorff-Heidepriem, H., Hoffmann, P., & Monro, T. M. (2015). Surface plasmon scattering in exposed core optical fiber for enhanced resolution refractive index sensing. *Sensors.*, *15*(10), 25090–25102.

Le, M. H., Jimenez, C., Chainet, E., & Stambouli, V. (2015). A label-free impedimetric DNA sensor based on a nanoporous SnO_2 film: Fabrication and detection performance. *Sensors.*, *15*(5), 10686–10704.

Lee, B., Park, J. H., Byun, J. Y., Kim, J. H., & Kim, M. G. (2018). An optical fiber-based LSPR aptasensor for simple and rapid in-situ detection of ochratoxin A. *Biosensors & Bioelectronics*, *102*, 504–509.

Lepinay, S., Staff, A., Ianoul, A., & Albert, J. (2014). Improved detection limits of protein optical fiber biosensors coated with gold nanoparticles. *Biosensors & Bioelectronics*, *52*, 337–344.

Li, C., Li, Z., Li, S. L., Zhang, Y. N., Sun, B. P., Yu, Y. H., et al. (2020). LSPR optical fiber biosensor based on a 3D composite structure of gold nanoparticles and multilayer graphene films. *Optics Express*, *28*(5), 6071–6083.

Li, J. Z., Liu, X., Sun, H., Wang, L. M., Zhang, J. Q., Deng, L., et al. (2020). An optical fiber sensor coated with electrospinning polyvinyl alcohol/carbon nanotubes composite film. *Sensors.*, *20*(23).

Lichtenberg, J. Y., Ling, Y., & Kim, S. (2019). Non-specific adsorption reduction methods in biosensing. *Sensors.*, *19*(11).

Lin, H. Y., Tsao, Y. C., Tsai, W. H., Yang, Y. W., Yan, T. R., & Sheu, B. C. (2007). Development and application of side-polished fiber immunosensor based on surface plasmon resonance for the detection of Legionella pneumophila with halogens light and 850 nm-LED. *Sensors and Actuators a-Physical*, *138*(2), 299–305.

Liu, C., Xu, B. J., Zhou, L., Sun, Z., Mao, H. J., Zhao, J. L., et al. (2018). Graphene oxide functionalized long period fiber grating for highly sensitive hemoglobin detection. *Sensors and Actuators B-Chemical*, *261*, 91–96.

Liu, L. L., Marques, L., Correia, R., Morgan, S. P., Lee, S. W., Tighe, P., et al. (2018). Highly sensitive label-free antibody detection using a long period fibre grating sensor. *Sensors and Actuators B-Chemical*, *271*, 24–32.

Liu, X., Yue, Z., Romeo, T., Weber, J., Scheuermann, T., Moulton, S., et al. (2013). Biofunctionalized anti-corrosive silane coatings for magnesium alloys. *Acta Biomaterialia*, *9*(10), 8671–8677.

Liu, Y., Cao, H., Yu, Y., & Chen, S. (2015). Corrosion protection of silane coatings modified by carbon nanotubes on stainless steel. *International Journal of Electrochemical Science*, *10*(4), 3497–3509.

Lobry, M., Lahem, D., Loyez, M., Debliquy, M., Chah, K., David, M., et al. (2019). Non-enzymatic D-glucose plasmonic optical fiber grating biosensor. *Biosensors & Bioelectronics*, 142.

Long, F., He, M. A., Zhu, A. N., Song, B. D., Sheng, J. W., & Shi, H. C. (2010). Compact quantitative optic fiber-based immunoarray biosensor for rapid detection of small analytes. *Biosensors & Bioelectronics*, *26*(1), 16–22.

Loyez, M., Albert, J., Caucheteur, C., & Wattiez, R. (2018). Cytokeratins biosensing using tilted fiber gratings. *Biosensors-Basel*, *8*(3).

Loyez, M., Lobry, M., Wattiez, R., & Caucheteur, C. (2019). Optical fiber gratings immunoassays. *Sensors.*, *19*(11).

Luo, B. B., Xu, Y. F., Wu, S. X., Zhao, M. F., Jiang, P. J., Shi, S. H., et al. (2018). A novel immunosensor based on excessively tilted fiber grating coated with gold nanospheres improves the detection limit of Newcastle disease virus. *Biosensors & Bioelectronics*, *100*, 169–175.

Maguis, S., Laffont, G., Ferdinand, P., Carbonnier, B., Kham, K., Mekhalif, T., et al. (2008). Biofunctionalized tilted Fiber Bragg Gratings for label-free immunosensing. *Optics Express*, *16*(23), 19049–19062.

Malachovska, V., Ribaut, C., Voisin, V., Surin, M., Leclere, P., Wattiez, R., et al. (2015). Fiber-optic SPR immunosensors tailored to target epithelial cells through membrane receptors. *Analytical Chemistry*, *87*(12), 5957–5965.

Mustapa, M. A., Abu Bakar, M. H., Kamil, Y. M., Syahir, A., & Mahdi, M. A. (2018). Biofunctionalized tapered multimode fiber coated with dengue virus NS1 glycoprotein for label free detection of anti-dengue virus NS1 IgG antibody. *IEEE Sensors Journal*, *18*(10), 4066–4072.

Nguyen, T. T., Bea, S. O., Kim, D. M., Yoon, W. J., Park, J. W., An, S. S. A., et al. (2015). A regenerative label-free fiber optic sensor using surface plasmon resonance for clinical diagnosis of fibrinogen. *International Journal of Nanomedicine*, *10*, 155–163.

Quero, G., Consales, M., Severino, R., Vaiano, P., Boniello, A., Sandomenico, A., et al. (2016). Long period fiber grating nano-optrode for cancer biomarker detection. *Biosensors & Bioelectronics*, *80*, 590–600.

Ribaut, C., Loyez, M., Larrieu, J. C., Chevineau, S., Lambert, P., Remmelink, M., et al. (2017). Cancer biomarker sensing using packaged plasmonic optical fiber gratings: Towards in vivo diagnosis. *Biosensors & Bioelectronics*, *92*, 449–456.

Rivero, P. J., Goicoechea, J., & Arregui, F. J. (2019). Layer-by-layer nano-assembly: A powerful tool for optical fiber sensing applications. *Sensors.*, *19*(3).

Saini, S. S., Stanford, C., Lee, S. M., Park, J., DeShong, R., Bentley, W. E., et al. (2007). Monolayer detection of biochemical agents using etched-core fiber Bragg grating sensors. *IEEE Photonics Technology Letters*, *19*(17–20), 1341–1343.

Sciacca, B., Francois, A., Hoffmann, P., & Monro, T. M. (2013). Multiplexing of radiative-surface plasmon resonance for the detection of gastric cancer biomarkers in a single optical fiber. *Sensors and Actuators B-Chemical*, *183*, 454–458.

Semwal, V., & Gupta, B. D. (2018). LSPR- and SPR-based fiber-optic cholesterol sensor using immobilization of cholesterol oxidase over silver nanoparticles coated graphene oxide nanosheets. *IEEE Sensors Journal*, *18*(3), 1039–1046.

Shabaneh, A., Girei, S., Arasu, P., Mahdi, M., Rashid, S., Paiman, S., et al. (2015). Dynamic response of tapered optical multimode fiber coated with carbon nanotubes for ethanol sensing application. *Sensors.*, *15*(5), 10452–10464.

Shevchenko, Y., Francis, T. J., Blair, D. A. D., Walsh, R., DeRosa, M. C., & Albert, J. (2011). In situ biosensing with a surface plasmon resonance fiber grating aptasensor. *Analytical Chemistry*, *83*(18), 7027–7034.

Shi, S., Wang, L. B., Su, R. X., Liu, B. S., Huang, R. L., Qi, W., et al. (2015). A polydopamine-modified optical fiber SPR biosensor using electroless-plated gold films for immunoassays. *Biosensors & Bioelectronics*, *74*, 454–460.

Shi, S., Wang, L. B., Wang, A. K., Huang, R. L., Ding, L., Su, R. X., et al. (2016). Bioinspired fabrication of optical fiber SPR sensors for immunoassays using polydopamine-accelerated electroless plating. *Journal of Materials Chemistry C., 4*(32), 7554–7562.

Sridevi, S., Vasu, K. S., Asokan, S., & Sood, A. K. (2015). Sensitive detection of C-reactive protein using optical fiber Bragg gratings. *Biosensors & Bioelectronics, 65*, 251–256.

Sridevi, S., Vasu, K. S., Jayaraman, N., Asokan, S., & Sood, A. K. (2014). Optical biosensing devices based on etched fiber Bragg gratings coated with carbon nanotubes and graphene oxide along with a specific dendrimer. *Sensors and Actuators B-Chemical, 195*, 150–155.

Stanford, C. J., Dagenais, M., Park, J. H., & DeShong, P. (2008). Real-time monitoring of siloxane monolayer film formation on silica using a fiber Bragg grating. *Current Analytical Chemistry, 4*(4), 356–361.

Steel, A. B., Levicky, R. L., Herne, T. M., & Tarlov, M. J. (2000). Immobilization of nucleic acids at solid surfaces: Effect of oligonucleotide length on layer assembly. *Biophysical Journal, 79*(2), 975–981.

Su, J. X., Dai, S. X., & Gan, N. (2020). Optimized Ge-As-Se-Te chalcogenide glass fiber sensor with polydopamine-coated tapered zone for the highly sensitive detection of p-xylene in waters. *Optics Express, 28*(1), 184–193.

Sun, D. D., Ran, Y., & Wang, G. J. (2017). Label-free detection of cancer biomarkers using an in-line taper fiber-optic interferometer and a fiber Bragg grating. *Sensors., 17*(11).

Tabassum, R., & Gupta, B. (2015). Performance analysis of bimetallic layer with zinc oxide for SP-based fiber optic sensor. *Journal of Lightwave Technology, 33*(22), 4565–4571.

Tan, R. X., Ibsen, M., & Tjin, S. C. (2019). Optical fiber refractometer based metal ion sensors. *Chemosensors, 7*(4).

Tang, Y. F., Long, F., Gu, C. M., Wang, C., Han, S. T., & He, M. (2016). Reusable split-aptamer-based biosensor for rapid detection of cocaine in serum by using an all-fiber evanescent wave optical biosensing platform. *Analytica Chimica Acta, 933*, 182–188.

Tao, M. M., Wang, A. H., Xu, L. N., Jin, Y. L., Cao, M., & Gu, N. (2016). Selective electroless silver plating of optical fiber probes with protruding tips. *Microsystem Technologies-Micro- and Nanosystems-Information Storage and Processing Systems, 22*(10), 2487–2491.

Tedeschi, L., Domenici, C., Ahluwalia, A., Baldini, F., & Mencaglia, A. (2003). Antibody immobilisation on fibre optic TIRF sensors. *Biosensors & Bioelectronics, 19*(2), 85–93.

Tong, K., Wang, F. C., Wang, M. T., Dang, P., Wang, Y. X., & Sun, J. R. (2018). D-Shaped photonic crystal fiber biosensor based on silver-graphene. *Optik., 168*, 467–474.

Tyagi, D., Mishra, S. K., Zou, B., Lin, C. C., Hao, T., Zhang, G., et al. (2018). Nano-functionalized long-period fiber grating probe for disease-specific protein detection. *Journal of Materials Chemistry B., 6*(3), 386–392.

Urrutia, A., Goicoechea, J., Rivero, P. J., Matias, I. R., & Arregui, F. J. (2013). Electrospun nanofiber mats for evanescent optical fiber sensors. *Sensors and Actuators B-Chemical, 176*, 569–576.

Usha, S. P., & Gupta, B. D. (2018). Urinary p-cresol diagnosis using nanocomposite of ZnO/MoS2 and molecular imprinted polymer on optical fiber based lossy mode resonance sensor. *Biosensors & Bioelectronics, 101*, 135–145.

Voisin, V., Pilate, J., Damman, P., Megret, P., & Caucheteur, C. (2014). Highly sensitive detection of molecular interactions with plasmonic optical fiber grating sensors. *Biosensors & Bioelectronics, 51*, 249–254.

Wang, R. Y., Xiang, Y., Zhou, X. H., Liu, L. H., & Shi, H. C. (2015). A reusable aptamer-based evanescent wave all-fiber biosensor for highly sensitive detection of Ochratoxin A. *Biosensors & Bioelectronics, 66*, 11–18.

Wang, R. Y., Zhou, X. H., Zhu, X., Yang, C., Liu, L. H., & Shi, H. C. (2017). Isoelectric bovine serum albumin: Robust blocking agent for enhanced performance in optical-fiber based DNA sensing. *ACS Sensors., 2*(2), 257–262.

Wang, Y. M., Pang, X. F., Zhang, Y. Y., & Wang, H. Z. (2009). Characterization of covalent immobilization on the surface of optical fibers by scanning electron microscopy and energy dispersive X-ray spectrometry. *Surface and Interface Analysis, 41*(10), 775–778.

Yildirim, N., Long, F., He, M., Gao, C., Shi, H. C., & Gu, A. Z. (2014). A portable DNAzyme-based optical biosensor for highly sensitive and selective detection of lead (II) in water sample. *Talanta, 129*, 617–622.

Zeni, L., Perri, C., Cennamo, N., Arcadio, F., D'Agostino, G., Salmona, M., et al. (2020). A portable optical-fibre-based surface plasmon resonance biosensor for the detection of therapeutic antibodies in human serum. *Scientific Reports, 10*(1).

Zhang, Q., Xue, C. Y., Yuan, Y. L., Lee, J., Sun, D., & Xiong, J. J. (2012). Fiber surface modification technology for fiber-optic localized surface plasmon resonance biosensors. *Sensors., 12*(3), 2729–2741.

Zheng, Y. F., Lang, T. T., Shen, T. T., & Shen, C. Y. (2018). Simple immunoglobulin G sensor based on thin core single-mode fiber. *Optical Fiber Technology, 41*, 104–108.

Zhou, W. C., Li, K. W., Wei, Y. L., Hao, P., Chi, M. B., Liu, Y. S., et al. (2018). Ultrasensitive label-free optical microfiber coupler biosensor for detection of cardiac troponin I based on interference turning point effect. *Biosensors & Bioelectronics, 106*, 99–104.

11

Evaluation of sensors

11.1 Diffraction limit

Several lenses have to be aligned in certain configurations inside optical or light microscopy (LM) systems to see cells and tissues. The main property of such lenses is to pass through the visible light and magnify the observing object. That objects can be of any origin, that is, (Grotjohann et al., 2011) biological or other transparent or nontransparent samples. LM in its regular/simple technical configuration does not affect the specimen's surface structure (Sezgin, 2017).

Despite the impressive ability of LM to see considerably small objects, there are physical phenomena that limit the lenses' optical resolution. This limitation is called the "diffraction limit," which has the properties such as lens misalignment and the diffraction of light. The diffraction limit of the LM was theoretically defined by Abbe (1873), which is proportional to the wavelength of the light being observed and inversely proportional to the numerical aperture (NA) of the objective lens. The formulation of Abbe's diffraction limit is given in Eq. 11.1 (Sezgin, 2017):

$$d = \frac{\lambda}{2\text{NAobj}} \tag{11.1}$$

where d is the minimum theoretical distance that equals the proportion of the wavelength λ of 500 nm (green light), divided by 2 multiplied to an objective lens with NA_{obj} of 1.0. Theoretically, it indicates the lens's apparent limitation, which has difficulty focusing on seeing objects less than 250 nm (Sezgin, 2017).

The endless curiosity of inventors, and constant research and development of the new microscopy methods and technologies toward overpassing diffraction limit, has resulted in the flourishing of the creation of several superresolution microscopy systems (SRMS). New SRMS methods allow researchers to investigate biological and biophysical events at the single-molecule level and beyond using fluorescent probes and labeling techniques (Khater, Nabi, & Hamarneh, 2020). The following section will cover several types of SRSM methods.

Optical Fiber Biosensors.
DOI: https://doi.org/10.1016/B978-0-12-819467-6.00011-1

11.2 Superresolution microscopy systems

SRMS, from their first introduction and development, starting from the last decades, had quickly gained as a critical research tool to study living matter (Bates, Huang, Dempsey, & Zhuang, 2007; Betzig et al., 2006; Huang, Wang, Bates, & Zhuang, 2008; Rust, Bates, & Zhuang, 2006). Tremendous progress in research during recent years, such as pharmacology and new fluorescent proteins/dyes/fluorophores development (Grotjohann et al., 2011), has helped to visualize, for example, cells in native condition at superior optical resolution (Wang & Fei, 2020). SRMS has also gained importance in understanding answers to the questions in biomedical engineering and biophysical properties of biomolecules (i.e., spatial organization, dynamics, and function) (Fei et al., 2015; Manley et al., 2008; Xu, Zhong, & Zhuang, 2013).

11.2.1 Photoactivated localization microscopy and stochastic optical reconstruction microscopy systems

The primary prerequisites for superresolution methods are that fluorescent agents' ability (i.e., fluorophores) has to be photoactivatable and photoswitchable. By applying fluorescent agents to specific wavelengths of light (i.e., laser light), they undergo an on and off switch process appearing between bright and dark emission states. Trigger light is maintained at even a reduced rate while superresolution illumination ensuring because only a single fluorophore is fluorescing at the moment inside a diffraction-limited range. (Fig. 11.1A) (Rust et al., 2006).

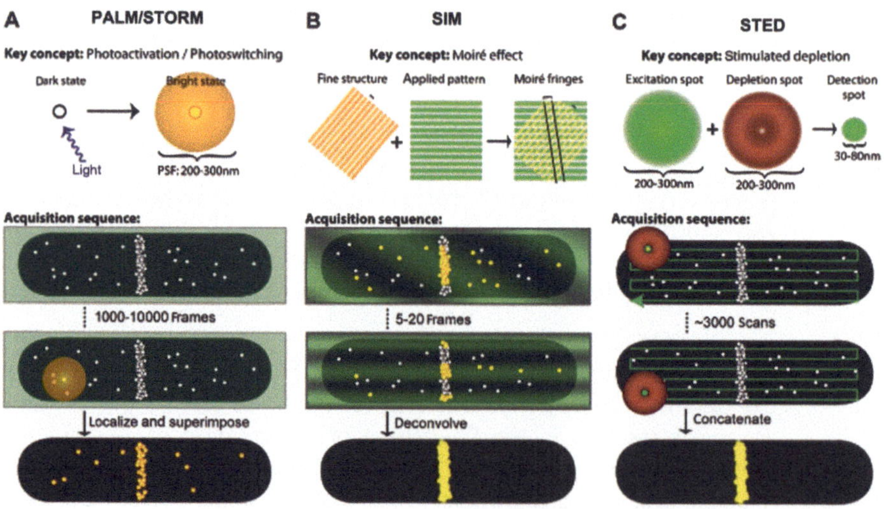

Figure 11.1 General schematic overview and image formation for various superresolution microscopy systems: (A) photoactivated localization microscopy (PALM) and stochastic optical reconstruction microscopy (STORM); (B) Structured illumination microscopy system; (C) Stimulated emission depletion (STED) microscopy system (Coltharp & Xiao, 2012).

By nanometer accuracy, these single molecules' positions are therefore determined by matching their energy curves with a Gaussian function that quantifies the point spread function (PSF) of the microscope. To reconstruct a superresolution shot, points collected from thousands of frames will then be superimposed. Fiducial beads are often applied on the specimen that track and adjust the level shift over that little lengthy acquisition period (Coltharp & Xiao, 2012).

Decreased amplification illumination (violet arrow) is applied using single-molecule localization methods such as photoactivated localization microscopy and stochastic optical reconstruction microscopy so that single molecules become stochastically stimulated and localized. The triggered molecule generates a diffraction-limited dot (diffuse yellow circle) that suits the Gaussian mechanism to identify the molecule's orientation with nanometer accuracy. Once hundreds or even thousands of molecules have indeed been identified, its coordinates become plastered to produce a superresolution snapshot (bottom) (Coltharp & Xiao, 2012).

11.2.2 Structured illumination microscopy system

Structured illumination microscopy (SIM) reaches superresolution through collecting precise spatial features from systemic interaction with fixed lighting sequences. As a sinusoidal emission sequence (Fig. 11.2B, green color) is introduced to a fluorescent specimen, the interference pattern is found. The diffraction-limited fringes of this interference process, named moiré fringes, supply knowledge on the specimen's underlying structural layout that cannot be examined with a classical LM system. By extending the concept of exposure patterns of varying positioning and orientation axes to much the same specimen (Fig. 11.2B), the specimen's subdiffraction-limited network resources can be derived from the Fourier transform of the corresponding waves (Coltharp & Xiao, 2012).

SIM employs the moiré effect, that effects when an illumination sequence (green dots) is distributed to a material with component models that are finer than that of the diffraction limit (e.g., closely spaced yellow dots or molecule positions).

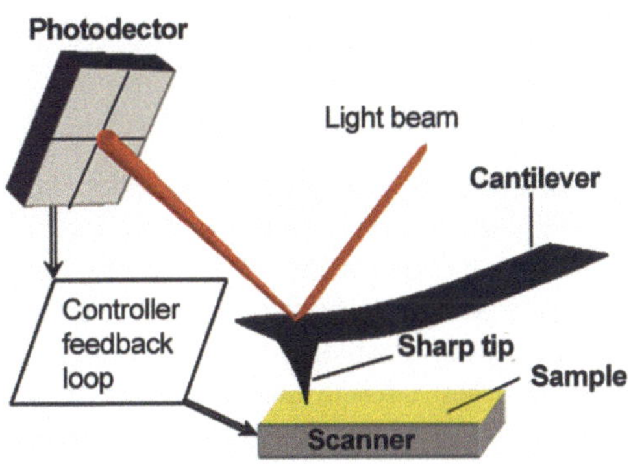

Figure 11.2 Schematic overview of principles of AFM (Pletikapic & DeNardis, 2017). *AFM*, Atomic-force microscopy.

Interference here between lighting design and the specimen induces moiré fringes (two of which should be viewed as directional black lines), which are also positioned further along than the accompanying specimen distance displaying subdiffraction-limited attributes. Several exposure patterns are added to the sample, and the physical knowledge obtained from the Fourier transformations within each pattern is utilized to create a superresolution picture (bottom). Since the emission of fluorophores (yellow circles) is diffraction-limited, the diffraction-limited parameters are excluded for consistency (Coltharp & Xiao, 2012).

11.2.3 Stimulated emission depletion microscopy system

The stimulated emission depletion (STED) microscopy method has an optical resolution above the diffraction boundary. In efforts to realize a high-resolution image, the fluorescent agent plays an important role. There are many other critical factors to get a STED picture. Initially, the fluorescent agent does have to be excited by laser light from the lowest energy (Switch OFF state) to the (Singlet) higher power (switch ON state). The second component of the mechanism is either de-excited (1) by laser beam, by stimulated emission (SE) or (2) by immediate fluorescence emission. Spontaneous effect can be observed over a relatively tiny amount of time in the next few nanoseconds following a stimulation of a fluorescent probe for a longer cycle of laser lightening (with photons) (with photons) (with photons). In other words, the fluorescence of a fluorescent probe during 4 ns of excited-state existence and 25 cm^2/J SE cross-section requires 10 MW/cm^2 of laser light intensity (Vicidomini, Bianchini, & Diaspro, 2018).

Triggered activated molecules that are with lower energy state in donut-shaped regions located around the central confocal location (Fig. 11.3C). Only molecules within 30–80 nm of the center of the excitation site are observed in this route. This saturation principle has been applied to fluorophore photoswitching by using a donut-shaped depletion pulse to turn fluorophores off rather than inducing emissions (Grotjohann et al., 2011). This method, known as the Reversible Saturable Optical Fluorescence Transitions (RESOLFT), reduces the adverse impact that the high-power depletion beam can have on cell viability because its RESOLFT depletion beam is being used at a much lower power (approximately 1 kW/cm^2) than with stimulated depletion laser (100–500 MW/cm^2) (Coltharp & Xiao, 2012).

Concentric stimulation and depletion lasers (green circle and red donut, respectively) are focused onto a specimen for STED scanning. While fluorophores are activated in the diffraction-limited excitation place (large green circle), the depletion beam (red donut) boosts molecules far beyond the central 30–80 nm region back to the ground while they emit photons, producing a superresolution of the PSF (small green circle). Such lasers are inspected to obtain a superresolution image across the specimen (bottom) (Coltharp & Xiao, 2012).

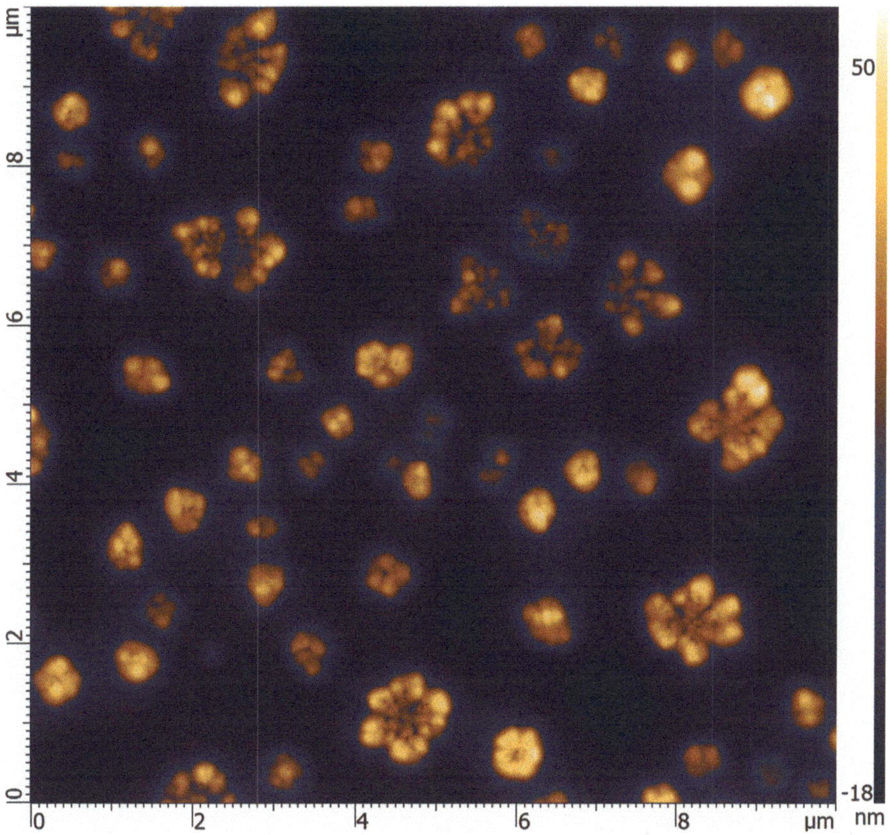

Figure 11.3 Nanoscopic AFM image of the processed herb Rhizoma Polygonati (Benassi et al., 2021). *AFM*, Atomic-force microscopy.

11.3 Atomic-force microscopy and application

11.3.1 Atomic-force microscopy

Since the development of atomic-force microscopy (AFM) in 1980 (Binnig, Quate, & Gerber, 1986), AFM gain massive popularity among researchers and professionals due to its simplicity and practicality being one of the high-resolution surface scanning microscopic techniques nowadays.

Due to its versatile application options in many fields, AFM can measure features sized from several nanometers and up to several hundred microns. Measurements can be done in the air and liquid environment to examine solid or soft biological surfaces without surface modification to the sample. This factor makes AFM more attractive comparing to electron microscopes (Johnson, Hilal, & Bowen, 2009).

AFM is a member of a family of scanning probe microscopy systems, with a primary goal to get nanometer (1–5 nm) scaled resolution topographical images, depends on the sharpness of the sensor's tip. Before real scanning using a cantilever, it is key to calibrate the spring constant of it. Later it will be used to sense the interactions between the probe and the surface being used to get a very high-resolution image of the sample. The main advantage of an AFM is that it provides direct images of biological specimens at subnanometer resolution under physiological conditions (Dufrene, 2004; Dufrene, 2008).

The sample is mounted on a piezoelectric scanner, which ensures 3D positioning with high accuracy. More detailed working principles of AFM are schematically illustrated in Fig. 11.2 (Pletikapic & DeNardis, 2017).

A specimen's location determines the following phases of AFM imaging on the XYZ directional movement of the piezoelectric scanner, which creates a 3D image with only a few nanometer resolution out over surface measurement duration. The 3D image is acquired through a laser light that shines on the top of the cantilever's outer surface, but this needs to be mirrored in the photodiode, illustrating the vibration of the spot from the curved cantilever. Across the deflection of its location from the cantilever, a difference includes its range between the tip and the instrument. A fixed gap is recovered with a feedback mechanism seen between the reference positioning device and the hard drive piezoelectric scanner. Recorded cantilever displacement variables are electronically processed to a quasi-3D dataset obtained. Consequently, AFM creates authentic –3D images of the specimen with a spatial resolution of 0.1 nm and a longitudinal dimension to 1 nm (Pletikapic & DeNardis, 2017).

11.3.2 Application of AFM in life science

Existing literature suggests the practicability of using AFM as an excellent nanoscopic tool to achieve unprecedented high-resolution of tiny forms and surface properties of living matter measured in the air or native conditions.

According to authors published in recent years (Bekmurzayeva et al., 2018; Benassi et al., 2021; Nurkesh et al., 2019; Sypabekova et al., 2019), the application of AFM in biotechnology, biomedical engineering, and biophysics has gained much practical popularity due to simplicity to work on and generate tremendous results.

According to Bekmurzayeva et al., the proposed research's central idea was a development of a biosensor based on chemically etched Fiber Bragg Grating for thrombin detection. This measurement's primary goal was to measure with high sensitivity of a shift in refractive index toward detection of thrombin. To do that, the surface of an etched fiber was modified with biologically active agents. Furthermore, after each step of biofunctionalized biomolecules onto the fiber surface, the AFM was used to demonstrate surface peculiarities.

Developed technology has excellent prospects in future clinical applications (Bekmurzayeva et al., 2018).

Another successful application of AFM in life science was to study the surface properties of carbon nanodots as potential agents in anticancer and imaging methodology. Moreover, proposed research results illustrate interesting results on the significant DNA damage induced by carbon dots based on prostate cancer cell lines. The obtained high-resolution AFM images show these dramatic transformations with the DNA molecule of cancer cells. The latter study results demonstrate the premier and an efficient, low-cost, and green nanomaterials are revealed for cancer therapy and anti-infection (Nurkesh et al., 2019).

According to Sypabekova et al., the authors conducted new and innovative research on detecting *Mycobacterium tuberculosis* secreted protein MPT64 using an interdigitated electrode to target an immunogenic protein as electrochemical impedance using capturing device. The AFM was a pivotal instrument to precisely measure the surface roughness of modified clinical samples by completing each technological step. The developed technology based on aptasensor helps to identify tuberculosis in a short amount of time (Sypabekova et al., 2019).

Also, in another excellent research, authors Benassi et al. (2021) studied various biochemical metabolism mechanisms with natural herbs, with processed Rhizoma Polygonati (RP). Chemically active molecules exhibited by the herbs product show an interesting phosphate-like process interlinked with the creation of flower-shaped assembly in a nanosize structure. Fig. 11.3 illustrates the application of AFM to the morphological study of flowery arranged clusters of RP (Benassi et al., 2021).

Moreover, herbs' phosphate-like activity prevents further cancer cell development through phosphatase indication by possibly crosstalk with kinases signaling or DNA damage by either directly binding or unwinding DNA that proved this idea by using AFM. As a result, authors proposed for the first time a concept of the neologism herbzyme, which is a combination of the herb and enzyme (Benassi et al., 2021).

11.4 Conclusion

This chapter presents a general overview of the modern line of the superresolution optical, fluorescent, and nanoscopic microscopies. The specific technical peculiarities, as well as their application fields, have also been discussed.

It is expected in the nearest future. Along with fast-growing developments, the science and technology accosted with the development of ultra-high-resolution microscopies will appear by combining or creating utterly new microscopic methodologies that will boost scientific discoveries across biomedical engineering, biophysics, and life sciences in general.

References

Abbe, E. (1873). Beiträge zur theorie des mikroskops und der mikroskopischen wahrnehmung. *Archive for Microscopic Anatomy*, *9*, 413–418.

Bates, M., Huang, B., Dempsey, G. T., & Zhuang, X. (2007). Multicolor super-resolution imaging with photo-switchable fluorescent probes. *Science (New York, N.Y.)*, *317*, 1749–1753.

Bekmurzayeva, A., Dukenbayev, K., Shaimerdenova, M., Bekniyazov, I., Ayupova, T., Sypabekova, M., ... Tosi, D. (2018). Etched fiber bragg grating biosensor functionalized with aptamers for detection of thrombin. *Sensors*, *18*, 4298.

Benassi, E., Fan, H., Sun, Q., Dukenbayev, K., Wang, Q., Shaimoldina, A., ... Xie, Y. (2021). Generation of particle assemblies mimicking enzymatic activity by processing of herbal food: the case of Rhizoma Polygonati and other natural ingredients in traditional Chinese medicine. *Nanoscale Advances*. Available from https://doi.org/10.1039/D0NA00958J, accepted.

Betzig, E., Patterson, G. H., Sougrat, R., Lindwasser, O. W., Olenych, S., Bonifacino, J. S., ... Hess, H. F. (2006). Imaging intracellular fluorescent proteins at nanometer resolution. *Science (New York, N.Y.)*, *313*, 1642–1645.

Binnig, G., Quate, C. F., & Gerber, Ch (1986). Atomic force microscope. *Physical Review Letters*, *56*, 930.

Coltharp, C., & Xiao, J. (2012). Superresolution microscopy for microbiology. *Cellular Microbiology*, *14*(12), 1808–1818.

Dufrene, Y. F. (2008). Atomic force microscope and chemical force microscopy of microbial cells. *Nature Protocols*, *3*, 1132–1138.

Dufrene, Y. F. (2004). Using nanotechniques to explore microbial surfaces. *Nature Reviews*, *2*, 451–460.

Fei, J., Singh, D., Zhang, Q., Park, S., Balasubramanian, D., Golding, I., & Vanderpool, C. K. (2015). RNA biochemistry. Determination of in vivo target search kinetics of regulatory noncoding RNA. *Science (New York, N.Y.)*, *347*, 1371–1374.

Grotjohann, T., Tesla, I., Leutenegger, M., Bock, H., Urban, N., Lavoie-Cardinal, F., ... Hell, S. (2011). Diffraction-unlimited all-optical imaging and writing with a photochromic GFP. *Nature*, *478*, 204–208. Available from https://doi.org/10.1038/nature10497.

Huang, B., Wang, W., Bates, M., & Zhuang, X. (2008). Three-dimensional super-resolution imaging by stochastic optical reconstruction microscopy. *Science (New York, N.Y.)*, *319*, 810–813.

Johnson, D., Hilal, N., & Bowen, W. R. (2009). *Basic principles of atomic force microscopy, atomic force microscopy in process engineering* (pp. 1–30). Elsevier BV. Available from https://doi.org/10.1016/b978-1-85617-517-3.00001-8.

Khater, I. M., Nabi, I. R., & Hamarneh, G. (2020). A review of super-resolution single molecule localization microscopy cluster analysis and quantification methods. *Patterns*, *1*(3), 100038.

Manley, S., Gillette, J. M., Patterson, G. H., Shroff, H., Hess, H. F., Betzig, E., & Lippincott-Schwartz, J. (2008). High-density mapping of single-molecule trajectories with photoactivated localization microscopy. *Nature Methods*, *5*, 155–157.

Nurkesh, A. A., Sun, Q., Fan, H., Dukenbayev, K., Tsoy, A., Altaikyzy, A., ... Xie, Y. (2019). Date pit carbon dots induce acidic inhibition of peroxidase and disrupt dna repair in antibacteria resistance. *Global Challenges*, *3*, 1900042.

Pletikapic, G., & DeNardis, N. I. (2017). Application of surface analytical methods for hazardous situation in the Adriatic Sea: Monitoring of organic matter dynamics and oil pollution. *Natural Hazards and Earth System Sciences*, *17*, 31–44.

Rust, M., Bates, M., & Zhuang, X. (2006). Sub-diffraction-limit imaging by stochastic optical reconstruction microscopy (STORM). *Nature Methods*, *3*, 793–796. Available from https://doi.org/10.1038/nmeth929.

Sezgin, E. (2017). Super-resolution optical microscopy for studying membrane structure and dynamics. *Journal of Physics: Condensed Matter*, *29*, 273001.

Sypabekova, M., Dukenbayev, K., Tsepke, A., Akisheva, A., Oralbayev, N., & Kanayeva, D. (2019). An aptasensor for the detection of Mycobacterium tuberculosis secreted immunogenic protein MPT64 in clinical samples towards tuberculosis detection. *Scientific Reports*, *9*, 16273.

Vicidomini, G., Bianchini, P., & Diaspro, A. (2018). STED super-resolved microscopy. *Nature Methods*, *15*(3), 173–182.

Wang, Y., & Fei, J. (2020). Continuous active development of super-resolution fluorescence microscopy. *Physical Biology*, *17*, 030401.

Xu, K., Zhong, G., & Zhuang, X. (2013). Actin, spectrin, and associated proteins form a periodic cytoskeletal structure in axons. *Science (New York, N.Y.)*, *339*, 452–456.

12

Medical devices and standards

12.1 Medical devices

Medical devices (MDs) are medical items intended by the manufacturer for human use and are intended for medical purposes. The medical instruments' primary aim is predominantly biologically, opposed to pharmaceutical items that function pharmacologically, immunologically, or metabolically (Medical devices, 2013).

MDs include implants, catheter products, injection, transfusion and dialysis, surgical technology for human use, software, automatic pacemakers, dental appliances, bandaging equipment, corrective lenses, x-ray machines, hospital equipment, laboratory diagnostics, and in vitro diagnostic instruments, as well as other devices. MDs are often known to be items containing or are covered with a drug or a substance that is considered medicinal products or components of a medicinal product if used in isolation and may be annexed to the therapeutic device by working on the body (Medical devices, 2013).

12.2 Biocompatibility of medical devices

An obligatory part of the conformity assessment is the biological examination or biopsy inspection of a medical system (Medical devices biocompatibility, 2021).

The statement "First, not harm" embodies the principle—threads dispersed across medical culture—that prevention is first and foremost in health treatment. This principle is defended because policymakers have set up regulatory agencies in medical matters to preserve public health. Patients' safety is protected by ensuring that no damage can be done to new MDs is also a call for companies (Jorgensen, 2018).

Despite all precautions, it is important to take an implant immediately after implantation into consideration in advance. For instance, it can cause a life-threatening fever or infection because it is not clean and sterile. There are many harmful outcomes on a broader time span, ranging from local tissue inflammation to cancer

Optical Fiber Biosensors.
DOI: https://doi.org/10.1016/B978-0-12-819467-6.00012-3

that can result from substance problems. Biocompatibility analysis is intended to check potential side effects on medical equipment that a patient may have and make sure the system is not dangerous first (Jorgensen, 2018).

A complex and emerging topic, which is the cornerstone of international standardization—ISO 10993, is the biocompatibility of MDs. The first section of ISO 10993-1 gives a description of materials' biocompatibility and the possible risk reduction strategy. The other chapters discuss risk mitigation subjects from sample processing to animal experiments to how a toxicological risk evaluation can be conducted. United States Food and Drug Administration (FDA) typically accepts ISO 10993 for MDs submitted for commercial approval and has recently issued a guide to how it advises the implementation of ISO 10993 (Jorgensen, 2018).

Biocompatibility presentation should be performed in three steps: to evaluate the device components, identify possible hazards, and recommend future assessments and monitoring for the risks found based on patient interaction with the device.

The *first* is a biological evaluation plan (BEP). This offers good internal documentation of the methodology used to resolve biocompatibility as an early risk evaluation outlined in ISO 10993-1.

Second, a range of approaches for mitigating the possible threats found in BEP will be used to analyze and validate the apparatus. These threats (and related trials) are those mentioned in ISO 10993-1 Annex A.

This is mostly determined by using the following mixture:

- Modern biological studies in vivo or in vitro.
- The toxicological risk evaluation is accompanied by chemical testing.
- Written review focused on knowledge from research literature and the therapeutic application of products.

Third, all research findings and written assessments must be summarized in the FDA's Capstone Biological Evaluation Report. Compared with more static biocompatibility techniques that pursued a strategy free of device-based content awareness from the checkbox, contemporary strategies may be misleading due to an obvious uncertainty against the uninitiated (Jorgensen, 2018).

12.3 Biocompatibility of medical devices, testing, and risk assessment steps

12.3.1 Evaluating the biocompatibility of medical devices

The primary objective for all medical equipment producers is to give patients extra value while eliminating biological risks. It ensures that foreign regulatory authorities meet strict biocompatibility research criteria such that the devices are medically acceptable to use until they are commercially available (Biocompatibility testing, 2021, ISO Standard 10993, 2018).

The anticipated function of an MD or substance that comes into contact with the patient's body should be achieved without causing any detrimental impact on a patient. Like mutagenic, possible adverse reactions can vary from short-term (acute) to long-term (chronic) body allergic events. Therefore the relationship of the system and the tissue, the cells, or the patient's body fluids is usually tested on the medical instruments for biological examination and biocompatibility checking. A biocompatibility evaluation is predominantly aimed to safeguard patients from significant biological threats (Biocompatibility testing, 2021; ISO Standard 10993, 2018).

12.3.2 Biological evaluation of medical devices under ISO 10993 standard

The International Standard Organization (ISO) is responsible for developing the key regulatory criteria for nonclinical biocompatibility and testing of medical instruments, especially the ISO 10993 series. Analogs domestic and regional requirements, however, provide additional tests and factors and separate international and national test papers to be incorporated into safety and feasibility assessment (Schuh & Funk, 2019).

The biological risk evaluations performed for MDs are outlined in ISO 10993 and the product-specific guidelines, while the selection of functional testing is device specific (Medical devices biocompatibility, 2021).

ISO 10993-1 standard, Biological evaluation of medical devices—Part 1: A risk control appraisal and testing, provides a mechanism for assessing the necessary biocompatibility precautions to undertake a biological examination. The essential assessments are focused on the form and intended usage of MDs or products and the extent and period of association between the body and the MD. The following subsection will describe an assessment for biological effects from the exposure of an MD or material to the human body, including testing (Biocompatibility testing, 2021; ISO Standard 10993, 2018).

12.3.3 Risk assessment steps and test requirements by ISO, FDA, and ASTM

Biocompatibility monitoring tests medical equipment compliance with a biological environment as an essential part of the bio-risk evaluation. It explores the relationship between the system in contact with different forms of living cells and tissues subjected to the device (Biocompatibility testing, 2021; ISO Standard 10993, 2018).

Table 12.1 reviews the relevant bio-risk assessment tests to help producers fulfill the criteria of biocompatibility tests of the ISO, FDA, and American Society for Testing and Materials (ASTM) (Biocompatibility testing, 2021; ISO Standard 10993, 2018).

Table 12.1 Biocompatibility testing requirements by ISO, FDA, and ASTM (Biocompatibility testing, 2021; ISO Standard 10993, 2018).

Type of risk assessment	ISO standard nomenclature	Brief description
Cytotoxicity	10993-5	Cytotoxicity estimations are done to assess the common harmfulness level of the therapeutic gadget or fabric on cell culture through in vitro elution and agarose overlay strategies.
Genotoxicity	10993-3 and FDA	Genotoxicity estimations are required to check the nearness of poisons that can affect the hereditary fabric of cells. According to ISO standard 10993-3 (2018) control, gene transformation should go through the bacterial mutagenicity test/bacterial invert change test. Chromosomal harms through in vitro chromosomal distortion measure through mouse lymphoma measure and/or in vivo DNA harm through in vitro/in vivo chromosomal distortions test and in vitro/in vivo erythrocyte micronucleus examinations.
Hemocompatibility	10993-4 and ASTM	Hemocompatibility assessments are facilitated to examine blood-contacting restorative devices' impacts on blood and blood components through hematology and thrombosis tests.
Irritation	10993-10	Bothering testing evaluates the therapeutic gadget for skin fractiousness through, i.e., essential skin, visual, intracutaneous reactivity tests, and in vitro skin aggravation tests.
Sensitization	10993-10	Sensitization evaluations are conducted to assess conceivable antagonistic cutaneous responses of the resistant framework to the restorative gadget through in vivo and in vitro testing strategies.
Systemic effects of systemic toxicity and pyrogenicity	10993-11 and ASTM	Intense to constant systemic poisonous quality tests assess the impacts of therapeutic gadgets in vivo. Pyrogenicity measurements are carried out to test for material-mediated fever-causing compounds called pyrogens that affect patients when they contact the restorative gadget.
Implantation	10993-6	Implantation examinations assess restorative devices' impacts on the encompassing living tissue at both plainly visible and infinitesimal levels.
Chemical characterization	10993-18	Chemical inquire about should be conducted to recognize extractable and leachable sums that move from a helpful contraption when utilized or challenged.
Toxicological risk assessment	10993-17	A toxicological hazard appraisal of extractable and leachable makes a difference measure-related dangers based on introduction and secure admissions dosage.
Sterility testing	11737 series	Bioburden assessment, as portion of sterility testing, makes a difference decide the populace of microorganisms on a therapeutic gadget that has not been sterilized.
Sterile barrier system	11607 and EN 868 series	Sterile obstruction estimations are required to approve a restorative device's bundling framework to guarantee the gadget keeps up its sterility and aseptic quality some time recently utilize.

12.4 Biocompatibility of metallic nanoparticles and application in cancer therapy

Technology of materials is a diverse area of substance vital to MD invention. It is also essential for material engineers to be aware of the new technical advancements (Boutrand, 2012).

Composite technologies must fulfill demanding specifications for durability, scale, biocompatibility, and biostability. In particular, the interest in nanoparticles and biodegradable polymers for MDs has risen rapidly in recent years. Due to its exceptional optical clarity, controllable porosity, chemical inertness, and biocompatibility, nanoparticles are attractive. The production of nanoparticles for the delivery of targeted drugs is an intensive field of study. The supply of poorly soluble materials over the blood–brain barrier is one significant application (Boutrand, 2012).

Designed biodegradable polymers are desirable because of their ability to retain and distribute drugs on-site in a regulated manner as they degrade (Boutrand, 2012).

12.4.1 Biocompatible silver, gold, and silver/gold alloy nanoparticles for enhanced cancer therapy

In the previous recent years, in the literature, flourish a significant trend of application metal-based nanoparticles (NPs). In particular, silver NPs (AgNPs), gold NPs (AuNPs), and their alloys have biomedical applications for tumor detection.

In present days, the aim of nanooncology is today to diagnose cells without side effects, to track them, and to treat them. The paper's authors explain the microbiota fermentation for hepatoprotection toward diethylnitrosamine (DEN)-induced liver cancer in the design Sprague Dawleys (SD) rat with biocompatible nanoparticles of silver and gold. Their alloys are used. Centered on in vivo tests, tumor decreases in animals treated with nanoparticles (a decrease of $<45\%$ to 65%) were observed in vivo studies. Finally, the results demonstrate the potential activities against DEN-induced liver cancer of AgNPs, AuNPs, and Ag/AuNPs broadly and may be potential candidates for effective nanodrug development (Shanmugasundaram, Radhakrishnan, Gopikrishnan, Kadirvelu, & Balagurunathan, 2017).

12.4.2 Express label-free and real-time detection of cancer cells using gold nanoparticles and optical fiber aptasensor

Circulating tumor cell (CTC) detection is an essential target of oncological diagnosis and care because CTCs are crucial to the malignancy in cancer progression and at very low doses. Authors propose to track metastatic breast cancer cells a fiber-wide plasma aptasensor with several narrowband wavelength resonances. As per the research reported, the bioreceptor chosen and immobilized for optical fiber's surface was a particular aptamers to mammaglobin-A enzyme. In vitro assays confirm that label-free and real-time detection of cancer cells occurs within 5 minutes, while the other use of functionalized AuNPs allows a twofold amplification of the biosensor response. The findings indicate that fiber-optic sensors are critical for identifying cells at low levels and, particularly, throughout the sense of malignant tumors in early stages (Loyez et al., 2020).

12.4.3 Biomedical application of fiber-optic biosensor device for rapid detection of COVID-19

To recognize infected persons, particularly immunocompromised cases, the quick and cheap diagnosis of COVID-19 is, according to the authors, necessary for stopping the disease's propagation through local transmission. As an alternative to reverse transcription polymerase chain reaction, antibody-based diagnostic markers have minimal assistance with such an immense sense of false positiveness. The researchers report using our single-stage, wash-free identification of SARS-CoV-2 virus particles directly in the salival sample using a limited sample pretreatment platform for field-deployable/portable fiber-optic absorbance biosensors (Murugan, Bhatia, Sai, & Satija, 2020).

12.5 Conclusion

Finally, this chapter dealt with a comprehensive review of biocompatibility and MD risk management concerns. Moreover, the application of internationally recognized ISO standards regulating biocompatibility and their requirements and detailed steps had been discussed. Besides, the application of metallic nanoparticles toward tumor detection and the use of optical fibers for COVID-19 detection had been discussed.

References

Biocompatibility testing. (2021). https://www.tuvsud.com/en/industries/healthcare-and-medical-devices/medical-devices-and-ivd/medical-device-testing/chemical-or-biological-testing-of-medical-devices/biocompatibility-testing.

Boutrand, J.-P. (Ed.), (2012). *Biocompatibility and performance of medical devices*. Woodhead Publishing.

ISO Standard 10993. (2018). *Biological evaluation of medical devices — Part 1: Evaluation and testing within a risk management process*. https://www.iso.org/obp/ui#iso:std:iso:10993:-1:ed-5:v2:en.

Jorgensen, M. (2018). *Biocompatibility of medical devices is a complex and evolving subject. Here's what you need to know*. https://www.mddionline.com/testing/brief-introduction-medical-device-biocompatibility.

Loyez, M., Hassan, E., Lobry, M., Liu, F., Caucheteur, C., Wattiez, R., ... Albert, J. (2020). Circulating cancer cell detection using an optical fiber Aptasensor. *Proceedings SPIE 11361, Biophotonics in Point-of-Care, 113610L*.

Medical devices. (2013). https://www.bfarm.de/EN/MedicalDevices/_node.html.

Medical devices biocompatibility. (2021). https://www.scc-gmbh.de/eu-services/medical-devices/biological-evaluation-medical-devices-biocompatibility.

Murugan, D., Bhatia, H., Sai, V. V. R., & Satija, J. (2020). P-FAB: A fiber-optic biosensor device for rapid detection of COVID-19. *Transactions of the Indian National Academy of Engineering*, *5*, 211–215.

Schuh, J. A. C. L., & Funk, K. A. (2019). Compilation of international standards and regulatory guidance documents for evaluation of biomaterials, medical devices, and 3-D printed and regenerative medicine products. *Toxicologic Pathology*, *47*, 3.

Shanmugasundaram, T., Radhakrishnan, M., Gopikrishnan, V., Kadirvelu, K., & Balagurunathan, R. (2017). Biocompatible silver, gold and silver/gold alloy nanoparticles for enhanced cancer therapy: In vitro and in vivo perspectives. *Nanoscale*, *9*, 16773.

III

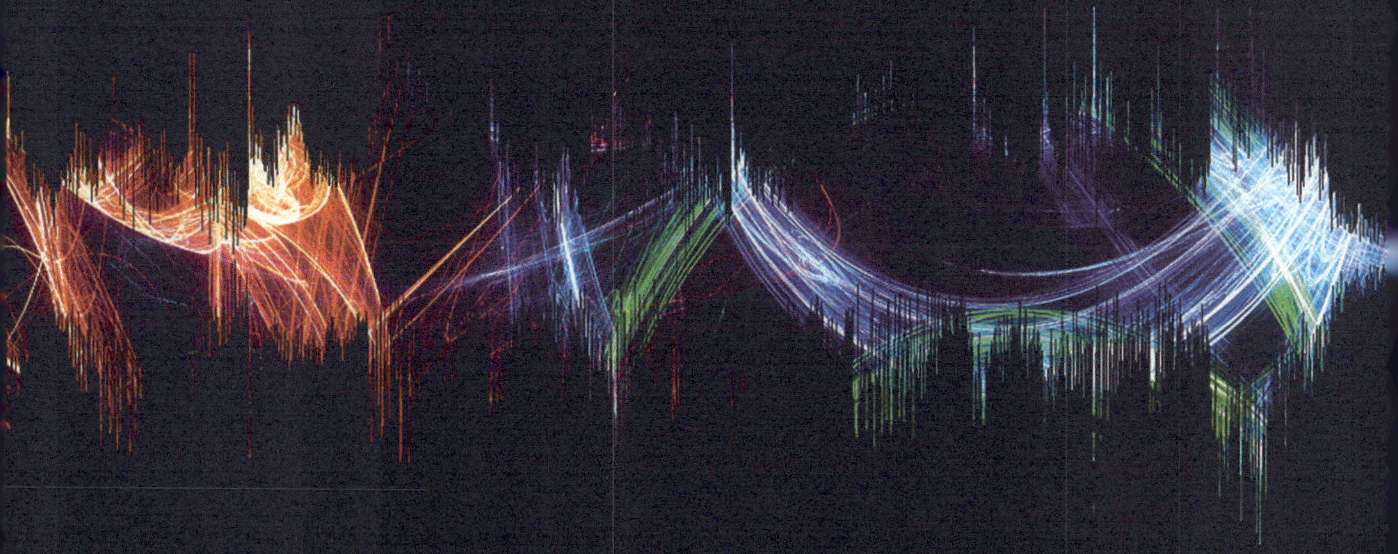

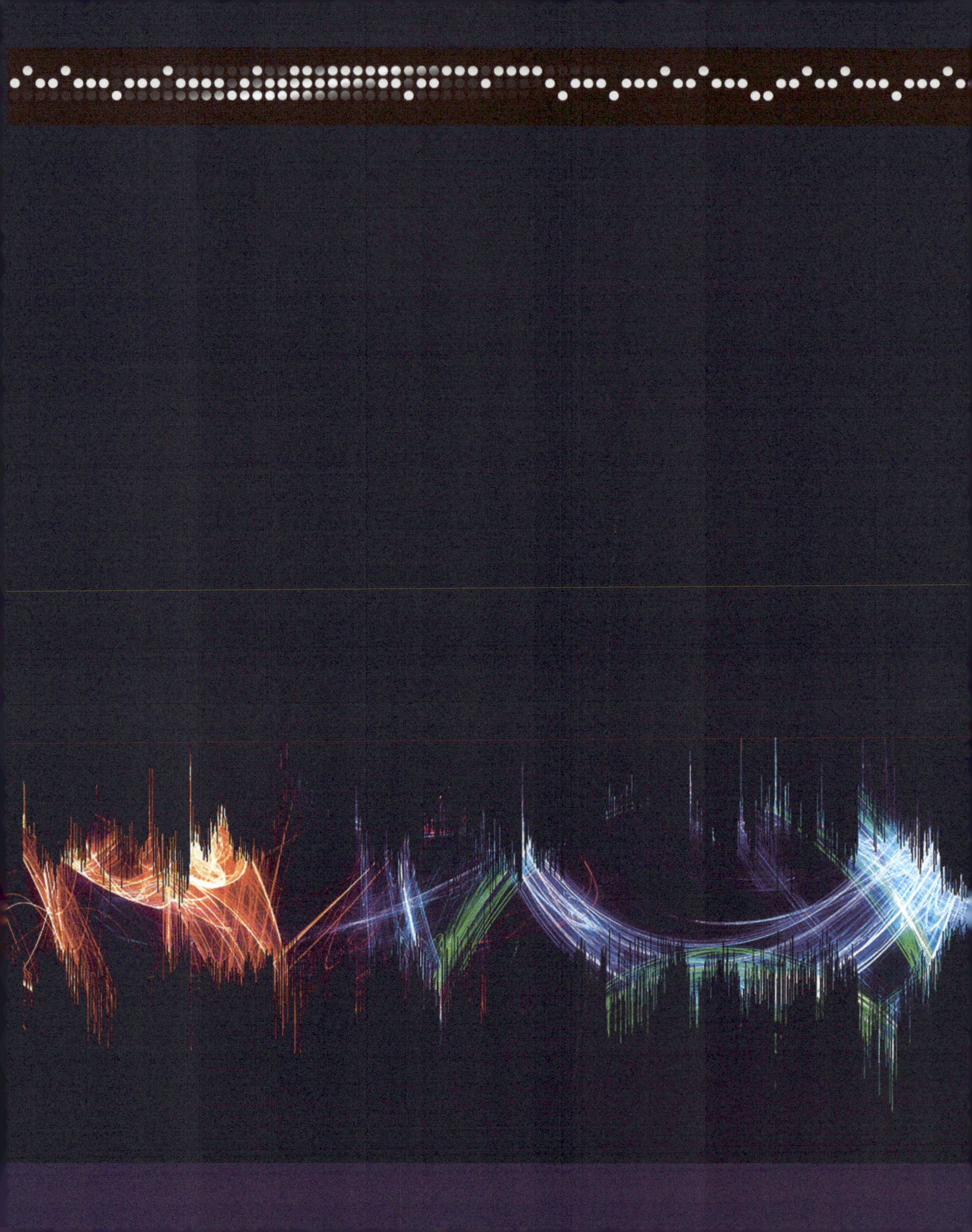

13

Analyte and sample detection

13.1 Glucose sensing using optical fiber sensor

Glucose is a ubiquitous source of energy for cells. Glucose level is increased in diabetes mellitus, a "silent epidemic," and monitoring its level is important in this disease (Kadashetti et al., 2015). High glucose level associated with diabetes increases a risk of cardiovascular disorders, neurological issues, kidney failure, and eyesight loss (Khan, Watekar, & Kang, 2018). Glucose is the most detected analyte among all biosensors including optical fiber biosensors; the type of optical fiber used and their performance is presented in Table 13.1. Some of the studies did not use specific ligands against glucose while others covered the fiber with glucose sensitive materials. Many other studies rely on enzymes: glucose oxidase (GOx) or glucose dehydrogenase as a ligand. Conversion of glucose by GOx results in the formation of gluconic acid and hydrogen peroxide; and refractive index (RI) of the solution changes inducing change in the signal in optical fiber [e.g., resonance wavelength shift in transmission in case of long period fiber grating (LPFG)]. One of the studies using excessively tilted fiber Bragg grating (FBG) and GOx had better performance (in terms of thermal cross-talk, linearity, and accuracy) than previously reported LPFG-based sensor (Luo, Yan, Sun, Li, & Zhang, 2014). Another sensor, dual-peak LPFG had higher sensitivity than both of the previous systems (excessively tilted FBG and LPFG) (Badmos et al., 2017). Sensitivity of a graphene oxide–coated biosensor showed to be influenced by the amount of immobilized enzyme and pH of the solution (Xu, Huang, Ding, & Cai, 2020). An indirect approach of glucose determination was proposed by Zhang et al. (2018), where hydrogen peroxide produced due to GOx activity (i.e., when glucose binds) etches silver coating of tilted fiber Bragg grating (TFBG), which leads to lowering of surface plasmon resonance (SPR) attenuation and correlates with glucose levels. Physiologically relevant glucose concentrations were detected in serum using this sensor.

Enzyme-based biosensors have a drawback in being very sensitive to temperature and pH change (Lobry et al., 2019); therefore, other systems based on affinity of

Optical Fiber Biosensors.
DOI: https://doi.org/10.1016/B978-0-12-819467-6.00013-5

Table 13.1 Optical fiber biosensors for glucose sensing.

Optical fiber	Ligand	Concentration range	Performance		References
			LOD	Sensitivity	
Dual peak LPFG80-μm-cladding B/Ge codoped SMF	GOx	0.1–3.2 mg/mL	0.1 mg/mL[a]	7.12 ± 0.12 nm/(mg/mL) 12.21 ± 0.19 nm/(mg/mL)	Badmos et al. (2017)
U-shaped	GOx	0.1%–0.5% (w/v)		2.899 nm/%	Chen, Li, Wu, and Chiang (2018)
Fabry–Perot interferometry	Glucose sensitive dye	1 μM–1 M		3.25 nm/mM	Khan et al. (2018)
Side-polished low-index polymer	–	0%–5% (w/v)		0.46 nm/mM	Cao et al. (2018)
TFBG–SPR	Concanavalin A	10^{-7} M	10^{-6} to 10^{-4} M		Lobry et al. (2019)
Exc. tilted FBG	GOx	0.1–5 mg/mL		0.298 nm/(mg/mL)	Luo et al. (2014)
Multimode plastic fiber	GOx	10 nM–100 mM	10 nM		Pahurkar, Tamgadge, Gambhire, and Muley (2015)
TFBG–SPR	GOx	0–12 mM		0.5 dB/mM	Zhang et al. (2018)

[a]*Inferred.*

Exc., excessively; *GOx*, glucose oxidase.

glucose to other molecules rather than enzymatic conversion are developed. This includes the use of a lectin protein (Concanavalin A), which has four binding sites to bind four glucose molecules (Lobry et al., 2019). Glucose-sensitive materials employed for glucose sensing include membranes that are doped with glucose sensitive dyes (Khan et al., 2018) or hydrogel with glucose-sensitive moieties (3-phenylboronic acid) (Tierney, Falch, Hjelme, & Stokke, 2009).

13.2 Sensing metal ions using optical fiber sensor

Heavy metals (metals with densities $>5\ g/cm^3$) are widely produced by various human activities causing pollution of aquatic and terrestrial ecosystems and negatively affect human health (Oehme & Wolfbeis, 1997). Several studies have used optical fiber (both as intrinsic and extrinsic optical fiber sensors) as a transducer for detection of metals including heavy metals. One of the earliest studies used the ability of metal ions to inhibit enzyme activity (urease), pH strip as a transducer (pH increases as the urea is converted to ammonia and carbon dioxide by the enzyme), and optical fiber bundle together with spectrometer to measure the change of reflection at a certain wavelength as the analyte concentration changes. Several heavy metal ions including Hg(II), Ag(I), Cu(II), Ni(II), Zn(II), Co(II), and Pb (II) were analyzed this way (Kuswandi, Andres, & Narayanaswamy, 2001). Later examples include direct functionalization of optical fiber with metal chelating/sensitive materials and the sensitivity of optical fibers toward RI change. A comprehensive review on the sensors based on optical fiber refractometers for metal ion detection is available (Tan, Ibsen, & Tjin, 2019). Optical fiber coated with a polymer containing complexing agent (calixeren) able to bind heavy metals of interest. Binding of metal ions with the agent changes the absorption properties; and as a result light power transmitted along the fiber changes. Cations of copper(II), cobalt(II), and cadmium(II) with limit of detection (LOD) of 1, 10^{-3}, and $10^{-4}\ \mu M$, respectively, were detected by the sensor (Benounis, Jaffrezic-Renault, Halouani, Lamartine, & Dumazet-Bonnamour, 2006). Bioavailable forms of mercury and arsenic were detected in the soil using cladding-etched optical fiber and bacterial cells grown directly on its surface (Ivask et al., 2007). Biosensor based on mercury ion–selective film incorporated in microfluidic system showed similar results as a reference method (cold vapor atomic absorption spectrometry) while analyzing river samples (Nuriman & Kuswandi, 2011). An LOD of 0.7 nM was achieved for localized surface plasmon resonance (LSPR) biosensor for specific detection of mercury ions (Jia, Bian, Sun, Tong, & Xia, 2018). Cadmium ions were detected by LSPR biosensor with nanoparticles and chelating agent (phytochelatins) immobilized on optical fibers. The biosensor showed high sensitivity, stability, and reproducibility (Lin & Chung, 2009). Kumar et al. developed cadmium-specific recombinant bacterial strain as ligands to detect cadmium ions with an LOD of $5\ \mu g/L$ (Kumar, Verma, & Singh, 2017).

13.3 Sensing other small analytes using optical fiber biosensor

Different optical fiber structures functionalized with specific recognition elements were employed to detect a variety of targets as shown in Table 13.2. These include ascorbic acid detection by enzyme-based system reaching sensitivity of 8.3 nm/mM and LOD of 51.94 μM (Zhu et al., 2020). A range of important biomarkers were detected by different settings based on optical fibers including cholesterol (Razo-Medina, Trejo-Duran, & Alvarado-Mendez, 2018; Semwal & Gupta, 2018), amino acids (Sharma, Semwal, & Gupta, 2019), urea (Botewad, Pahurkar, & Muley, 2018), triacylglycerides (Baliyan,

Table 13.2 Optical fiber biosensors for small molecule detection.

Small molecule	Importance[1]	Setup used Range measured	LOD	References
Triacylglyceride	Increased in coronary heart disease and hyperlipoprotenimia	LPFGTemp. controlled 0–7 mM	0.2 mM	Baliyan et al. (2016)
L-Arginine	Biomedical research and food production	Plastic-clad quartz fiber SPR5–500 nM	0.005 μM	Fan and Wang (2020)
Urea	Congestive heart, urinary tract obstruction, gastrointestinal disorders, chronic or acute renal failure, burns, dehydration, starvation, shock, malnutrition, little dietary protein in the diet, liver diseases, hepatic failure, nephritic syndrome, and cachexia	MM plastic cladded silica core 100 nM–100 mM	100 nM[2]	Botewad et al. (2018)
Sucrose	Food industry and healthcare	LSPR4°Bx to 33°Bx		Chauhan, Punjabi, Sharma, and Mukherji (2016)
Ascorbic acid	Food industry and healthcare	Periodically tapered SMF10 μM–1 mM	51.94 μM	Zhu et al. (2020)
Cholesterol	Hypertension, coronary heart disease, arteriosclerosis, brain thrombosis, lipid metabolism dysfunction along with myocardial infarction	LSPR 0–10 mM	1.131 mM	Semwal and Gupta (2018)
Taurine	Proper central nervous system functioning, maintaining liver functions, cardiovascular health, reproductive well being	LSPR 0–0.1 mM	53 μM	Sharma et al. (2019)
Melamine	Low toxicity but chronicle administration of high concentration can induce kidney damage	Multimode fiber SPR	4.3×10^{-11} M	Shrivastav and Gupta (2016)

[1] Mostly according to the reference.

[2] Indirectly measured; °Bx—degree Brix where 1 degree is 1 g of sucrose in 100 g of solution.

Sital, Tiwari, Gupta, & Sharma, 2016), and ferritin (Peterson, Cunningham, & Andrade, 2014). A "fight-or-flight" hormone, cortisol was detected in an artificial saliva by a lossy mode resonance (LMR) optical fiber biosensor coated with nanocomposite material (molecular imprinting of ZnO and polypyrrole) (Usha, Shrivastav, & Gupta, 2017). Optical fiber biosensors are not only capable of using liquid media (blood, urea, juice, etc.) but were employed for sensing targets in gaseous form. Thus bioreporter bacteria–coated optical fibers were used to monitor air toxicity (chloroform, toluene, and compounds from paint) (Eltzov, Pavluchkov, Burstin, & Marks, 2011). Zeolite-coated LPFG demonstrated an ability to distinguish isopropanol from organic vapor (Zhang, Tang, Dong, Wei, & Xiao, 2009). In another study, the swelling ability of a resin (Novolac) due to exposure to ethanol or methanol vapor was used. This changes RI of polymer optical fiber making it sensitive to vapor pressure (Morisawa, Amemiya, Kohzu, Liang, & Muto, 2001).

Optical fiber biosensors for toxin proteins detection go back as early as 1990s when botulinum toxin (Ogert, Brown, Singh, Shriverlake, & Ligler, 1992), ricin (Narang, Anderson, Ligler, & Burans, 1997), and enterotoxin B (King et al., 1999) were detected. Later, small toxins were also frequently chosen as analyte of interest. Thus ochratoxin A, a widespread food toxin which is toxic to nerve, liver, kidneys, fetus, and immune system, was detected by aptamer-based biosensor (Wang, Xiang, Zhou, Liu, & Shi, 2015). Another study used LSPR system to build biosensor capable of analyzing real grape juice samples for the presence of this toxin (Lee, Park, Byun, Kim, & Kim, 2018).

The use of fiber as a transducer offers a possibility of remote sensing of environmental contaminants. Molecules which could be sensed by optical fiber biosensors include explosives as trinitrotoluene, which is detected by molecularly imprinted polymer-coated plastic fiber (Cennamo et al., 2013). Simultaneous detection of microcystin-LR and trinitrotoluene was achieved by immobilizing two antibodies specific to the compounds (Long et al., 2010). Phenolic compounds such as catechol, *m*-cresol, phenol, and 4-chlorophenol were detected by fiber coated with enzyme-entrapped gel (Singh, Mishra, & Gupta, 2013). Another highly toxic compound, *p*-cresol, was measured on optical fiber–based LMR sensor (Usha & Gupta, 2018).

Detecting DNA molecules is important in genetic disorders diagnosis, determining pathogen infection and ensuring good safety. DNA sensing was achieved by optical fiber biosensors based on different configurations (Table 13.3). Very often, complementary nature of its structure is utilized; DNA complementary to the target is immobilized and hybridization of the probe DNA (target) is measured. Bertucci et al. were able to detect gene from a genetically modified soy without amplification (Bertucci et al., 2015). Moreover, this was possible when the target DNA was with other nontarget DNA molecules in the media.

Table 13.3 Optical fiber biosensors for DNA detection.

Optical fiber used	Ligand	Target DNA (Probe)	Sensitivity LOD	References
MOF	Peptide nucleic acid complementary to RR gene	RR gene (genomic DNA)	1%	Bertucci et al. (2015)
Dual peak LPFG	Complementary to target	15 nt	4 nM	Chen et al. (2015)
Etched FBG	Complementary to target	20 nt	0.7 μg/mL	Dagenais et al. (2005)
PCF	Complementary to target	22 nt	5 nM	Gao et al. (2016)
Etched FBG	Complementary to *dnaK* gene of *Escherichia coli*	DNA from *dnaK* gene	29 nm/RIU	Chryssis et al. (2005)
Narrow bandwidth LPFG	Complementary to target	15 nt	10%/ μM10 nM	Delgado-Pinar et al. (2017)

nt, Nucleotides; *RR*, roundup ready soy (genetically modified organism).

13.4 Protein sensing

Protein is a biomolecule, which is involved in many processes in a living cell. The structure of the protein is determined by the different amino acid sequences encoded by the genetic information. The 3D structure of different proteins varies and hence their function within the cells. The chain of amino acids is called a polypeptide where each amino acid is held by a peptide bond. One or several long polypeptide chains can fold to make a functional protein. Proteins perform vast majority of works including catalyzing metabolic reactions (enzymes), immune response (antibodies), DNA replication, transportation, signaling (biomarkers), and structural support (Fig. 13.1). In medical biosensing field, proteins in the form of biomarkers are being used as an indicator for a specific type of disease or a condition. The abnormal levels of protein or an altered protein therefore can be used as an analyte and hence detected using various biosensing platforms. Most of the proteins are temperature sensitive, therefore the detection of such proteins should be done at optimal to protein temperatures (usually from ambient temperatures to 37°C). The chemical composition and hence 3D structure of each protein is different from one another. Therefore the specific selection is one of the key factors in developing biosensors. Some proteins might have similar structure but different functions. Distinguishing the similarity is another aspect that needs to be taken into consideration during biosensor development. Since proteins are the key players in a living organism, its detection and at the same time quantification level is important for point of care and personalized testing.

An important aspect in biosensor development is sensing the protein in a real case scenario (blood, urine, saliva, and tissue) or at least in an environment that

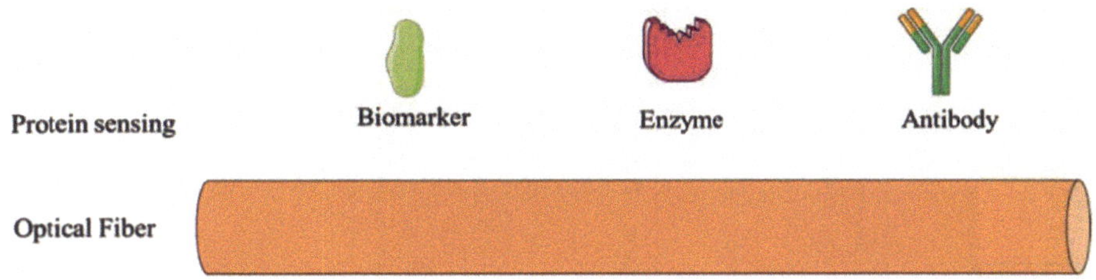

Figure 13.1 Different protein types used as an analyte on optical fiber–based biosensors.

mimics the real samples. The complexity of the clinical samples should not interfere with the sensitivity and the specificity of the biosensing device in other words the sensor should be able to distinguish the protein amongst a pool of other proteins. The biosensor development usually starts with detecting the protein in a buffer prepared in the laboratory. The chemical composition of the buffer usually facilitates the stability of the protein and hence ensures the creation of an ideal environment for the protein detection. This step is usually performed to identify the limit of detection of the sensor, that is, the lowest concentration of the protein that can be reliably detected. Next, to test the specificity of the sensor, the detection of other proteins that have similar and/or different structure from the target protein, dissolved in the same buffer is performed to identify if they bind the surface of the sensor or not. These proteins are usually called controls or control proteins. In most of the cases, control proteins do bind the surface nonspecifically up to a certain threshold; however, the signal from control proteins is usually much lower than the target protein. Therefore such nonspecific binding should be accounted during the data analysis process. Thirdly, once the biosensors pass the above two steps, the target protein is then dissolved in a spiked samples such as serum, urine, etc. The target protein detection in spiked samples starts from low to high concentrations. This step is important since it shows the binding ability of the sensor to the target protein in a rich medium. Rich medium consists of various biomolecules from large molecular complexes, cell debris as well as small molecules and ions. To eliminate larger molecular complexes, filtering of the sample through a membrane filter can be performed. In addition, the dilution of the sample in a buffer can be performed. The dilution factor of the sample differs from one study to another. And the last and the most important aspect is testing the sensor in real sample and/or environment and further validation. The results obtained from spiked sample measurements, that is concentration correlation curve, could be used to describe the results obtained from real sample measurement.

Table 13.4 briefly summarizes currently available optical fiber–based biosensors for protein detection. Most of the optical fiber–based biosensors for protein detection made use of TFBG fiber exhibiting an SPR phenomenon. Such biosensors have been widely used for the detection of biomarkers such as C-reactive

Table 13.4 Currently available optical fiber–based biosensors for protein detection.

Fiber type and modification	Receptor	Analyte (protein)	Fiber surface modification	Detection limit	References
FBG etched	CRP antibody	CRP	1. Conjugation of CRP antibody via graphene oxide through EDC/NHS activation 2. Target protein detection	0.01 mg/L	Sridevi, Vasu, Asokan, and Sood (2015)
	Aptamer-NH_2	Thrombin	1. Silanisation with APTES 2. Crosslinking aptamers via glutaraldehyde 3. Blocking with BSA 4. Target protein detection	10 nM 0.075–0.110 nM	Bekmurzayeva et al. (2018) (Sypabekova et al., 2019)
TFBG excitation of SPR(50 nm Au)Tilt angle 10°	Aptamer-SH		1. Aptamer conjugation via S–S bond 2. Protein detection	22.6 nM	Shevchenko et al. (2011)
TFBG tilt angle 20°	Biotinylated BSA	Anti-BSA	1. Polyacrylic-acid film generation 2. Conjugation of biotinylated BSA probes via avidin–biotin interactions 3. Target protein detection	86–87 μg/L	Maguis et al. (2008)
TFBG excitation of SPR, LSPR(50 nm Au, 13 nm AuNPs)Tilt angle 20°	1 Aptamer-SH2 Aptamer-SH	Thrombin	1. Aptamer conjugation via S–S bond 2. Target protein detection	1 nM	Lao et al. (2019)
TFBG excitation of SPR, LSPR(30 nm Au nanocages)Tilt angle 10°	Biotin	Avidin	1. Silanisation with APTMS 2. Crosslinking cysteamine via glutaraldehyde 3. Conjugation of Au nanocages 4. 11-Mercaptoundecanoic acid (MUA) formation, EDC/NHS activation and protein conjugation 5. Target protein detection	8–11 pM	Lepinay, Staff, Ianoul, and Albert (2014)
TFBG excitation of SPR(50 nm Au)Tilt angle 10°	Boronic acid	Glycoprotein	1. (3-((11-mercaptoun-decanamido) methyl) phenyl) boronic acid 2. Blocking with BSA 3. Target protein detection	15.56 nM	Zhang et al. (2017)
TFBG excitation of SPR(2–3 nm Cr, 30 nm Ag) depositionTilt angle 20°		Proteinurea		1.5×10^{-3} mg/mL	Guo et al. (2016)
TFBG excitation of SPR(35 nm Au)Tilt angle 7°	Aptamer-SH	HER-2 (Human Epidermal Growth Factor Receptor-2)	1. Aptamer conjugation via S–S bond 2. Blocking with MCH 3. Target protein detection	10^{-12} g/mL	Lobry et al. (2020)

TFBG excitation of SPR(50 nm Au)Tilt angle 20°	Aquaporin 2 antibody	Aquaporin 2	1. MUA formation, EDC/NHS activation and antibody conjugation 2. Target protein detection	1.5 ng/mL	Han et al. (2017)
TFBG excitation of SPR(50 nm Au)Tilt angle 6°	(a) Biotin(b) Transferrin antibody	(a) Streptavidin (b) Transferrin	a. Biotinylated thiol formation (mercaptoundecylhexaethyleneoxy biotin amide) b. 6-Mercaptohexanoic acid formation, EDC/NHS activation and transferrin conjugation	(a) 2 pM(b) 10^{-6} g/mL	Voisin, Pilate, Damman, Megret, and Caucheteur (2014)
TFBG excitation of SPR(50 nm Au)Tilt angle 7° TFBG excitation of SPR(5 nm Au)Tilt angle 7° TFBG excitation of SPR35 nm AuTilt angle 7° TFBG excitation of SPR35 nm Au by ELP (electroless plating) Tilt angle 7° TFBG tilt angle 7°	CK17 antibody	Cytokeratin	1. Mercaptopoly(ethylene glycol) carboxylic acid formation, EDC/NHS activation and antibody conjugation 2. Blocking with BSA 3. Target protein detection 1. Silanisation with APTMS 2. Blocking with BSA 3. Target protein detection	10^{-10} g/mL $\leq 10^{-12}$ g/mL $\sim 10^{-12}$ g/mL $\sim 10^{-11}$ g/mL $\sim 10^{-9}$ g/mL	Caucheteur, Loyez, Gonzalez-Vila, and Wattiez (2018), Loyez, Albert, Caucheteur, and Wattiez (2018), Loyez et al. (2019), and Ribaut et al. (2017)
TFBG, tilt angle 20°	Aquaporin 2 antibody	Aquaporin 2	Au coating, 11-Mercaptoundecanoic acid formation, EDC/NHS activation and antibody conjugation	1.5 ng/mL	Khan et al. (2018)
TFBG, tilt angle 6°	Transferrin antibody	Transferrin	Au coating, 6-Mercaptohexanoic acid formation, EDC/NHS activation and antibody conjugation	10^{-6} g/mL	Voisin et al. (2014)
LPG periodicity 110 μm	IgM antibody	Antihuman IgM	Poly(allylamine hydrochloride)/gold-coated silica nanoparticles, 11-Mercaptoundecanoic acid (11-MUA) formation, EDC/NHS activation and antibody conjugation, blocking with BSA	22 pg/mm^2	Liu et al. (2018)

protein, thrombin, proteinurea, cytokeratin (CK), etc. In all of the cases, a thin metal layer, usually Au, is deposited on the surface of the TFBG fiber that is used for the generation of SPR as well as to immobilize the specific receptors. The recent work by Loyez et al. (2019) targeted the immediate diagnosis of lung cancer in distal bronchial tree. The group manufactured a minimally invasive TFBG optical fiber imbedded inside the catheter. The set-up was consisted of optical fiber grating connected to the optical interrogator through a light polarizer. The device was designed to detect cancer cell surface biomarker CK17 by functionalizing the surface of the fiber with CK17-specific antibodies. Ex vivo studies on freshly resected human lobectomies showed that the device is capable of detecting the biomarker and hence distinguish healthy patient samples from diseased ones. The device could also give an information on the stiffness of the tissue enabling the correct positioning of the catheter. The device was validated in in vivo studies in anesthetized pig lungs corresponding to the results obtained in ex vivo studies.

Another protein biomarker named aquaporin for nephrotic syndrome was detected by TFBG optical fiber via the antibodies immobilized on the fiber surface (Han et al., 2017). The protein was also detected in rat urine samples with a real-time intensity change difference between the control group and the diseased group. The sensor had a sensitivity of 1.5 ng/mL in an in-site detection and a possibility to be easily placed in a hypodermic needle to allow similar measurements in vivo.

13.5 Bacterial cell detection

Bacterial cells are important targets for detection and identification since they are the common cause of many infectious diseases. The common process of bacterial cell detection includes microscopy, biochemical analysis, and cell culture. Due to its limitations such as costly, time consuming procedure and the need in trained personnel facilitated the emergence of point of care and portable biosensing devices including optical fiber–based biosensors. The detection of bacterial cells is important in the fields such as public health, medicine, food safety, and security.

The development of biosensors for the whole cell detection is somehow a challenging task. First of all, size of the cell is much larger (micrometer) than the size of the protein (nanometer) and exhibits different shapes (rod, spherical, and spiral shaped) and hence the fluidic system and/or cell detection mechanism needs to be well thought unlike detecting smaller molecules such as proteins. Secondly, the surface of the bacterial cell is complex covered with different surface epitopes which can lead to nonspecific interactions with the sensor surface (Ahmed, Rushworth, Hirst, & Millner, 2014). Bacterial cell contains two outer layers: cell wall and cell membrane. The outer layer of the bacterial cell is called cell wall, which is composed of a polymer matrix named peptidoglycan. Depending on the structure and the thickness of the cell wall, bacterial cell is classified into two groups: Gram positive and Gram negative bacteria. The outer lipid membrane of Gram negative bacteria contains lipopolysaccharides (LPS) and peptidoglycan wall surrounding Gram positive bacteria contains extra components such as lipids, surface proteins, and glycoproteins. The specific cell wall associated with surface proteins, LPS, glycoproteins, and peptidoglycan is the main targets for the recognition. The specific recognition could be facilitated by receptors such as carbohydrate-binding proteins, antibodies, and synthetic short oligonucleotides (aptamers) that are selected against whole bacteria or either against specific cell surface proteins and viruses that bind particular bacterial cells. Biosensors based on bacterial recognition should offer high specificity, discrimination between viable and nonviable cells, inexpensive, small, easy to operate and label free, with little or no sample preparation. The sample preparation usually involves bacterial cell culturing, centrifugation, and cell resuspension.

The detection of bacterial cells is possible on different types of optical fibers. For instance, Srinivasan et al. showed the detection of *Escherichia coli* bacteria on FBG fibers by immobilizing antibodies specific to the bacterium (Srinivasan, Umesh, Murali, Asokan, & Siva Gorthi, 2017). *E. coli* bacteria are associated with the pathogenesis of several diseases involving the intestine, bladder, and kidneys. The study nicely showed the shift in the reflected Bragg wavelength, which was used to dynamically monitor the antibody immobilization of FBG fiber and interaction of *E. coli* with the functionalized fiber. The use of antibodies, however, has some limitations such as high price, stability, and cross-binding to other bacteria, which may result in false positives (Balasubramanian, Sorokulova, Vodyanoy, & Simonian, 2007). In addition, the detection of live bacterial cells add an extra obstacle in creating a good biosensor. To distinguish viable cells from nonviable ones, Tripathi et al. used T4 bacteriophage as a bioreceptor for the detection of *E. coli* bacteria (Tripathi et al., 2012). Bacteriophage is a type of virus that infects the live bacteria. T4 bacteriophage was covalently immobilized on an etched LPG fiber with a reliable detection of *E. coli* at concentrations as low as 10^3 cfu/mL.

13.6 Human cell detection

Unlike bacterial cell, human cells do not contain a cell wall and contain only cell membrane. The cell membrane contains specific imbedded surface proteins and carbohydrate sugar chains. To detect human cells, the cells first need to be grown or cultured on special media followed by harvesting. Harvesting is the process where a special chemical is added to detach the cell from the surface. Harvested cells are then centrifuged at a certain speed and sometimes fixed. After the centrifugation, the number of resuspended cells is counted. For concentration-dependent analysis, the stock solution is serial diluted and detected. To remove unbound cells, the surface of the fiber is usually washed followed by signal recording. Other cell lines closely related to the target cell line can be used as a control to show the specificity toward the target cell.

Human cell detection is based on the same principle where the detection is achieved by immobilizing-specific receptors that can specifically bind a cell in interest. The receptor could bind a specific feature of the cell, such as surface proteins. The receptors in the form of antibodies or aptamers could be selected against that protein which is only present on particular cell type. Like in other biosensing platforms, the key of developing a successful biosensor is the specific interaction between the bioreceptor and the cell in interest. An example of such bioreceptor is aptamer called MAMA2 specifically selected against mammaglobin protein present on breast cancer cells (Fig. 13.2). By immobilizing the MAMA2 aptamer on the surface of the TFBG-based optical fiber biosensor, it was possible to detect circulating breast cancer cells (MDA-MB-415) with an LOD of 49 cells/mL. The additional use of aptamer-coated Au nanoparticles allowed a twofold amplification of the biosensor response with an LOD 10 cells/mL (Loyez et al., 2020). The application of Au nanoparticles facilitated the generation of local SPR and hence increasing the detection threshold. The biosensor presented a good specificity result as compared to other breast cancer cell lines which do not express mammaglobin proteins (MCF-10A and HEK-2). This study demonstrated the feasibility of optical fiber–based biosensors for label free, sensitive, and specific detection of the cells.

Another study demonstrated specific single cell-sensing in real time and for targeting membrane proteins in intact cells on an Au-coated TFBG fibers (Malachovska et al., 2015). Antibodies against membrane proteins served as bioreceptors. The developed sensor was able to monitor, in real time, the specific attachment of single intact cells in concentrations from 3×10^6 cells/mL. In this work, nonfunctionalized optical fiber served as a control. Some studies involving cell detection used standard laboratory glass microscope coverslips as incubation chambers whereas other preferred to design a microfluidic system which closely mimics the blood vessels. In addition to detection, characterization techniques such as atomic force microscopy, confocal microscopy and/or scanning electron microscopy can be used to visualize the cell that bound the fiber surface. The most relevant methods for optical fiber biosensors for detection of cells are listed in Table 13.5.

13.7 Performance of biosensors

Temperature is an important parameter to consider when building an optical fiber biosensor since optical fiber. Many of the optical fiber structures used in biosensor fabrication can be sensitive to temperature including FBG, side-polished fibers, photonic crystal fiber, and tapered (Roriz, Silva, Frazao, & Novais, 2020). Maintaining constant temperature throughout the measurements is important since such parameters as resonance wavelength (e.g., in LPFG-based platform) is

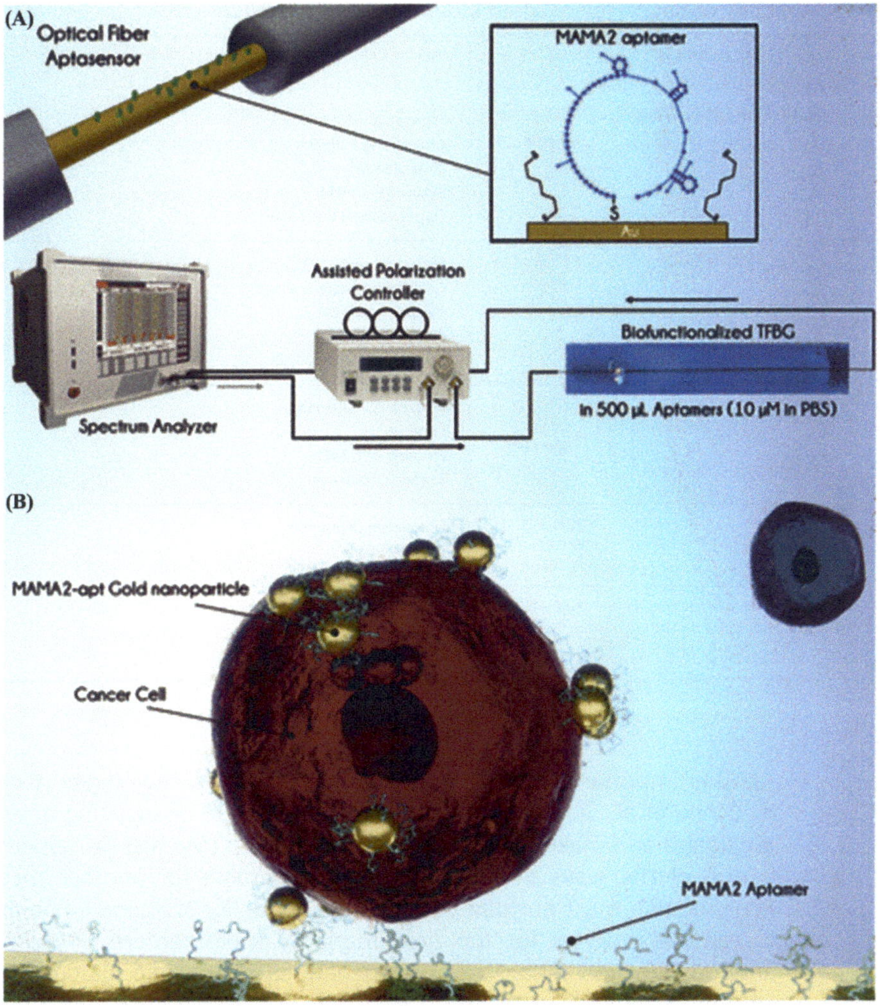

Figure 13.2 (A) Presentation of the experimental setup, using gold-coated TFBGs biofunctionalized with thiolated aptamers and blocked with mercaptohexanol. The optical fiber is connected to a spectrum analyzer and a polarization controller. Liquid samples are added to the sensing area into a low-bind gut container to ensure total immersion of the grating while limiting the needed volumes to 500–800 μL. (B) Artistic view of the target cancer cells interacting with aptamers (the same MAMA2 aptamers) immobilized on the optical fiber surface and functionalized gold nanoparticles (representation not to scale). Source: *Adapted from Loyez, M., Hassan, E. M., Lobry, M., Liu, F., Caucheteur, C., Wattiez, R., ... Albert, J. (2020). Rapid detection of circulating breast cancer cells using a multiresonant optical fiber aptasensor with plasmonic amplification.* ACS Sensors, *5(2), 454–463.*

a strong function of temperature. Especially built flow cells with a thermocouple and thermometric feedback control unit can be used for such purposes (Baliyan et al., 2016).

Table 13.5 Summary of optical fiber–based biosensors used for cell detection.

Fiber type and modification	Receptor	Analyte	Surface modification	Detection limit	References
FBG	*E. coli* antibody	*E. coli* bacteria	1. Silanisation with APTES 2. Crosslinking antibody via glutaraldehyde 3. Blocking with BSA 4. Target bacteria detection		Srinivasan et al. (2017)
LPG etched	Bacteriophage	*E. coli* bacteria	1. Silanisation with APTES 2. Crosslinking bacteriophage via glutaraldehyde 3. Blocking with BSA 4. Target bacteria detection	10^3 cfu/mL	Tripathi et al. (2012)
TFBG excitation of SPR, LSPR(50 nm Au, 10 nm AuNPs)Tilt angle 8°	Aptamer-SH (mammaglobin-A)	Circulating breast cancer cell	1. Aptamer conjugation via S–S bond 2. Blocking with MCH 3. Target cell detection	49 cells/mL	Loyez et al. (2020)
TFBG excitation of SPR (50 nm Au)	Fibronectin	NIH-3T3 fibroblast cell density	1. Fibronectin deposition 2. Cell seeding		Shevchenko et al. (2014)
TFBG excitation of SPR (50 nm Au)Tilt angle 5–8°	Epidermal growth factor receptor (EGFR) antibody	Epithelial cells	1. Conjugation of antibody via Dojindo's carboxylic acid 2. Target cell detection	3×10^6 cells /mL	Malachovska et al. (2015)

Another important characteristics of biosensor are its regeneration and reusability (Zhou et al., 2018). Regeneration often refers to dissociating of analyte from the ligand and making ligand site available again (Morales & Halpern, 2018). It is one of the ways to make the sensor reusable for another measurement. Regeneration must not damage the binding ability of ligand while making sure to remove analytes for the next round of measurement. Protein bound to antibody-covered surface can be regenerated with acidic solutions such as glycine buffers (pH 2–2.3) (Zhou et al., 2018). Regeneration of the sensor can also be done using 1% sodium dodecyl sulfate which was used to disrupt the binding of IgG and anti-IgG (Chiavaioli et al., 2018). Baseline signal can be recorded after regeneration (Chiavaioli et al., 2018). Metal ions can be regenerated from the surface while maintaining the activity of the enzyme (ligand) with L-cysteine (Kuswandi et al., 2001).

Stability and durability of the fabricated biosensor dictate whether it can be repeatedly used in real-life applications and over reduces the cost of analysis (Pahurkar et al., 2015). The stability of the sensors (LSPR covered with GNP; prior to antibody functionalization) can be tested by measuring the RI in testing solutions for 2 weeks with the interval of 2 days (Cao, Tu, Sun, & Grattan, 2013). In other cases, the stability of biosensor was analyzed by testing the analyte measurement every 2 days

Table 13.6 Testing specificity of optical fiber biosensors.

Target analyte	Species used in specificity tests	Comments	References
Hg^{2+}	Pb^{2+}, Fe^{2+}, Mg^{2+}, Zn^{2+}, Ca^{2+}, and Cu^{2+}	Interfering ions No significant interferences to target detection	Jia et al. (2018)
Cd^{2+}	Pb^{2+} Zn^{2+} $CrO_4{}^{2-}$	Same concentration as target (10 ppb)	Cai et al. (2020)
Ochratoxin A	Aflatoxin B1 Aflatoxin B2 Deoxynivalenol Chloramphenicol	Other toxins 0.01 nM	Wang et al. (2015)
Ochratoxin A	Zearalenone Ochratoxin B	Other toxins	Lee et al. (2018)
Urea	Glucose Ascorbic acid L-Alanine L-Arginine Their combination with target in PBS	Interfering substances No response	Botewad et al. (2018)
Tryacylglyceride	Urea (42 mg/dL) Glucose (150 mg/dL) Ethanol (80 mg/dL) Added to target analyte All physiological concentrations	Interfering substances No response	Baliyan et al. (2016)
Glucose	Urea Ascorbic acid Lactic acid Fructose Sucrose	Interfering substances 10 mM each Lower signal	Pahurkar et al. (2015)
Glucose	Na^{+}, K^{+}, Ca^{2+}, Mg^{2+}, Cl^{-}, HCO^{3-}, $HPO_4{}^{2-}$ Ascorbic acid Fructose Urea Sucrose		Xu et al. (2020)
ssDNA	Noncomplementary ssDNA	Small signal change 100 nM, 50 nM, 25 nM, 10 nM, 5 nM, 2.0 nM, 1.0 nM	Gao et al. (2016)
Glutamate	Taurine, creatinine, and lactate	Negligible signal 0–10 mM	Semwal and Gupta (2018)
Dopamine	Serotonin 5-HT (10^{-6} M) Urea (10^{-3} M) Glucose (10^{-3} M) Vitamin C (10^{-3} M)	Interfering molecules with high concentrations	Hu et al. (2018)
Cardiac troponin	CRP, IgG, and PSA	Same concentration as target analyte (10 fg/mL) Lower response	Zhou et al. (2018)

(Continued)

Table 13.6 Continued

Target analyte	Species used in specificity tests	Comments	References
His-Mccs	Trypsin BSA HSA	Also His-tagged as a target	Ravikumar, Chen, Jayaraman, Poh, and Chan (2018)
IgG	Rabbit IgG Human IgG BSA	1 mg/mL	Zheng, Lang, Shen, and Shen (2018)
Peptide His-MccS	Trypsin BSA HSA	All with high histidine content Significantly lower dip shift	Ravikumar et al. (2018)
Cell	A431 cell line OCM1 cell line	Overexpressed receptor Negative expression	Malachovska et al. (2015)

BSA, Bovine serum albumin; *CRP*, C-reactive protein; *His-Mccs*, hexa-histidine tagged microcin; *HSA*, human serum albumin; *IgG*, immunoglobulin G; *PSA*, prostate-specific antigen.

over the period of 30 days (Botewad et al., 2018). Stability of an enzyme-based glucose biosensor was tested for the period of 50 days and was found stable for 36 days. This was performed by measuring one specific concentration every day and storing the sensor at 4°C after each use for the period (Pahurkar et al., 2015). Measuring the same concentration of analyte three (Fan & Wang, 2020) and up to five times (Baliyan et al., 2016) using the sensor with the same surface chemistry can be done to demonstrate its stability.

Carefully designing control experiments is crucial for adequate evaluation of biosensor performance. For this, sensor not functionalized with the ligand can be a good candidate to show that analyte of interest is binding the ligand and not other moieties on the surface. Thus LPFG not functionalized with the ligand was used to check RI cross-sensitivity in analyte detection (Badmos et al., 2017). In another study, U-bent optical fiber without the ligand was used to check the effect the sensing layer has on the measurement of the analyte (Chen et al., 2018).

Specificity of biosensor should also be evaluated to ensure that it can be used to measure the target of interest with minimal interference from other substances. Testing specificity can be achieved by probing different analytes, which are either closely related to the analyte of interest (similar structure and properties) or are interfering substances in the media where they are usually present. Some examples of the testing specificity of optical fiber biosensors are shown in Table 13.6. These include using molecules closely related in both structure and properties (fructose and sucrose in glucose sensing), interfering ions, and small molecules or proteins present in the blood or urea. Serum albumins (BSA and HSA) are among proteins widely used in specificity studies due to their abundance in serum. When cells are used as analytes of interest, cells having the target receptor expressed (if target is extracellular protein) and cells having negative expression can be used as was demonstrated in Malachovska et al. (2015).

References

Ahmed, A., Rushworth, J. V., Hirst, N. A., & Millner, P. A. (2014). Biosensors for whole-cell bacterial detection. *Clinical Microbiology Reviews, 27*(3), 631–646.

Badmos, A. A., Sun, Q. Z., Sun, Z. Y., Zhang, J. X., Yan, Z. J., Lutsyk, P., ... Zhang, L. (2017). Enzyme-functionalized thin-cladding long-period fiber grating in transition mode at dispersion turning point for sugar-level and glucose detection. *Journal of Biomedical Optics, 22*(2).

Balasubramanian, S., Sorokulova, I. B., Vodyanoy, V. J., & Simonian, A. L. (2007). Lytic phage as a specific and selective probe for detection of Staphylococcus aureus—A surface plasmon resonance spectroscopic study. *Biosensors & Bioelectronics, 22*(6), 948–955.

Baliyan, A., Sital, S., Tiwari, U., Gupta, R., & Sharma, E. K. (2016). Long period fiber grating based sensor for the detection of triacylglycerides. *Biosensors & Bioelectronics, 79*, 693–700.

Bekmurzayeva, A., Dukenbayev, K., Shaimerdenova, M., Bekniyazov, I., Ayupova, T., Sypabekova, M., ... Tosi, D. (2018). Etched fiber Bragg grating biosensor functionalized with aptamers for detection of thrombin. *Optics & Laser Technology Under review, 18*(12).

Benounis, M., Jaffrezic-Renault, N., Halouani, H., Lamartine, R., & Dumazet-Bonnamour, I. (2006). Detection of heavy metals by an optical fiber sensor with a sensitive cladding including a new chromogenic calix 4 arene molecule. *Materials Science & Engineering C-Biomimetic and Supramolecular Systems, 26*(2–3), 364–368.

Bertucci, A., Manicardi, A., Candiani, A., Giannetti, S., Cucinotta, A., Spoto, G., ... Corradini, R. (2015). Detection of unamplified genomic DNA by a PNA-based microstructured optical fiber (MOF) Bragg-grating optofluidic system. *Biosensors & Bioelectronics, 63*, 248–254.

Botewad, S. N., Pahurkar, V. G., & Muley, G. G. (2018). Fabrication and evaluation of evanescent wave absorption based polyaniline-cladding modified fiber optic urea biosensor. *Optical Fiber Technology, 40*, 8–12.

Cai, S. S., Pan, H. X., Gonzalez-Vila, A., Guo, T., Gillan, D. C., Wattiez, R., & Caucheteur, C. (2020). Selective detection of cadmium ions using plasmonic optical fiber gratings functionalized with bacteria. *Optics Express, 28*(13), 19740–19749.

Cao, S. Q., Shao, Y., Wang, Y., Wu, T. S., Zhang, L. F., Huang, Y. J., ... Wang, Y. P. (2018). Highly sensitive surface plasmon resonance biosensor based on a low-index polymer optical fiber. *Optics Express, 26*(4), 3988–3994.

Cao, J., Tu, M. H., Sun, T., & Grattan, K. T. V. (2013). Wavelength-based localized surface plasmon resonance optical fiber biosensor. *Sensors and Actuators B-Chemical, 181*, 611–619.

Caucheteur, C., Loyez, M., Gonzalez-Vila, A., & Wattiez, R. (2018). Evaluation of gold layer configuration for plasmonic fiber grating biosensors. *Optics Express, 26*(18), 24154–24163.

Cennamo, N., D'Agostino, G., Galatus, R., Bibbo, L., Pesavento, M., & Zeni, L. (2013). Sensors based on surface plasmon resonance in a plastic optical fiber for the detection of trinitrotoluene. *Sensors and Actuators B-Chemical, 188*, 221–226.

Chauhan, S. K., Punjabi, N., Sharma, D. K., & Mukherji, S. (2016). A silicon nitride coated LSPR based fiber-optic probe for possible continuous monitoring of sucrose content in fruit juices. *Sensors and Actuators B-Chemical, 222*, 1240–1250.

Chen, X., Liu, C., Hughes, M., Nagel, D., Hine, A., & Zhang, L. (2015). EDC-mediated oligonucleotide immobilization on a long period grafting optical biosensor. *Journal of Biosensors and Bioelectronics, 6*(2). Available from https://doi.org/10.4172/2155-6210.1000173.

Chen, K. C., Li, Y. L., Wu, C. W., & Chiang, C. C. (2018). Glucose sensor using U-shaped optical fiber probe with gold nanoparticles and glucose oxidase. *Sensors, 18*(4). Available from https://doi.org/10.3390/s18041217.

Chiavaioli, F., Zubiate, P., Del Villar, I., Zamarreno, C. R., Giannetti, A., Tombelli, S., ... Baldini, F. (2018). Femtomolar detection by nanocoated fiber label-free biosensors. *ACS Sensors, 3*(5), 936–943.

Chryssis, A. N., Saini, S. S., Lee, S. M., Yi, H. M., Bentley, W. E., & Dagenais, M. (2005). Detecting hybridization of DNA by highly sensitive evanescent field etched core fiber Bragg grating sensors. *IEEE Journal of Selected Topics in Quantum Electronics, 11*(4), 864–872.

Dagenais, M., Chryssis, A. N., Yi, H., Lee, S. M., Saini, S. S., & Bentley, W. E. (2005). Optical bio-sensors based on etched fiber Bragg gratings. *Conference on Optoelectronic Integrated Circuits VII, Spie-Int Soc Optical Engineering*, 214–224, San Jose, CA.

Delgado-Pinar, M., Shi, Q., Poveda-Wong, L., Delgado-Pinar, E., Xu, B. J., Zhao, J. L., ... Andres, M. V. (2017). Oligonucleotide-hybridization fiber-optic biosensor using a narrow bandwidth long period grating. *IEEE Sensors Journal, 17*(17), 5503–5509.

Eltzov, E., Pavluchkov, V., Burstin, M., & Marks, R. S. (2011). Creation of a fiber optic based biosensor for air toxicity monitoring. *Sensors and Actuators B-Chemical, 155*(2), 859–867.

Fan, X. C., & Wang, Q. (2020). Sensitive determination of arginine based on hydrogen bonding by a surface plasmon resonance (SPR) sensor. *Instrumentation Science & Technology, 48* (2), 196–211.

Gao, R., Lu, D. F., Cheng, J., Jiang, Y., Jiang, L., Xu, J. D., & Qi, Z. M. (2016). Fiber optofluidic biosensor for the label-free detection of DNA hybridization and methylation based on an in-line tunable mode coupler. *Biosensors & Bioelectronics, 86*, 321–329.

Guo, T., Liu, F., Liang, X., Qiu, X. H., Huang, Y. Y., Xie, C., ... Albert, J. (2016). Highly sensitive detection of urinary protein variations using tilted fiber grating sensors with plasmonic nanocoatings. *Biosensors & Bioelectronics, 78*, 221–228.

Han, L. Z., Guo, T. A., Xie, C., Xu, P., Lao, J. J., Zhang, X. J., ... Guan, B. O. (2017). Specific detection of aquaporin-2 using plasmonic tilted fiber grating sensors. *Journal of Lightwave Technology, 35*(16), 3360–3365.

Hu, W. J., Huang, Y. Y., Chen, C. Y., Liu, Y. K., Guo, T. A., & Guan, B. O. (2018). Highly sensitive detection of dopamine using a graphene functionalized plasmonic fiber-optic sensor with aptamer conformational amplification. *Sensors and Actuators B-Chemical, 264*, 440–447.

Ivask, A., Green, T., Polyak, B., Mor, A., Kahru, A., Virta, M., & Marks, R. (2007). Fibre-optic bacterial biosensors and their application for the analysis of bioavailable Hg and As in soils and sediments from Aznalcollar mining area in Spain. *Biosensors & Bioelectronics, 22*(7), 1396–1402.

Jia, S., Bian, C., Sun, J. Z., Tong, J. H., & Xia, S. H. (2018). A wavelength-modulated localized surface plasmon resonance (LSPR) optical fiber sensor for sensitive detection of mercury(II) ion by gold nanoparticles-DNA conjugates. *Biosensors & Bioelectronics, 114*, 15–21.

Kadashetti, V., Baad, R., Malik, N., Shivakumar, K. M., Vibhute, N., Belgaumi, U., ... Pramod, R. C. (2015). Glucose level estimation in diabetes mellitus by saliva: A bloodless revolution. *Romanian Journal of Internal Medicine, 53*(3), 248–252.

Khan, M. R. R., Watekar, A. V., & Kang, S. W. (2018). Fiber-optic biosensor to detect pH and glucose. *IEEE Sensors Journal, 18*(4), 1528–1538.

King, K. D., Anderson, G. P., Bullock, K. E., Regina, M. J., Saaski, E. W., & Ligler, F. S. (1999). Detecting staphylococcal enterotoxin B using an automated fiber optic biosensor. *Biosensors & Bioelectronics, 14*(2), 163–170.

Kumar, S., Verma, N., & Singh, A. K. (2017). Development of cadmium specific recombinant biosensor and its application in milk samples. *Sensors and Actuators B-Chemical, 240*, 248–254.

Kuswandi, B., Andres, R., & Narayanaswamy, R. (2001). Optical fibre biosensors based on immobilised enzymes. *Analyst, 126*(8), 1469–1491.

Lao, J. J., Han, L. Z., Wu, Z., Zhnag, X. J., Huang, Y. Y., Tang, Y., & Guo, T. (2019). Gold nanoparticle-functionalized surface plasmon resonance optical fiber biosensor: In situ detection of thrombin with 1 nM detection limit. *Journal of Lightwave Technology, 37*(11), 2748–2755.

Lee, B., Park, J. H., Byun, J. Y., Kim, J. H., & Kim, M. G. (2018). An optical fiber-based LSPR aptasensor for simple and rapid in-situ detection of ochratoxin A. *Biosensors & Bioelectronics, 102*, 504–509.

Lepinay, S., Staff, A., Ianoul, A., & Albert, J. (2014). Improved detection limits of protein optical fiber biosensors coated with gold nanoparticles. *Biosensors & Bioelectronics, 52*, 337–344.

Lin, T. J., & Chung, M. F. (2009). Detection of cadmium by a fiber-optic biosensor based on localized surface plasmon resonance. *Biosensors & Bioelectronics, 24*(5), 1213–1218.

Liu, L. L., Marques, L., Correia, R., Morgan, S. P., Lee, S. W., Tighe, P., ... Korposh, S. (2018). Highly sensitive label-free antibody detection using a long period fibre grating sensor. *Sensors and Actuators B-Chemical, 271*, 24–32.

Lobry, M., Lahem, D., Loyez, M., Debliquy, M., Chah, K., David, M., & Caucheteur, C. (2019). Non-enzymatic D-glucose plasmonic optical fiber grating biosensor. *Biosensors & Bioelectronics, 142*, 111506.

Lobry, M., Loyez, M., Hassan, E. M., Chah, K., DeRosa, M. C., Goormaghtigh, E., ... Caucheteur, C. (2020). Multimodal plasmonic optical fiber grating aptasensor. *Optics Express, 28*(5), 7539–7551.

Long, F., He, M. A., Zhu, A. N., Song, B. D., Sheng, J. W., & Shi, H. C. (2010). Compact quantitative optic fiber-based immunoarray biosensor for rapid detection of small analytes. *Biosensors & Bioelectronics, 26*(1), 16–22.

Loyez, M., Albert, J., Caucheteur, C., & Wattiez, R. (2018). Cytokeratins biosensing using tilted fiber gratings. *Biosensors-Basel, 8*(3), 74.

Loyez, M., Hassan, E. M., Lobry, M., Liu, F., Caucheteur, C., Wattiez, R., ... Albert, J. (2020). Rapid detection of circulating breast cancer cells using a multiresonant optical fiber aptasensor with plasmonic amplification. *ACS Sensors, 5*(2), 454–463.

Loyez, M., Larrieu, J. C., Chevineau, S., Remmelink, M., Leduc, D., Bondue, B., ... Caucheteur, C. (2019). In situ cancer diagnosis through online plasmonics. *Biosensors & Bioelectronics, 131*, 104–112.

Luo, B. B., Yan, Z. J., Sun, Z. Y., Li, J. F., & Zhang, L. (2014). Novel glucose sensor based on enzyme immobilized 81 degrees tilted fiber grating. *Optics Express, 22*(25), 30571–30578.

Maguis, S., Laffont, G., Ferdinand, P., Carbonnier, B., Kham, K., Mekhalif, T., & Millot, M. C. (2008). Biofunctionalized tilted fiber Bragg gratings for label-free immunosensing. *Optics Express, 16*(23), 19049–19062.

Malachovska, V., Ribaut, C., Voisin, V., Surin, M., Leclere, P., Wattiez, R., & Caucheteur, C. (2015). Fiber-optic SPR immunosensors tailored to target epithelial cells through membrane receptors. *Analytical Chemistry, 87*(12), 5957–5965.

Morales, M. A., & Halpern, J. M. (2018). Guide to selecting a biorecognition element for biosensors. *Bioconjugate Chemistry, 29*(10), 3231–3239.

Morisawa, M., Amemiya, Y., Kohzu, H., Liang, C. X., & Muto, S. (2001). Plastic optical fibre sensor for detecting vapour phase alcohol. *Measurement Science and Technology, 12*(7), 877–881.

Narang, U., Anderson, G. P., Ligler, F. S., & Burans, J. (1997). Fiber optic-based biosensor for ricin. *Biosensors & Bioelectronics, 12*(9–10), 937–945.

Nuriman., Kuswandi, B., & Verboom, W. (2011). Optical fiber chemical sensing of Hg(II) ions in aqueous samples using a microfluidic device containing a selective tripodal chromoionophore-PVC film. *Sensors and Actuators B-Chemical, 157*(2), 438–443.

Oehme, I., & Wolfbeis, O. S. (1997). Optical sensors for determination of heavy metal ions. *Mikrochimica Acta, 126*(3–4), 177–192.

Ogert, R. A., Brown, J. E., Singh, B. R., Shriverlake, L. C., & Ligler, F. S. (1992). Detection of clostridium-botulinum toxin-A using a fiber optic-based biosensor. *Analytical Biochemistry, 205*(2), 306–312.

Pahurkar, V. G., Tamgadge, Y. S., Gambhire, A. B., & Muley, G. G. (2015). Glucose oxidase immobilized PANI cladding modified fiber optic intrinsic biosensor for detection of glucose. *Sensors and Actuators B-Chemical, 210*, 362–368.

Peterson, R. D., Cunningham, B. T., & Andrade, J. E. (2014). A photonic crystal biosensor assay for ferritin utilizing iron-oxide nanoparticles. *Biosensors & Bioelectronics, 56*, 320–327.

Ravikumar, R., Chen, L. H., Jayaraman, P., Poh, C. L., & Chan, C. C. (2018). Chitosan-nickel film based interferometric optical fiber sensor for label-free detection of histidine tagged proteins. *Biosensors & Bioelectronics, 99*, 578–585.

Razo-Medina, D. A., Trejo-Duran, M., & Alvarado-Mendez, E. (2018). Cholesterol biosensor based on a plastic optical fibre with sol-gel: structural analysis and sensing properties. *Journal of Modern Optics, 65*(3), 348–352.

Ribaut, C., Loyez, M., Larrieu, J. C., Chevineau, S., Lambert, P., Remmelink, M., ... Caucheteur, C. (2017). Cancer biomarker sensing using packaged plasmonic optical fiber gratings: Towards in vivo diagnosis. *Biosensors & Bioelectronics, 92*, 449–456.

Roriz, P., Silva, S., Frazao, O., & Novais, S. (2020). Optical fiber temperature sensors and their biomedical applications. *Sensors, 20*(7), 2113.

Semwal, V., & Gupta, B. D. (2018). LSPR- and SPR-based fiber-optic cholesterol sensor using immobilization of cholesterol oxidase over silver nanoparticles coated graphene oxide nanosheets. *IEEE Sensors Journal, 18*(3), 1039–1046.

Sharma, P., Semwal, V., & Gupta, B. D. (2019). A highly selective LSPR biosensor for the detection of taurine realized on optical fiber substrate and gold nanoparticles. *Optical Fiber Technology, 52*, 101962.

Shevchenko, Y., Camci-Unal, G., Cuttica, D. E., Dokmeci, M. R., Albert, J., & Khademhosseini, A. (2014). Surface plasmon resonance fiber sensor for real-time and label-free monitoring of cellular behavior. *Biosensors & Bioelectronics, 56*, 359–367.

Shevchenko, Y., Francis, T. J., Blair, D. A. D., Walsh, R., DeRosa, M. C., & Albert, J. (2011). In situ biosensing with a surface plasmon resonance fiber grating aptasensor. *Analytical Chemistry, 83*(18), 7027–7034.

Shrivastav, A. M., & Gupta, B. D. (2016). SPR and molecular imprinting-based fiber-optic melamine sensor with high sensitivity and low limit of detection. *IEEE Journal of Selected Topics in Quantum Electronics, 22*(4). Available from https://doi.org/10.1109/JSTQE.2015.2478876.

Singh, S., Mishra, S. K., & Gupta, B. D. (2013). SPR based fibre optic biosensor for phenolic compounds using immobilization of tyrosinase in polyacrylamide gel. *Sensors and Actuators B-Chemical, 186*, 388–395.

Sridevi, S., Vasu, K. S., Asokan, S., & Sood, A. K. (2015). Sensitive detection of C-reactive protein using optical fiber Bragg gratings. *Biosensors & Bioelectronics, 65*, 251–256.

Srinivasan, R., Umesh, S., Murali, S., Asokan, S., & Siva Gorthi, S. (2017). Bare fiber Bragg grating immunosensor for real-time detection of *Escherichia coli* bacteria. *Journal of Biophotonics, 10*(2), 224–230.

Sypabekova, M., Korganbayev, S., Gonzalez-Vila, A., Caucheteur, C., Shaimerdenova, M., Ayupova, T., ... Tosi, D. (2019). Functionalized etched tilted fiber Bragg grating aptasensor for label-free protein detection. *Biosensors & Bioelectronics, 146*, 111765.

Tan, R. X., Ibsen, M., & Tjin, S. C. (2019). Optical fiber refractometer based metal ion sensors. *Chemosensors, 7*(4), 63.

Tierney, S., Falch, B. M. H., Hjelme, D. R., & Stokke, B. T. (2009). Determination of glucose levels using a functionalized hydrogel-optical fiber biosensor: Toward continuous monitoring of blood glucose in vivo. *Analytical Chemistry, 81*(9), 3630–3636.

Tripathi, S. M., Bock, W. J., Mikulic, P., Chinnappan, R., Ng, A., Tolba, M., & Zourob, M. (2012). Long period grating based biosensor for the detection of Escherichia coli bacteria. *Biosensors & Bioelectronics, 35*(1), 308–312.

Usha, S. P., & Gupta, B. D. (2018). Urinary p-cresol diagnosis using nanocomposite of ZnO/ MoS_2 and molecular imprinted polymer on optical fiber based lossy mode resonance sensor. *Biosensors & Bioelectronics, 101*, 135–145.
Usha, S. P., Shrivastav, A. M., & Gupta, B. D. (2017). A contemporary approach for design and characterization of fiber-optic-cortisol sensor tailoring LMR and ZnO/PPY molecularly imprinted film. *Biosensors & Bioelectronics, 87*, 178–186.
Voisin, V., Pilate, J., Damman, P., Megret, P., & Caucheteur, C. (2014). Highly sensitive detection of molecular interactions with plasmonic optical fiber grating sensors. *Biosensors & Bioelectronics, 51*, 249–254.
Wang, R. Y., Xiang, Y., Zhou, X. H., Liu, L. H., & Shi, H. C. (2015). A reusable aptamer-based evanescent wave all-fiber biosensor for highly sensitive detection of Ochratoxin A. *Biosensors & Bioelectronics, 66*, 11–18.
Xu, B., Huang, J., Ding, L. Y., & Cai, J. (2020). Graphene oxide-functionalized long period fiber grating for ultrafast label-free glucose biosensor. *Materials Science & Engineering C-Materials for Biological Applications, 107*, 110329.
Zhang, J., Tang, X. L., Dong, J. H., Wei, T., & Xiao, H. (2009). Zeolite thin film-coated long period fiber grating sensor for measuring trace organic vapors. *Sensors and Actuators B-Chemical, 135*(2), 420–425.
Zhang, Y., Wang, F., Qian, S. Y., Liu, Z. X., Wang, Q., Gu, Y. Y., ... Peng, W. (2017). A novel fiber optic surface plasmon resonance biosensors with special boronic acid derivative to detect glycoprotein. *Sensors, 17*(10), 2259.
Zhang, X. J., Wu, Z., Liu, F., Fu, Q. Q., Chen, X. Y., Xu, J., ... Albert, J. (2018). Hydrogen peroxide and glucose concentration measurement using optical fiber grating sensors with corrodible plasmonic nanocoatings. *Biomedical Optics Express, 9*(4), 1735–1744.
Zheng, Y. F., Lang, T. T., Shen, T. T., & Shen, C. Y. (2018). Simple immunoglobulin G sensor based on thin core single-mode fiber. *Optical Fiber Technology, 41*, 104–108.
Zhou, W. C., Li, K. W., Wei, Y. L., Hao, P., Chi, M. B., Liu, Y. S., & Wu, Y. H. (2018). Ultrasensitive label-free optical microfiber coupler biosensor for detection of cardiac troponin I based on interference turning point effect. *Biosensors & Bioelectronics, 106*, 99–104.
Zhu, G., Agrawal, N., Singh, R., Kumar, S., Zhang, B. Y., Saha, C., & Kumar, C. (2020). A novel periodically tapered structure-based gold nanoparticles and graphene oxide—Immobilized optical fiber sensor to detect ascorbic acid. *Optics and Laser Technology, 127*, 106156.

14

Emerging topics in optical fiber biosensors

14.1 Packaging toward in vivo, real-time detection

A key advantage of optical fiber biosensors (OFBs) over other technologies, such as microelectromechanical sensors, field-effect transistors, or conductometric sensors, is the capability to work at a rapid detection rate and in a miniature form factor. Over recent years, this capability has been exploited for the fabrication of biological sensors, as well as sensors that combine the biochemical detection with physical parameters (e.g., tactile sensors or breathing rate analysis), that are packaged in a way that ensure in vivo operation, or the application in contact with the patient undergoing diagnostic (Loyez et al., 2019). In this section, we discuss solutions that have been proposed for endoscopic catheters, urologic devices, and percutaneous needles, which represent the most important case scenarios for OFB devices.

14.1.1 Endoscopic devices

Endoscopy, from the Greek root "*endon*"—inner and "*skopeo*"—to see, is a procedure used in medicine to inspect inside specific parts of the body (Kuipers & Haringsma, 2005). Originally, endoscopy has been mainly referred to as an imaging method: while noncontact imaging methods based on X-ray, magnetic resonance, ultrasound, or positron emission perform an external analysis of body parts, endoscopy is a more invasive procedure as it requires a device (endoscope) inserted within the body. By using a minimally invasive device, such as a guidewire, an externally coupled light source, and an appropriate set of lenses, the endoscope can visualize and magnify small parts of tissues, cavity, and inner parts of the organs under analysis. This method is very popular in the analysis of the gastrointestinal tract with procedures such as colonoscopy or esophagogastroduodenoscopy (Kim & Kim, 2017), for the diagnostic of some respiratory diseases, and more recently for diagnostic of solid tumors.

Modern devices for endoscopy couple the original imaging capability with biosensors, to perform a multiparameter diagnostic that substantially improve the

Optical Fiber Biosensors.
DOI: https://doi.org/10.1016/B978-0-12-819467-6.00014-7

efficiency and the variety of detection. Through the last decade, several research group designed endoscopic devices suited for diagnostic that incorporate fiber optic sensors. One of the most important results has been presented by Arkwright et al. from CSIRO (Commonwealth Scientific and Industrial Research Organisation), Australia, where the research team fabricated prototypes suited for colonoscopy (Arkwright, Underhill, et al., 2009) and a solid-state manometer for the analysis of the upper digestive apparatus (Arkwright, Blenman, et al., 2009). Here, the endoscopy devices combine imaging and an array of fiber Bragg gratings (FBGs): through a radiological label mounted around the device, it is possible to estimate the device positioning during the insertion, while the diagnostic is performed with an array of pressure-sensing FBGs that estimate and localize pressure events such as food swallowing in the esophagus. The work of CSIRO paved the road to endoscopic devices that enhance the diagnostic capabilities through the use of fiber optic sensors.

While the analysis of the digestive apparatus involves mainly the detection of physical parameters, the research recently presented by Loyez et al. (2019) introduces optical fiber biosensing in medical endoscopy, for cancer diagnostic. The packaging and application of this system is shown in Fig. 14.1. In this work, the authors have designed a minimally invasive endoscope that embeds

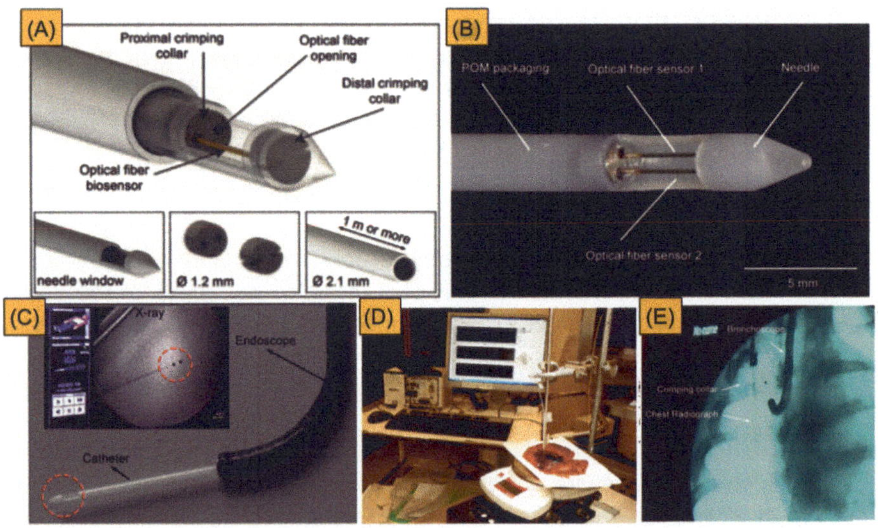

Figure 14.1 Design and application of an endoscopic device embedding plasmonic tilted FBG biosensors for the in situ diagnostic of cancer cells. (A) Design of the device packaging within an endoscopic device. (B) Picture of the optical fiber biosensing endoscope. (C) Photograph of the packaged device and its insertion facilitated by a radiomarked label using X-ray imaging. (D) Application of the endoscopy in ex vivo cancer cells detection. (E) Example of application of the endoscope in lung cancer identification. Source: *Adapted from Loyez, M., Larrieu, J. C., Chevineau, S., Remmelink, M., Leduc, D., Bondue, B., . . . Caucheteur, C. (2019). In situ cancer diagnosis through online plasmonics.* Biosensors and Bioelectronics, 131, *104–112, reproduced with permission.*

a pair of tilted FBG biosensors, functionalized for the detection of a type of cytokeratins that is expressed on the surface of cancer cells. Hence, through the insertion of the endoscope in the lung tissue by a proper device that allows the contact between the fiber and the healthy or tumoral tissue, it is possible to diagnose a difference in response that quantifies the specific biomarker concentration, providing a tool for in situ cancer detection at early stage. The system was tested ex vivo on a number of health and tumor tissue samples.

The sketch of the device is shown in Fig. 14.1A. The catheter has inner/outer diameter of 1.2/1.6 mm, and made of polyoxymethylene (POM), a thermoplastic that is particularly used in medical devices as it combines stiffness in the direction of insertion while preserving the flexural capability to navigate to the sensing point. The plastic of the catheter is terminated with a conical section, to facilitate the penetration through the tissue. In proximity of the tip, a window is obtained in the inner tubular section of the catheter, to host the active part of the sensing device [a plasmonic tilted fiber Bragg gratings (TFBG)]; this lateral fence allows exposing the sensor in contact with the surrounding tissue, and therefore performing a localized detection. This window has a 4 mm length and has two crimps that fix the optical fibers in place. The proximal crimp has two holes, which allows the fibers to pass through, being held in place by a medical-grade glue. The distal crimp has a similar cavity of 0.25 mm diameter, with a pattern that allows the fibers in place. The whole packaging, shown in Fig. 14.1 in schematic and photographically in Fig. 14.2, is then inserted in a bronchoscope, which performs imaging and navigation. This endoscopic device, encapsulating the inner POM catheter, is semiflexible as shown in Fig. 14.3, and allows a bending around the direction perpendicular to the insertion to reach the target region.

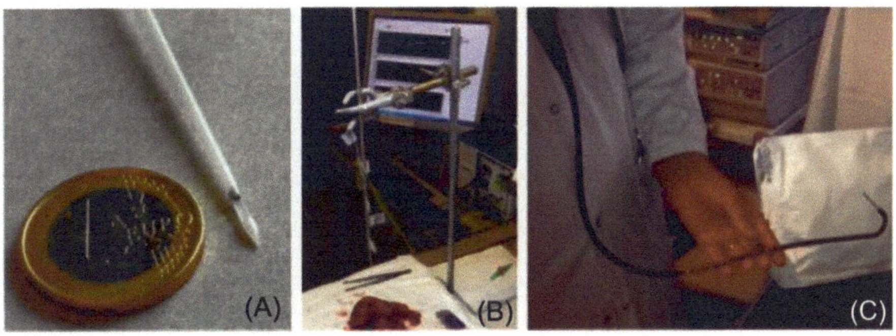

Figure 14.2 Design of a tilted FBG biosensor packaging for medical analysis. (A) View of the packaged sensing tip within a plastic tubular device. (B) Picture of the test condition, inserting the sensor in contact with the tissue under investigation. (C) Photo of the sensor packaged in the channel of an endoscope. Source: *From Guo, T., González-Vila, Á., Loyez, M., & Caucheteur, C. (2017). Plasmonic optical fiber-grating immunosensing: A review.* Sensors, *17(12), 2732.*

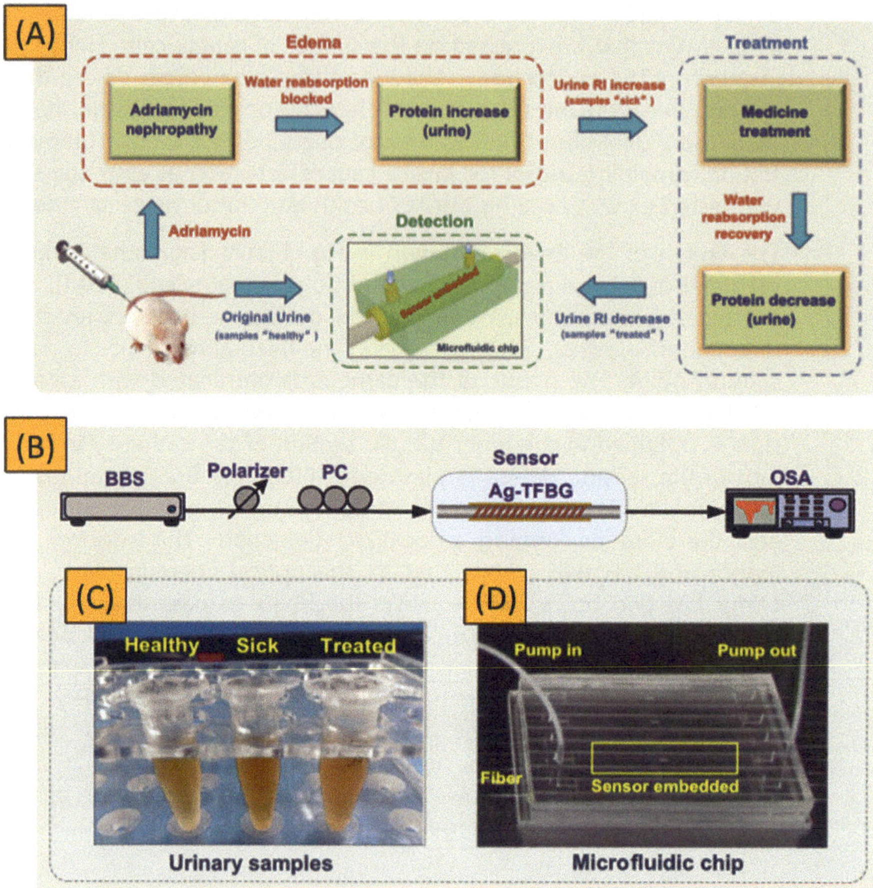

Figure 14.3 Diagnostic of urinary diseases using an optical fiber biosensor functionalized for urinary protein detection. (A) Sketch of the concept of the work, whereas healthy, sick, and treated samples of urine are obtained from mice; (B) scheme of the interrogation system; (C) photographs of urinary samples, characterized by a different refractive index; and (D) photograph of a microfluidic chip where the urine samples are circulated, hosting the fiber biosensor for detection. Source: *From Guo, T., Liu, F., Liang, X., Qiu, X., Huang, Y., Xie, C., . . . Albert, J. (2016). Highly sensitive detection of urinary protein variations using tilted fiber grating sensors with plasmonic nanocoatings.* Biosensors and Bioelectronics, *78, 221–228, reproduced with permission.*

The sensor reported by Loyez et al. has been functionalized for the detection of CK17 cytokeratins, which is a biomarker for lung cancer. With the packaging reported in Loyez et al. (2019), the semiflexible bronchoscope has been inserted ex vivo in samples of health and tumoral lung tissues, to evaluate a difference in response. The experiments have been reported on tissues, as reported in Fig. 14.1D: the needle has been inserted in the tissue from the vertical direction, placing the window hosting the two optical fibers in contact with the tissue undergoing the analysis. Several samples of adenocarcinoma, squamous cells carcinoma, and healthy tissues have been tested, each measuring a different intensity change of the TFBG sensors, which allows a discrimination of health and tumoral cells on the base of CK17 content.

The endoscopic device has also been tested in vivo, to show the capacity to perform a real-time measurement in animals. The experiments have been carried out on one anesthetized pig, inserting the endoscope in the bronchial region through X-ray guidance, as shown in Fig. 14.1E. The sensors measured the response to CK17 levels over a 5-minute period, showing a stable detection of the spectral levels.

A similar endoscopic packaging was reported in 2017 by Guo et al. and is shown in Fig. 14.2. The packaging has a similar form factor, that is a cylindrical cross-section of POM material with a conical tip, and a window where the optical fiber sensor is inserted. This packaging, mounted within the channel of an endoscope for testing tissue samples and other media, has also been used to test for phosphate buffer saline, and to analyze the spectral changes into liquid analytes. An application of this packaging has been presented by Ribaut et al. (2017), in the frame of cancer diagnostic using CK17 biomarkers. Overall, endoscopic design of fiber optic biosensors paves the road to multifunctional devices (Gono, 2008), whereas the diagnostic element can be combined with other sensing and imaging features such as cancer thermotherapies and shape sensing tools for accurate insertion of the medical device (Khan et al., 2019).

14.1.2 Urologic diagnostic

The diagnostic of urinary diseases using optical fiber sensors has been reported in recent years, making use of both pressure sensors (Poeggel et al., 2015) and biosensors. The detection of urinary protein variations using a plasmonic tilted FBG biosensor has been reported by Guo et al. (2016).

The sketch of this work is reported in Fig. 14.3, using a plasmonic TFBG as sensing element. The essence of the work is the real-time detection of the protein content of urine, which is lower in healthy subjects and tends to rise when renal disfunctions are present. The increase of protein excretion in urine is a marker for chronic kidney disease, and it can be diagnosed by inspecting urine samples using a precision biosensor. The method reported by Guo et al. is based on real-time detection of the refractive index (RI) figure of a urine sample, with values ranging from 1.3400 to 1.3408 that cover the range of healthy samples up to diagnosed renal diseases. Samples have been obtained from rats, following the concept in Fig. 14.3A: rats have been divided into three groups corresponding to healthy (no adriamycin nephropathy), sick (presence of adriamycin nephropathy), and treated (adriamycin nephropathy treated with Zhenwutang treatment). Urinary samples, as shown in Fig. 14.3C, have been collected and preserved; the detection system, based on a plasmonic TFBG, has been integrated on a chip.

The sensing system, operating in transmission, has been embedded in a microfluidic chip for the detection having multiple channels, as shown in Fig. 14.3D. The chip was made of PDMS and incorporating channels with 200 μm width and 150 μm height. Sensors have been fixed to the channels using an UV-sensitive adhesive. The active region for sensing is 20 mm along the chip direction, detecting a sample of 35 μL volume. The samples of urine were injected through the channels by an electrically controlled pumping system. The device reported by Guo et al. serves the purpose of rapid detection system for urinary analyte through a low-cost chip. This result was further extended by Han et al. (2017) for a more specific detection of protein, functionalizing the sensor for Aquaporin-2 detection with high precision.

A solution to perform real-time sensing in urology has been proposed by Poeggel et al. (Poeggel et al., 2015) and is shown in Fig. 14.4. This prototype was reported for urodynamic sensing, detecting in real time the pressure during urine infusion and urination processes using a pair of fiber optic sensors for the diagnostic of bladder outlet obstruction (Poeggel et al., 2014) using an optical fiber pressure and temperature sensor. Since the sensing tips are designed using a low-finesse extrinsic fabry-perot interferometer (EFPI) sensor, this architecture can be extended for RI sensing on each sensing fiber. The solution proposed by Poeggel et al. serves two purposes, and for this reason, it has two outlets: one channel is connected to a SmartDyn medical system that infuses a calibrated amount of saline solution within the patient's bladder, to mimic the bladder filling process at a rapid rate; the second channel contains the sensing fibers, which are then connected to the interrogator. For this purpose, a Y-junction is used to combine the two outlets: the optical output is closed using epoxy for plastic sealing to prevent leaks and maintaining the sensors in liquid, while the other outlet is connected to the pumping end of the urodynamic machine. The flexible hollow catheter is made of silicon rubber and has diameter of 5 Fr (equal to 1.67 mm); a Vygon Nutrisafe-2 model has been used for this work. The catheter tip is enclosed, but a series of side holes allows the

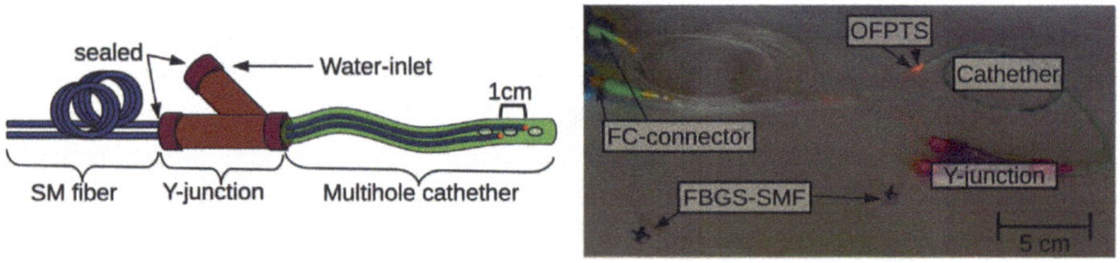

Figure 14.4 Prototype of a urodynamic flexible catheter, incorporating fiber optic sensors for real-time detection. (A) Sketch of the catheter and (B) photo of the catheter with embedded sensors; the tip is illuminated with red light. Source: *From Poeggel, S., Duraibabu, D., Tosi, D., Leen, G., Lewis, E., McGrath, D., . . . Mirone, V. (2015). Differential in vivo urodynamic measurement in a single thin catheter based on two optical fiber pressure sensors.* Journal of Biomedical Optics, 20*(3), 037005, reproduced with permission.*

liquid analyte to penetrate in the inner part of the needle and come in contact with the sensing region.

The system proposed by Poeggel et al. is designed for urodynamic pressure analysis, but it can also be extended to biosensing as the side holes allow a direct contact between the sensor and the liquid analyte sample. The friction exerted by the bladder on the catheter during the insertion is dissipated on the rubber exterior part of the catheter, hence the sensors enclosed inside the catheter are protected. The sensors are also glued to the connector that allows leaving the sensor in place without the use of crimps or other locking elements. The fixation point is external to the patient, which improves the biocompatibility as the portion of the catheter inserted in the bladder does not contain any glued parts or any fixation points.

14.1.3 Percutaneous devices

Percutaneous medical devices are inserted into inner organs or other tissues by piercing through the skin through a needle puncture, and then positioning the device into position by trespassing multiple layers of tissue. Percutaneous needles are used in several cardiovascular, diagnostic, anesthetic, and cancer treatment tasks (Gupta & Madoff, 2007). The two most significant applications of optical fiber sensors embedded in percutaneous devices are based on the epidural space identification (Beisenova, Issatayeva, Tosi, & Molardi, 2018), which serves as a guidance tool for a clinician to correctly identify the epidural space through the analysis of the insertion of the needle, and in supporting cancer diagnostic and treatment by inspecting in situ the alterations of the tissue (Beisenova et al., 2019). Percutaneous sensors can work both in depth within the tissue or close to the skin surface. In case of deep-seated sensing, the form factors include syringe-shaped tips, Chiba needles with a 45 degrees tip for improved tissue penetration, and Tuohy needles with a 90 degrees bent tip that ensures the penetration into the tissue as well as the delivery of fluid from an externally mounted syringe into the tissue. For shallow insertion, instead, miniaturized form factors have been reported having only the fiber sensor vested with a light coating as protective jacket.

Liao et al. reported in 2008 a sensing system designed to operate in close proximity to the skin, for the long-term monitoring of analytes (Liao et al., 2008); the architecture of this system, labeled *sencil* (sensory cilia) is shown in Fig. 14.5, as the sensor is designed to have the size and depth of insertion of human hair. The sensor reported in this work has been functionalized for glucose detection in vivo, measuring interstitial glucose concentration by fluorescence analysis, although the setup can be extended to measurement of analytes at infrared wavelengths.

The packaging of the sencil consists of an optical fiber with a 100 μm diameter, terminated with a hydrogel compound that allows it to pierce through the skin

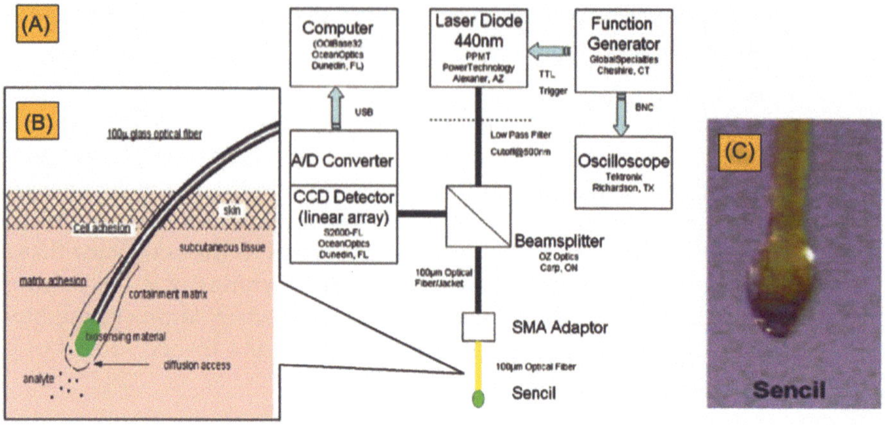

Figure 14.5 Prototype of a percutaneous *sencil* (sensory cilia) for glucose monitoring; the sensor is fabricated around a 100-μm optical fiber for operating under the skin layer. (A) Interrogation system and setup; (B) view of the sensor design and its positioning; and (C) picture of a sencil. Source: *From Liao, K. C., Hogen-Esch, T., Richmond, F. J., Marcu, L., Clifton, W., & Loeb, G. E. (2008). Percutaneous fiber-optic sensor for chronic glucose monitoring in vivo.* Biosensors and Bioelectronics, *23(10), 1458–1465, reproduced with permission.*

and fix the sensor in the location with a stiff fixation. The method used for the hydrogel solution is based on an UV-induced polymerization, which attaches to the biosensing matrix. The precursor, mostly based on polyethylene glycol acrylate, is prepared and stirred. By dipping the optical fiber into the precursor, under UV spot light, and repeating the process multiple times, the fiber gets polymerized at the tip which allows forming a round-shaped coating on the fiber tip, as shown photographically in Fig. 14.5C. By increasing the exposure time of the fiber into the polymeric precursor, it is possible to thicken the fiber tip, hence making the sensor more robust when inserted in place. The work of Liao et al. reports the results of different prototypes that have been tested for glucose sensing on mice, performing long-term sensing through multiple stencils inserted in position.

A work that proposes a percutaneous OFB for cancer diagnostic has been proposed by Liao, Chiu, Fan, Tseng, and Lu (2016), and Fan, Chiu, Lin, Liao, and Liao (2016). This system is based on a customized fiber-optic biosensor made of a bundle of fiber microcapillaries connected to an interrogation system, for the monitoring of the chemotherapy agent induced tumor apoptosis. The authors fabricated a percutaneous device inserted in a syringe applicator that is formed by a bundle of two multimode optical fibers with 200 μm diameter with a cladding of 10 μm, and two capillaries of 50/186 μm inner/outer diameter. The two fibers and two capillaries have been mounted in a cross-shaped section, housed in a tubular syringe. This setup allows combining sensing with the two OFBs, and the delivery of treatment via the two hollow capillaries. By connecting the fiber outputs to a spectrophotometer, the authors have been able to perform a real-time apoptosis detection in cells both in vitro and in vivo, using the outer end of the syringe to penetrate through the tissue.

14.2 Minimal architectures for single-mode fiber biosensing

An emerging trend in optical fiber biosensing is the possibility of engineering sensing probes that have a simplified fabrication process, which therefore keep an eye on the suitability for high-volume fabrication. Devices based on gratings and interferometers usually require multiple fabrication steps, and their performances depend substantially on the quality of the fabrication process as well as on the parameters of the structures. For example, gratings require a laser-based inscription in the fiber core and are often paired with other fabrication methods (etching, tapering, and polarization control); interferometers require multiple splicing methods and fiber polishing; tapers require a furnace with a pulling stage, and in general have a very low success rate for fabrication. In general, several methods that achieve remarkable performances are based on manufacturing methods that require multiple steps and often a low throughout. Surface plasmon resonance (SPR)-based structures represent an easy method for in-fiber sensing that achieves high performance while having a reproducible and easy manufacturing. However, they usually operate with multimode fibers and in the visible spectral range (where fibers carry $\gtrsim$10 times more propagating modes than in the third optical window), and therefore cannot take advantage of the high precision single-mode telecom fibers. In addition, SPR sensors operate in transmission, and therefore require additional components for obtaining a reflection probe.

In very recent times, there has been a substantial interest in developing OFBs based on single-mode telecom fibers operating around 1550 nm as reflection-based probes, but having a substantially simpler fabrication method. This way, we can combine the accurate detection of telecom-based components [e.g., the power stability of single-mode fibers (SMFs)] with a minimalistic and well repeatable approach for fabrication, suitable for high-volume manufacturing, while having similar performances. In general, this type of minimalistic biosensors do not achieve the same levels of reflectivity of gratings (close to 100%) or interferometers (few %); however, using a light detector with a great power sensitivity, it is possible to still achieve a reliable spectral detection, interrogating one or more devices. The key to access this minimalistic detectors is therefore the use of an optical backscatter reflectometer (Froggatt & Moore, 1998) (Luna OBR4600 interrogator, for all the sensors described in this chapter), which detects optical power values in the range of hundreds of fW. On the other hand, the fabrication processes are simple and scalable as the reflective probe is fabricated with simple structures having marginal values of reflectivity.

14.2.1 Reflector-less biosensors

The first architecture for a reflective probe has been demonstrated in a preliminary way in 2018 (Sypabekova et al., 2018) and subsequently extended for thrombin sensing application by Sypabekova et al. (Sypabekova, Aitkulov, Blanc, & Tosi, 2020) in 2020. This type of architecture is labeled as *reflector-less* biosensor because there is no reflective element fabricated in the fiber, but rather the reflected light arises from the Rayleigh scattering that is naturally present in any optical fiber. The principle of operation of a reflector-less biosensor can be synthesized as an etched FBG sensor without the grating element itself; we have described in Section 3.2 the working principle of an etched FBG, and it is based on the change of effective refractive index of the optical fiber in the exposed region, due to the exposure of the core to the surrounding analyte. The change of n_{eff} is transduced to a wavelength shift that applies to the Bragg wavelength of the grating; as such, we obtain an RI-dependent wavelength change that is applied to the FBG spectrum. If we remove the grating from an etched FBG, we would still observe the two phenomena induced in the light propagation: a change of the effective refractive index n_{eff} and a substantial evanescent wave loss occurring in the sensing region. However, we would not have the *fingerprint* of the spectrum, due to the lack of a reflective element.

The Rayleigh scattering, however, is present in any glass optical fiber and is one of the loss factors that is accounted along the propagation (Agrawal, 2011). When light is incident on the glass crystal structure of the fiber, due to the several defects and inhomogeneities of the material, a tiny portion of the light is reflected backwards. Elastic scattering effects (Rayleigh, Mie) induce reflective events that occur at the same wavelength of the incident light and can be detected with an optical backscatter reflectometer (OBR) interrogator in the frequency domain (Froggatt & Moore, 1998). Unlike the previously described sensing methods, the spectral fingerprint of the Rayleigh scattering is not a well-defined spectrum characterized by one or more peaks, but it is rather similar to a random signal since the defects in the fibers are unequally distributed in size, shape, location, and density. Each portion of the fiber therefore returns a different Rayleigh spectral signal that identifies the specific location; this is known as the *signature* of the fiber. When the fiber is exposed to a physical change, for example through a change of temperature or strain, the spectral signature shifts and we can detect the amount of wavelength change by performing a correlation between the reference and measured signatures; this operation is performed on each signature by the OBR.

Standard optical fibers are engineered to reduce the Rayleigh scattering as it is a loss factor that prevents long-distance transmission. When etched, the additional evanescent losses reduce the backscattered power below the limit of detection (LoD) of the OBR. Therefore we employ a custom-made fiber that is tailored to increase the Rayleigh scattering by a substantial amount. This fiber, manufactured by Universite' de Nice, France, has the core doped by an elongated MgO nanoparticles, which provide a substantial scattering level increase.

The prototype of a reflector-less biosensor, engineered for OBR operation and functionalized for thrombin sensing, is shown in Fig. 14.6. The system is based on an MgO nanoparticle-doped fiber wet-etched in hydrofluoric acid (HF) to

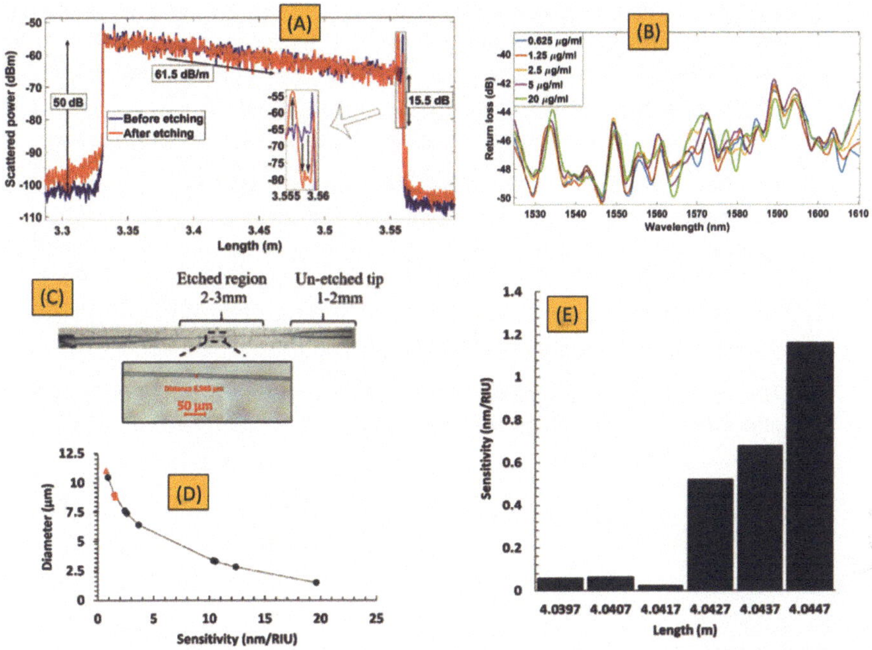

Figure 14.6 Concept and implementation of a reflector-less fiber optic biosensor based on a wet-etched MgO-doped fiber for protein sensing. (A) Backscattering power trace; (B) spectral signatures of the sensor for different protein levels; (C) photograph of a reflector-less sensor under microscope, with inset showing the inner diameter; (D) relationship between fiber diameter and sensitivity; and (E) relationship between the fiber location and the wavelength shift sensitivity. Source: *Adapted from Sypabekova, M., Aitkulov, A., Blanc, W., & Tosi, D. (2020). Reflector-less nanoparticles doped optical fiber biosensor for the detection of proteins: Case thrombin.* Biosensors and Bioelectronics, *165, 112365, reproduced with permission.*

reduce the cladding thickness. The high-scattering fiber is designed to have the same size of core and cladding of a standard SMF, and it can be spliced to any fiber using the standard recipe. Fig. 14.6A displays the power backscattered by the MgO fiber, before and after the etching process. At the transition between the SMF fiber and the MgO fiber, at 3.34 m, the backscattered power jumps by 50 dB; this is the scattering gain of the fiber. The fiber is etched in proximity of the tip, about 1–2 mm away from the end side; in the etched region, the losses account for 15.5 dB, in addition to the high losses of the MgO fiber (61.5 dB/m, two-way). Overall, the chart shows that despite the high propagation losses, the level of scattering measured in the etched region is higher than the SMF, and therefore the OBR can detect the spectral signatures.

The spectral signatures, measured for different protein levels (and therefore different RI values), are shown in Fig. 14.6B; it appears as a random signal, but having a slight wavelength shift that can be recorded using the mutual correlation method (Sypabekova et al., 2018). By calibrating the sensor for different RI values, given that the OBR performs a localized detection, we obtain a set of sensitivity values: the maximum value (1.2 nm/RIU for this sensor) is computed in correspondence of the thinnest part of the fiber, and we can therefore use this fiber portion for interrogation. By functionalizing the sensor for thrombin selective detection, the limit of the detection of this method approaches the nanomolar level.

Another key asset of reflector-less biosensors is that we can use a spatial division multiplexing network to simultaneously interrogate multiple sensors, on a single spectral scan. This approach has been reported by Ayupova et al. (2019), designing a prototype network of three sensing regions (two etched fibers for RI sensing and one temperature sensor). This architecture can be used for multiple analyte detection or for temperature compensation from RI measurements.

The key results are reported in Fig. 14.7. The system is based on an OBR interrogator and a network of splitters that separate each channel. Each fiber span is designed to

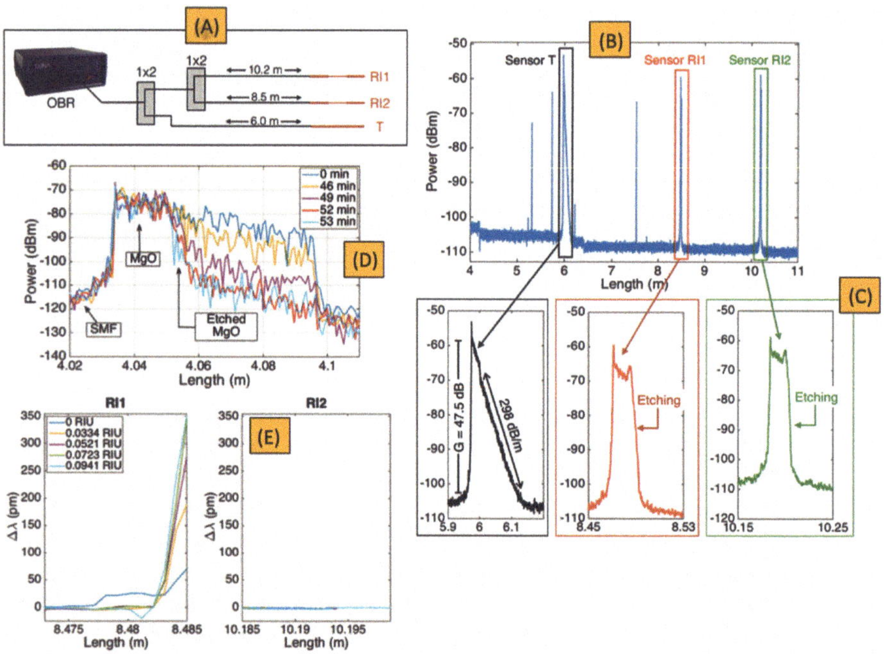

Figure 14.7 Multiplexed reflector-less biosensor. (A) Setup of the three-sensor multiplexing scheme based on spatial division multiplexing. (B) Scattering trace of the sensor network. (C) Insets show the scattering trace in proximity of each sensing element. (D) Scattering trace of an RI sensor during the fabrication, at various etching times. (E) Wavelength shift measured by two RI sensors (RI1 left and RI2 right), when an RI change is applied to RI1 sensor to prove the multiplexing operation. Source: *Adapted from Ayupova, T., Shaimerdenova, M., Korganbayev, S., Sypabekova, M., Bekmurzayeva, A., Blanc, W., ... Tosi, D. (2019). Fiber optic refractive index distributed multi-sensors by scattering-level multiplexing with MgO nanoparticle-doped fibers.* IEEE Sensors Journal, *20(5), 2504–2510, reproduced with permission.*

shift the location of each sensing region at a different length (6.0 m for the temperature sensor, 8.5 m for the RI1 sensor, and 10.2 m for the RI2 sensor). The inset in Fig. 14.7C shows the location of each sensor: the RI sensors have a high etching loss overlapping to the propagation losses, while the temperature sensor is a MgO fiber without etching. The analysis of the power traces during the fabrication shows how the etching process can be monitored: in proximity of the etched region, the losses grow during the etching process, as a result of the thinner fiber cladding. Multiplexing is proven by Fig. 14.7E: when RI changes are applied to RI1 sensor, they are displayed with a wavelength shift up to 350 pm (left chart), but no change is observed to the sensor RI2 (right chart).

Reflector-less biosensors can be an attractive technology for simple RI sensors: although fiber etching is not a rapid process, the availability of a multiplexing setup might allow parallel fabrication of tens of sensors simultaneously, and the sensitivity can be tuned during the calibration. By optimizing the fiber geometry and nanoparticle distribution, it is also possible to increase the sensitivity and tune the fiber losses.

14.2.2 Rapid fabrication of ball resonators

Another approach has been recently reported by Shaimerdenova, Ayupova, Sypabekova, and Tosi (2020), making use of a ball resonator with rapid fabrication recipe and an OBR interrogation system. The concept of the sensing system is to use a spherical tip resonator, but rather than illuminating it from the side to excite whispering gallery modes (Kosma, Zito, Schuster, & Pissadakis, 2013), it is interrogated using the OBR detecting the light in reflection.

The fabrication method, described in Fig. 14.8, is based on a CO_2 laser splicer using a rapid fabrication method. The ball resonator is fabricated on a pair of SMF, both cleaved on the tip. At first, the fibers are fused together; then, by pulling them, it is possible to fabricate a sphere on the fiber tip, having diameter around 500 μm. Fig. 14.8C shows the image of a ball resonator, which shows that the device shape is highly spherical. Four resonators have been reported in this work, with diameter ranging from 466 to 547 μm and ellipticity $e < 0.168$, as observed on the profilometry.

Unlike more traditional interferometers, the spectrum of a ball resonator has a weak reflectivity (return loss between −60 and −40 dB) due to the weakness of the wall reflectivity at the outer surface, and the spectral fingerprint is characterized by shallow reflectivity peaks that can be interrogated either in amplitude or in wavelength. The data reported in Shaimerdenova et al. (2020) report sensitivity values of 48.9−403.3 nm/RIU (wavelength shift detection) or 256.0−566.2 dB/RI (peak level amplitude) for the four resonators described in Fig. 14.8, detected for RI = 1.34.

The ball resonator is a rapid, replicable, and robust device with a wide surface for interaction. The RI sensitivity is compatible with other types of interferometers

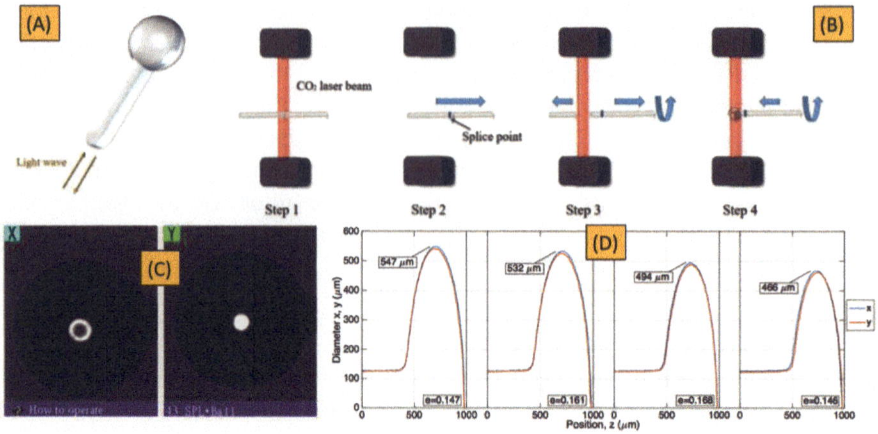

Figure 14.8 Schematic on the fabrication of ball resonator biosensors based on a rapid splicing recipe. (A) Concept of a ball resonator interrogated as a reflective interferometer. (B) Steps of fabrication of the resonator. (C) Pictures of the resonator along *x*/*y* axes. (D) Profilometry of four ball resonators fabricated with the splicing method. Source: *Adapted from Shaimerdenova, M., Ayupova, T., Sypabekova, M., & Tosi, D. (2020). Fiber optic refractive index sensors based on a ball resonator and optical backscatter interrogation.* Sensors, *20(21), 6199.*

such as single-multi-single-mode (SMS) or EFPI, but it can be achieved with a much simpler fabrication that involves only one splice and two cleaves; SMS, EFPI, and similar structures rely instead on fiber polishing and multiple splices at a calibrated distance, and are therefore harder in terms of fabrication process. The complexity of a ball resonator is instead within the interrogation, hence on the software that performs the spectral feature identification, spectral filtering, and peak tracking; we can therefore conclude that this type of devices shifts the complexity from the fabrication process to the process of interrogation of the sensor.

14.2.3 Shallow fiber tapers

As discussed in Section 6.3, the two main approaches for fiber tapering are based on performing a sharp adiabatic taper on the fiber tip down to $<< 10\ \mu m$ of thickness, which behaves as a modal interferometer, or fabricating a double taper which behaves as a Fabry-Perot cavity interferometer. The first approach leads to a very fragile sensor, as the fiber loses most of its mechanical strength (Sun, Sun, Guo, & Guan, 2018); in addition, this type of fabrication is hampered by the limits of glass fiber splicers, and therefore it is usually implemented by heating the fiber in a furnace while pulling it away at a constant rate with a micropositioner. The second method requires two splices and non-adiabatic tapers, and the distance between the two taper waists determines the free spectral range of the interferometer. The main complication is that in order to have a coherent structure, the two tapers have to be spliced in close proximity; for this reason, the fiber has to be tapered in two separate processes, hence complicating the fabrication.

However, using the OBR interrogator, it is possible to obtain a spectral response from a shallow taper, in which the ratio between the diameter of the waist and the original fiber cladding diameter is >20%. The working principle is based on the fact that the two sides of the taper waist can act as a weak pair of reflective mirrors; hence, a weak interferometery effect can be detected by interrogating the spectrum across the taper, in reflection. As for the previous sensors, rather than obtaining a clear reflective pattern, the spectrum appears with several features spread around the interrogation window, but with a detectable dependence on the surrounding RI.

To validate this concept, we fabricated a shallow adiabatic taper from an SMF, having diameter of approximately 25 μm in the waist section. The reflectivity of the taper is not sufficient to show an appropriate signal on a standard interrogator, but it can be resolved using an OBR to detect the spectrum, as shown in Fig. 14.9. The spectral envelope is formed by a sequence of peaks and valleys between −35 and

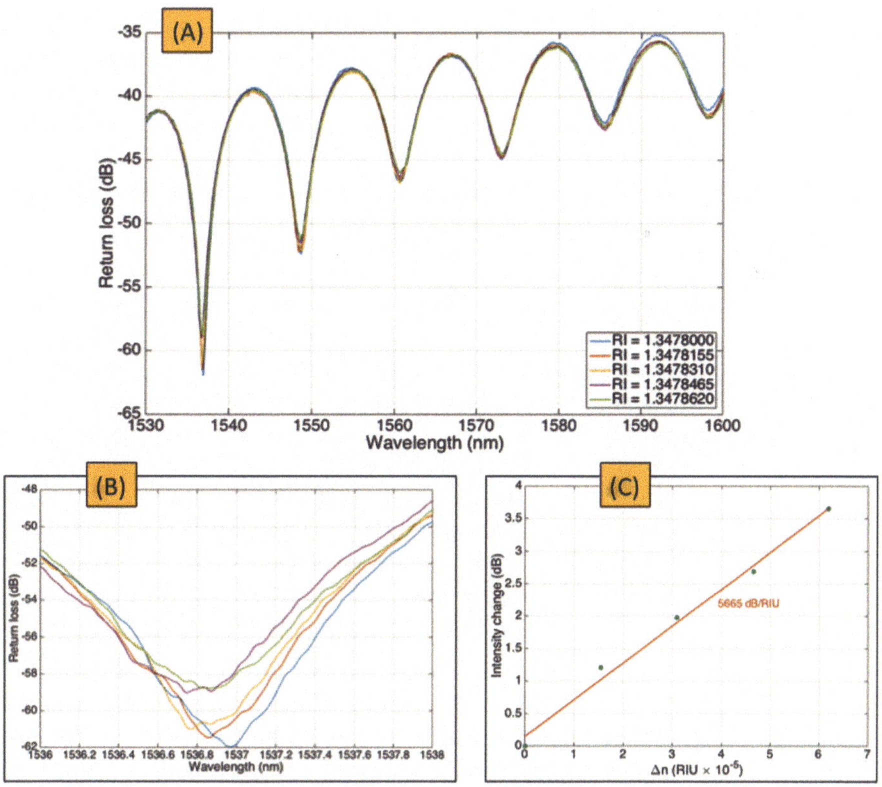

Figure 14.9 Characterization of the spectral characteristics of a shallow fiber taper interrogated with an OBR instrument. (A) Full spectrum of the taper for different RI values. (B) Inset of the spectrum around the valley by 1537 nm. (C) Estimation of the sensitivity, evaluated as 5665 dB/RIU by measuring the intensity change in the peak for different RI values.

−62 dB of return loss, with an envelope that changes when an RI variation is applied. The most sensitive point is around the valley at 1537 nm: by detecting the intensity change at the dip point, the sensitivity is estimated as 5665 dB/RIU, which is in line with several interferometers operating in the infrared wavelength range.

The possibility of using tapers is attractive from the biosensing perspective, as tapers have both a thin diameter and a small surface for interaction, hence showing a great biological responsivity (Kumar et al., 2019). Compared to etched fibers, they have a much stronger robustness to twists and torsions when the dimensions are similar, as the tapering process does not damage the crystal structure of the fiber in a significant way.

14.3 High-sensitivity low-limit sensors

One of the challenges of OFBs is the achievement of top-notch performance: fiber optics, particularly when operating with resonant phenomena, can provide exceptional values of sensitivity that translate in a low LoD. In this section, we discuss in details four architectures that achieve great performance: the first two works discuss numerical and experimental demonstration of sensitivity values of several tens of thousands of nm/RIU that are demonstrated in RI sensing; the other two works translate some of the performance levels in RI sensing into biosensors with a very low LoD, at the femtomolar concentration range.

14.3.1 Toward the 100,000 nm/RIU limit: mode transition in long-period grating

Long-period gratings (LPGs), described in Section 3.4, operate as transmission-based biosensors based on grating structures with a long pitch. The transmission spectrum collects several dips, each originating by a resonant LP mode provided at the core/cladding interaction; spectra are broad, with bandwidth that have tens of nanometers width, hence the structures are optimized to have an RI-sensitive mode within the wavelength range of the analyzer. As shown by Sypabekova et al. (2019) with tilted FBGs, the possibility of etching the fiber in proximity of the grating facilitates an increase of sensitivity in grating structures that excite cladding modes; this effect was used to obtain a ~15-fold increase of sensitivity in an etched-tilted FBG. A similar process is at the foundation of etched LPGs, in which the increase of sensitivity can bring this figure over the 10,000 nm/RIU level, in an effort for performing ultrasensitive detection.

To raise the sensitivity of an LPG, Smietana et al. proposed and experimentally implemented an LPG device based on a shallow etching of the fiber cladding, and a deposition of a thin aluminum oxide film; the main characteristics are shown in Fig. 14.10 (Śmietana, Koba, Mikulic, & Bock, 2016). To achieve the

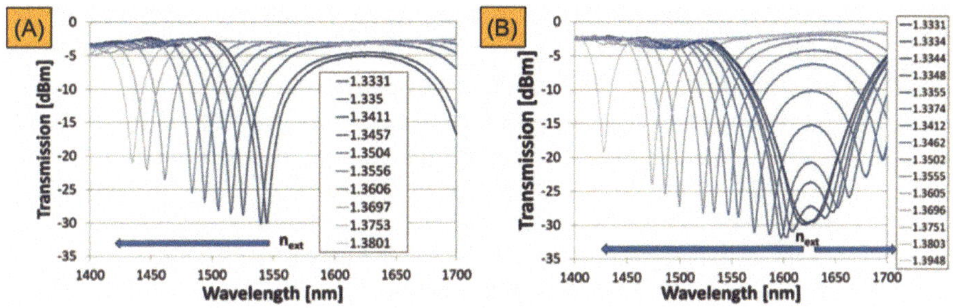

Figure 14.10 Properties of the transmission spectrum and sensitivity of an etched and thin-film–coated LPG operating near the dispersion tuning point, with LP_{09} and LP_{10} modes. (A) Spectrum of the LPG coated with 130 nm aluminum oxide layer. (B) Spectrum of the LPG etched and coated with aluminum oxide. Source: *Adapted from Śmietana, M., Koba, M., Mikulic, P., & Bock, W. J. (2016). Towards refractive index sensitivity of long-period gratings at level of tens of μm per refractive index unit: Fiber cladding etching and nano-coating deposition.* Optics Express, *24(11), 11897–11904, reproduced with permission.*

enhancement, two methods have been considered: (1) deposition of a 130 nm thick layer of aluminum oxide (Al_2O_3) around the LPG and (2) etching of the overlay and of the fiber using HF, to operate in the mode transition (MT) regime.

The use of metallic layers is known to enhance the performance of grating-based biosensors (Guo et al., 2017). This is shown in Fig. 14.10A, where a Al_2O_3-coated LPG is reported for different RI values. The central mode (LP_{09}) shifts toward the shorter wavelengths as the RI increases, and the intensity appears to decrease. When the LPG is both etched and coated, as shown in Fig. 14.10B, the transition between the LP_{09} and LP_{10} modes is substantially shortened. The spectrum appears with a single peak around 1610 nm, which progressively splits into two separate modes. The leftmost part of the spectrum shifts toward the short wavelengths as the external RI increases, while the rightmost spectral envelope shifts toward longer wavelengths, hence separating the behavior. This mode of operation, labeled as MT, can be achieved by reducing the fiber diameter to tune the resonance properties of the LPG (Del Villar, 2015). Rather than having a single mode that shifts unilaterally, we observe a split of the operating mode toward both direction, as the RI overcomes the 1.334 value.

The operation in MT regime unlocks an exceptional sensitivity. The sensitivity of aluminum oxide–coated LPGs ranges between 1000 and 5000 nm/RIU (black and gray curves), depending on the mode of operation, the thickness of the layer, and the surrounding RI value. Etched gratings instead allow achieving a much larger sensitivity figure, and in several portions achieving a >10,000 nm/RIU. The maximum value (40,000 nm/RIU) is observed for the LP_{10} mode of an LPG coated with 167 nm thick later around RI = 1.42. This value is, however, unpractical for sensing in water-based analytes. However, using LP_{09} mode for a 182 nm thickness layer, the sensitivity is 21,000 nm/RIU. Most importantly, the sensitivity appears to increase exponentially at the MT regime and flattens thereafter; hence, the LPG can be designed to have one resonant mode within the wavelength range of the interrogator, and tune the etching and deposition of the layer to obtain the MT for the target RI value of the analyte. The work of Smietana et al. experimentally demonstrates a sensing method that reliably overcomes the 10,000 nm/RIU threshold, maximizing the impact of resonant phenomena within the LPG.

The MT regime of an etched LPG has been numerically studied, and optimized, by Del Villar (2015). The resulting structure of a thin-film–coated LPG with etched fiber, assuming that the fiber is cylindrically and asymmetrically etched around its core, has been investigated using a numerical method that expands the coupled mode theory. The study has been performed varying both the fiber thickness and the grating pitch, and therefore allows a deeper optimization of the sensing structure.

For uncoated gratings, the structure behaves in a similar manner of a standard LPG, whereas all modes have a separate wavelength resonating in the device. When etched and coated with a coating of few hundreds of nanometers, instead, the MT can be observed. The sensitivity gets amplified by the MT effect, as when the surrounding RI increases, the wavelength shift appears to be larger than in normal LPG structures. The maximum of sensitivity, as shown in Fig. 14.11, is recorded when the overlapping mode begins the separation process: in this regime, the authors recorded a sensitivity of 143,000 nm/RIU, with an optimal grating having fiber diameter 34.8 μm and grating period 288.5 μm.

Overall, the mode-transition concept in LPGs can achieve extremely high values of sensitivity, observed both numerically (over 100,000 nm/RIU) and experimentally (up to 40,000 nm/RIU). Coupling the exceptional sensitivity with high-resolution detectors, it is possible to achieve extremely low LoD values for RI sensing. Theoretically, the concept appears to lead to very accurate biosensors, but the mode-transition LPG still has experimental drawbacks that limit the applications. Besides the operation as transmission device only, and the large bandwidth of the spectrum that impedes multiplexing, the etched-coated LPG appears to achieve extremely high values of sensitivity only when the structure is optimized by choosing the grating pitch, the fiber thickness, and the thickness of the film, altogether. The fabrication is therefore not a simple process, and the sensitivity can deviate from the high theoretical values as soon as the analyte RI falls off the optimal value. The other problem is the limit of the interrogator: for an interrogator having 100,000 nm/RIU sensitivity figure, a change of RI of 10^{-3} RIU would lead to a 100 nm wavelength shift, a value larger than the spectral window most of the interrogators operating in the infrared. For this reason, the main results

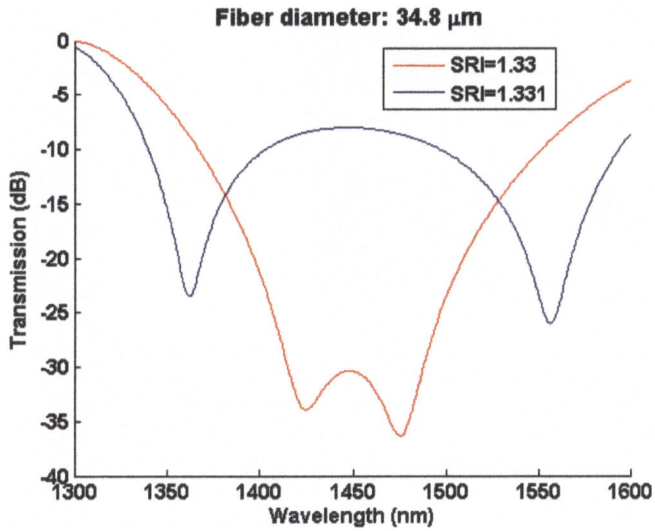

Figure 14.11 Simulated spectral characteristics for an etched LPG having fiber diameter 34.8 μm and grating period 288.5 μm. *LPG*, Long-period grating. Source: *Reprinted/Adapted with permission from © The Optical Society. Del Villar, I. (2015). Ultrahigh-sensitivity sensors based on thin-film coated long period gratings with reduced diameter, in transition mode and near the dispersion turning point.* Optics Express, *23(7), 8389–8398.*

presented so far make use of wideband optical spectrum analyzers and supercontinuum light sources, whereas the interrogators mostly used in sensing (spectrometers, FBG interrogators) cannot detect most of the wavelength shift patterns observed in mode-transitioning LPGs. Hence, this technology is mainly intended as a great asset for ultralow limits of detection, where the observed RI change is $\sim 10^{-4}$ or below.

14.3.2 Femtomolar concentration detection

The use of lossy mode resonance (LMR), in conjunction with fiber structures that induce a large amount of evanescent waves in the sensing point, can be exploited for the fabrication of high-resolution sensors. Chiavaioli et al. (2018) have recently presented a D-shaped fiber with an SnO_2 coating and a polarization controller, working at infrared wavelengths with a SMF, and performed femtomolar-level detection in a prototype setup.

The view of the system is shown in Fig. 14.12. The system makes use of a broadband light source connected to a linear polarizer. Then a polarization controller is used, to match the polarization parallel to the direction of the fiber vertical plane. The sensor is a D-shaped fiber, which is formed from a standard SMF by polishing the upper part of the cladding, as from Fig. 14.12B and C. The sensing region is then coated with a SnO_2 layer, sputtered on the surface

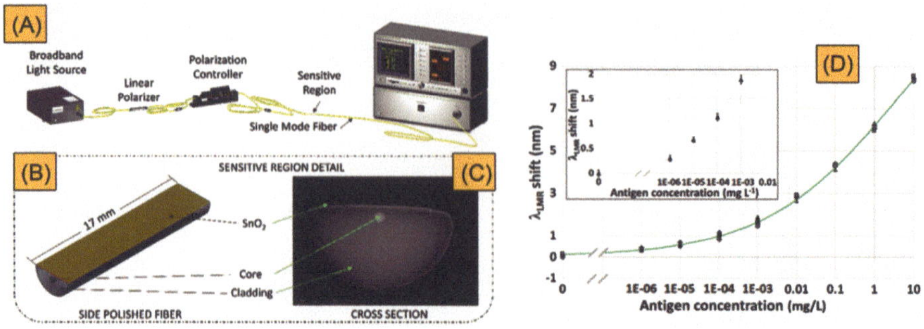

Figure 14.12 Femtomolar-level fiber optic biosensor based on lossy mode resonance on a D-shaped fiber. (A) Schematic of the working principle. (B) Sketch of the sensing fiber and coating. (C) Photograph of the fiber cross section. (D) IgG detection, reporting the lossy mode resonance wavelength change with respect to the antigen concentration. Source: *Adapted from Chiavaioli, F., Zubiate, P., Del Villar, I., Zamarreño, C. R., Giannetti, A., Tombelli, S., . . . Baldini, F. (2018). Femtomolar detection by nanocoated fiber label-free biosensors.* ACS Sensors, *3(5), 936–943, reproduced with permission.*

of the fiber. The spectra have been measured in the 1250–1700 nm range, with a resonance transmission dip at 1550 nm in correspondence to the third optical window.

The LMR effect induced in the structure allows a very sensitive shift of the transmission dip when the surrounding analyte changes. To test the efficiency of the sensor for a biological detection, the authors presented the case study of immunoglobulin G (IgG) detection, which is shown in Fig. 14.12D: the sensor responds according to a sigmoidal pattern (Chiavaioli, Gouveia, Jorge, & Baldini, 2017) as the concentration rises, with an estimated LoD of 0.15 ng/L corresponding to 1 fM.

Sansone, Macchia, Taddei, Torsi, and Giordano (2018) reported the fabrication of a fiber-optic biosensor optimized for high performance sensing of biotinylated bovine serum albumin (bBSA), using a concept based on photonic crystals–induced resonances in the UV–visible wavelength range. The key characteristics of the work are reported in Fig. 14.13.

The schematic of the working principle is shown in Fig. 14.13A. The photonic crystal is characterized by a wavelength-periodical dielectric constant, which induces a photonic bandgap phenomenon. The periodicity of the refractive index of the crystal, mounted on the tip of an UV–VIS fiber for spectrometry, results in a reflection spectrum characterized by reflective peaks. The spectral peaks at 505 nm is used by the authors as detection, measuring the normalized wavelength shift (Λ, equal to the ratio between the wavelength shift and the central wavelength at 503 nm). The LoD of bBSA, as reported in Fig. 14.13C, is around 1 fM, with the sensor spanning the 1 fM–10 nM concentration range.

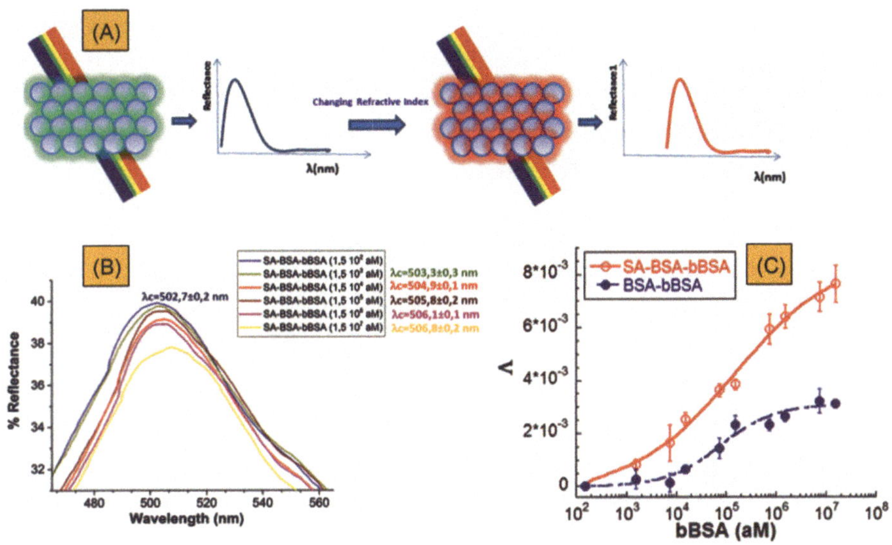

Figure 14.13 Detection of bBSA at femtomolar concentration level using a functionalized photonic crystal on a UV–VIS fiber. (A) Schematic of the working principle. (B) Spectra observed for different concentration levels. (C) Response of the sensor at different concentration values. Source: *Adapted from Sansone, L., Macchia, E., Taddei, C., Torsi, L., & Giordano, M. (2018). Label-free optical biosensing at femtomolar detection limit.* Sensors and Actuators B: Chemical, *255, 1097–1104, reproduced with permission.*

14.4 Cells sensing using multiresonant gratings

OFBs have been designed to detect several analytes that span from proteins, to enzymes, antibody/antigens, molecules among others. Cells detection has been reported in literature, usually performed with SPR sensors operating in visible wavelengths and with multimode fibers (Zhao, Tong, Xia, & Peng, 2019). The recent work of Loyez et al. (2020) instead aims at bringing the advantageous properties of power stability, accuracy, and detection resolution of the sensors operating with telecom fibers, onto the detection of circulating breast cancer cells using the a plasmonic grating structure.

The concept of this work is reported in Fig. 14.14. The sensing device is a tilted FBG inscribed in an SMF. After the grating fabrication, a 50 nm thick gold layer was fabricated around the fiber. Cells detection was implemented through a process of biofunctionalization: aptamers (MAMA2) have been evaluated after a previous selectivity study, and immobilized on the fiber surface for 60 minutes at 10 μM concentration. To excite narrowband resonances in the infrared, the method of gold nanoparticles has been used to induce localized SPR (Zhao et al., 2019). As from Fig. 14.14, the gold nanoparticles bind to the cell surface, inducing several SPR modes.

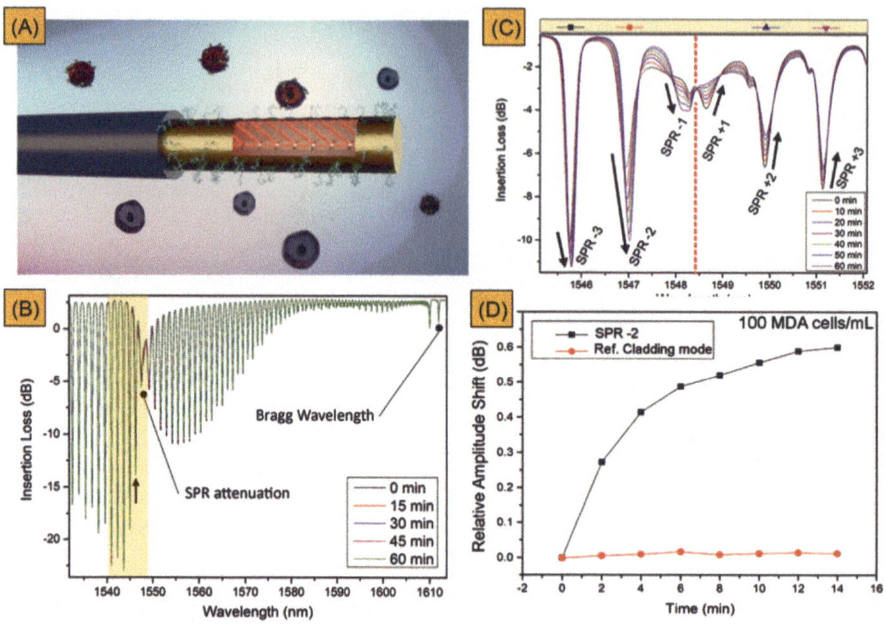

Figure 14.14 Detection of circulating breast cancer cells using a multiresonant plasmonic SPR-tilted FBG structure biofunctionalized with aptamers. (A) Schematic of the sensing system and of the fiber functionalization. (B) Spectrum of the sensor during the biofunctionalization, with 60 minutes duration. (C) Spectrum of the sensing device over 60 minutes of aptamer immobilization. (D) Shift of the interrogated plasmonic mode, with respect to the reference cladding mode, over 14 minute of detection at 100 cells/mL. Source: *Adapted from Loyez, M., Hassan, E. M., Lobry, M., Liu, F., Caucheteur, C., Wattiez, R., . . . Albert, J. (2020). Rapid detection of circulating breast cancer cells using a multiresonant optical fiber aptasensor with plasmonic amplification.* ACS Sensors, *5(2), 454–463, reproduced with permission.*

The analysis of the plasmonic TFBG device shows a multiresonant pattern: alongside the cladding modes of the grating that are visible in Fig. 14.14C, the modulation offered by the localized SPR effect induces several fringes toward the shorter (labeled SPR −1, −2, −3 in the figure) or longer (SPR + 1, + 2, + 3) wavelengths. This modulation is exploited for the detection: the mode SPR −2 offers the higher sensitivity, while other modes closer to the Bragg wavelength have a much smaller amplitude change. Here, the gold nanoparticles introduce an amplification of the sensitivity, which results in a larger amplitude shift at the detection (about twofold amplification, as estimated in the work with respect to a plasmonic TFBG without surface gold nanoparticles). Cells detection has been performed in a fluidic chamber, at various concentrations with an LoD estimated at 49 cells/mL). The wavelength shift traces, observed in Fig. 14.14D, observe a growing trend that stabilizes after 12 minutes, while most of the response (about 80%) is observed in the first 5 minutes.

14.5 Combining optical and electrochemical interrogation

Several lab-on-chip technologies combine electrical and optical methods of detection, to perform complex analytical diagnostic (Chen & Shamsi, 2017). This opportunity has been usually limited to free-space optical sensors, miniaturizing light-emitting diode sources and photodetectors around or within the chip, complementing the analytical and detection tools provided by electrochemical sensors, such as field-effect transistors. Complementing electrical technologies, SPR sensors have also been reported thanks to the generation of biocurrents in thin-film substrates. A recent work from Smietana et al., reproduced in Fig. 14.15, image from Śmietana et al. (2020) displayed with permission, combines a fiber-optic sensor with an electrochemical interrogation method. The approach proposed in this work is based on a sensor-on-chip and an LMR approach measuring the spectrum transmitted through the sensing region. The sensor is coated with indium tin oxide (ITO). The optical fiber sensors have undoubtedly better performance, in terms of sensitivity and LoD, with respect to electrical sensors; they also can interrogate a very low amount of analyte, which makes it compatible with the microfluidic channel of a chip. Electrochemical sensors, on the other side, perform better in terms of selectivity for biorecognition tasks, particularly when working with complex analytes, thanks to their capability to discriminating through separation processes. By combining the two methods, we can extract more information out of a lab-on-chip detection device.

The system proposed by Smietana et al. is based on a microfluidic chip, with an inner multimode silica fiber coated with a thin ITO film (350 nm thickness). The sensor operates using the LMR phenomenon, observed at visible wavelengths; light from a broadband tungsten light source is input into the large core fiber having 400 μm core diameter, and detected with an UV–VIS spectrometer on the transmission side. The measurement cell was connected with electrical wiring from the fiber core, through a network of three electrodes (working, counter, and reference) and performing electrochemical measurements with a potentiostat. This arrangement allows simultaneously performing two measurements: (1) transmission spectra at visible light and (2) cyclic voltammetry with a rapid scan rate (20 mV/s) for an electrical potential (E) ranging from -1 to $+1.5$ V.

The LMR sensor, like all OFBs, is sensitive to the RI change with a sensitivity ranging from 320 to 800 nm/RIU; this can be measured monitoring the LMR wavelength or the intensity of the light at the 630 nm spectral line. The application of the potential E has the effect of changing the RI of the analyte: changes of E result in a composition change of the ITO layer, which is an n-type semiconductor and therefore results in a positive change of the RI in proximity of the overlay when an increasing voltage is applied. This effect is

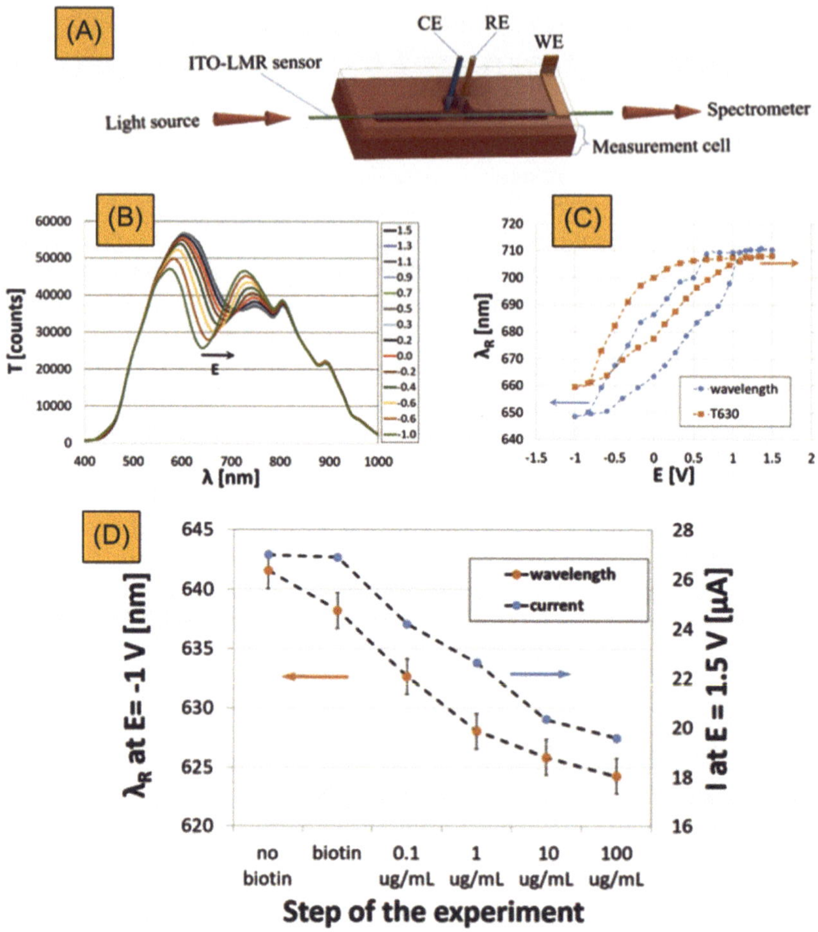

Figure 14.15 Prototype of an ITO-coated lossy mode resonance sensor on chip, using a cooperative optical-electrochemical interrogation approach. (A) Schematic of the sensor on chip, where the light source–spectrometer system is complemented with the electrochemical detection on the electrodes (*WE*, working electrode; *RE*, reference electrode; *CE*, counter electrode). (B) Spectrum of the fiber optic sensor at visible wavelengths for different values of the electric potential *E* applied (−1 to + 1.5 V). (C) Shift in resonance wavelength and amplitude at 630 nm wavelength for various values of electric potential *E*. (D) Biotin detection: the chart reports the lossy mode resonance (left) and output current (right) for different concentration levels. Source: *Adapted from Śmietana, M., Koba, M., Sezemsky, P., Szot-Karpińska, K., Burnat, D., Stranak, V., ... Bogdanowicz, R. (2020). Simultaneous optical and electrochemical label-free biosensing with ITO-coated lossy-mode resonance sensor.* Biosensors and Bioelectronics, 154,*112050, reproduced with permission.*

shown in Fig. 14.15B: the transmission spectral shifts toward the longer wavelengths for growing values of *E*. As shown in Fig. 14.15C, cyclic voltammetry charts of the OFBs are reported, whereas the LMR resonance and the intensity at 630 nm are reported for growing and decreasing values of *E*. Finally, the

LMR resonance wavelength and the current at 1.5 V potential are reported for different binding events of biotin, with density up to 0.1 mg/mL; the electrochemical interrogation is responsive at the higher concentration, while the optical interrogation has a lower detection limit.

Overall, the experimental work reported by Smietana et al. provides an important case study of lab-on-chips in which the optical fiber biosensing analysis is cooperative with the electrical interrogation, exploiting the electrooptic properties of the ITO thin film coating.

14.6 Discussion and conclusion

In this chapter, we discussed advanced concepts and emerging trends in the field of OFBs. While OFBs are themselves an emerging technology, which is progressing along the technology readiness scale, the several working principles and devices have achieved reliable and repeatable detection. Yet, scientists should look at the potential challenges that arise from the key performance factors, develop sensors from an application-driven perspective and with an eye on the industrialization of the technologies.

In Fig. 14.16, we report in a schematic view the main trends and open challenges for OFBs. We identify four key drivers: (1) manufacturing of the sensing devices, and related challenges; (2) sensing performance; (3) packaging, which allows working in situ and therefore position OFB as a technology competing also with biopsy devices, rather than only with bulk optics biosensors; and (4) applications that biosensors can target.

Manufacturing is the key toward volume production of sensors. While OFB cannot achieve a fabrication throughput similar to transistors or on-chip devices, we can apply methods consolidated in the fabrication of other technologies (e.g., diffraction lenses or fiber terminations) that have a much deeper industrialization stage than most of the fiber-optic sensing devices. In this area, the effort on *minimalistic* sensors is aimed at the reuse of well-established devices with manufacturing time of few seconds for an optical use. The works presented in this chapter, proposed by the authors, run along this path: for example, tapers are common in optical tweezers (Liu et al., 2017), while spherical tip resonators are common for microscopy diffractive lenses (Shen & Huang, 2009). The advanced splicers allow parallel fabrication of these devices with consolidated recipes. Reflector-less biosensors appear as the hardest device of this class, but by changing the fiber standards, we might be able to work on this technology without even the fabrication of a device, relying purely on Rayleigh scattering. The complexity shifts from the fabrication to the hardware/software methods used to interrogate the sensors; however, that would allow maintaining a disposable use of the sensors, necessary for many applications.

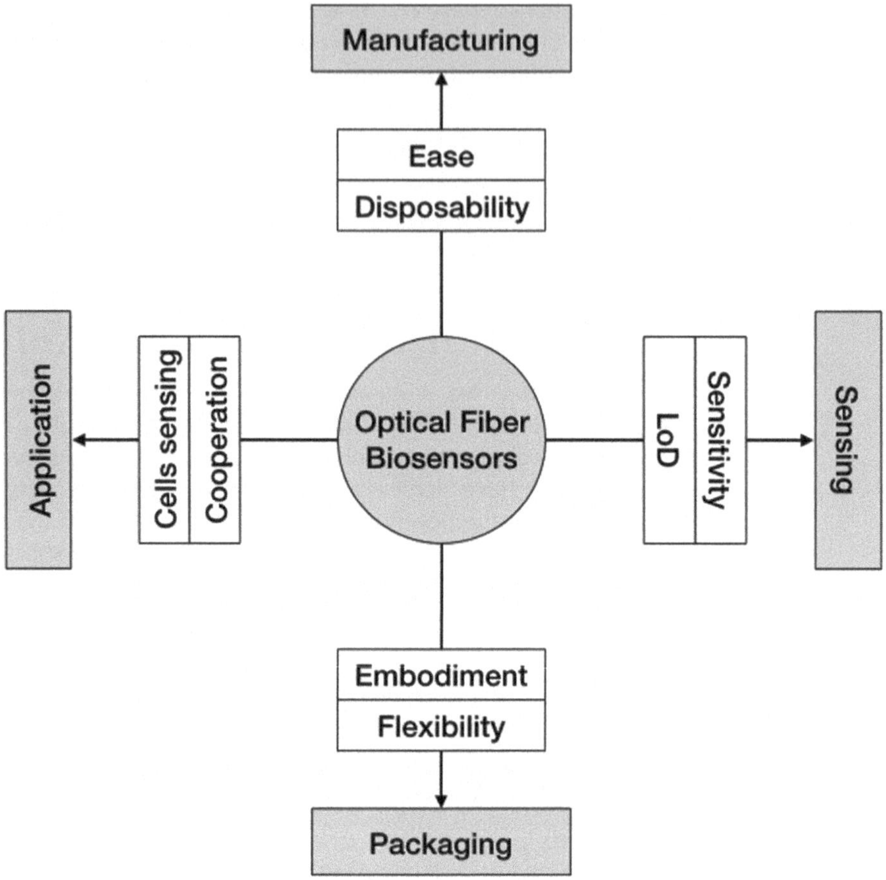

Figure 14.16
Sketch of the main trends and emerging topics in optical fiber biosensors.

The aspect of sensing performance, in current research, appears to influence the typologies of devices used for sensing. Minimalistic sensors approach tens up to hundreds of nm/RIU, whereas the use of LMR or specially tuned LPGs has proven to consistently beat the 10,000 nm/RIU figure. Over this limit, the interrogators would run out of spectral range but certainly the trend is to maximize the sensitivity to minimize the LoD, reaching picomolar, femtomolar, and down to the attomolar range. Such sensors would not be able to perform a reliable detection over many decades of concentrations, but certainly would serve the purpose of brining biosensors in areas where the analytes are such in small amount that traditional biosensors would struggle to detect. Clearly, here we observe a trade-off between the complexity of the sensing device and its manufacturability in large number and repeatable performance; but overall, the challenge of expanding the performance is certainly very concurrent in today's research.

Packaging is instead one of the aspects that current research is turning around. The works presented in this chapter fill the bridge between a lab-based sensing technology and a working device, capable of a reliable measurement in situ in real time. Here, the key principle is to stand on the shoulder of giants, by relying on medical devices that are commercially available and finding a method to embody the optical fiber in the device, making sure that the sensing capabilities are well maintained. This effort is beginning to prove successful in biosensing devices, whereas percutaneous devices and other types of medical devices (such as urologic or wearable) are running at a slower pace in this direction. In general, rigid and semiflexible packages are more suitable for hosting OFBs because the device is not only performing the insertion task but also protecting the inner fiber and delivering it to the treatment site. Flexible devices, such as those used in bladder analysis or the wearable devices that monitor respiration through elastic bands (Gong et al., 2019), instead pose a bigger threat as the fiber is subjected to much larger mechanical stress during operation. A great emphasis is given however on this research by several groups that are adapting commercial devices to biosensing functions.

Finally, a look at application shows that OFBs are mature in detecting in several common conditions, namely antibody/antigen pair (thanks to the favorable surface chemistry of the fiber coating), silanization (which is well established on the glass fiber surface), and in aptasensors. The emerging areas involve instead cells sensing, which is hampered by the optical size of cells and by the geometry of devices, and on lab-on-chip microfluidic technologies, where as shown in the previous section the optical fiber technology can complement electrochemical sensing for a cooperative interrogation.

References

Agrawal, G. P. (2011). Nonlinear fiber optics: Its history and recent progress. *Journal of the Optical Society of America B, 28*(12), A1–A10.

Arkwright, J. W., Blenman, N. G., Underhill, I. D., Maunder, S. A., Szczesniak, M. M., Dinning, P. G., & Cook, I. J. (2009). In-vivo demonstration of a high resolution optical fiber manometry catheter for diagnosis of gastrointestinal motility disorders. *Optics Express, 17*(6), 4500–4508.

Arkwright, J. W., Underhill, I. D., Maunder, S. A., Blenman, N., Szczesniak, M. M., Wiklendt, L., ... Dinning, P. G. (2009a). Design of a high-sensor count fibre optic manometry catheter for in-vivo colonic diagnostics. *Optics Express, 17*(25), 22423–22431, Dec 7.

Ayupova, T., Shaimerdenova, M., Korganbayev, S., Sypabekova, M., Bekmurzayeva, A., Blanc, W., ... Tosi, D. (2019). Fiber optic refractive index distributed multi-sensors by scattering-level multiplexing with MgO nanoparticle-doped fibers. *IEEE Sensors Journal, 20*(5), 2504–2510.

Beisenova, A., Issatayeva, A., Sovetov, S., Korganbayev, S., Jelbuldina, M., Ashikbayeva, Z., ... Tosi, D. (2019). Multi-fiber distributed thermal profiling of minimally invasive thermal ablation with scattering-level multiplexing in MgO-doped fibers. *Biomedical Optics Express, 10*(3), 1282–1296.

Beisenova, A., Issatayeva, A., Tosi, D., & Molardi, C. (2018). Fiber-optic distributed strain sensing needle for real-time guidance in epidural anesthesia. *IEEE Sensors Journal, 18*(19), 8034–8044, Aug 13.

Chen, S., & Shamsi, M. H. (2017). Biosensors-on-chip: A topical review. *Journal of Micromechanics and Microengineering, 27*(8), 083001.

Chiavaioli, F., Gouveia, C. A., Jorge, P. A., & Baldini, F. (2017). Towards a uniform metrological assessment of grating-based optical fiber sensors: From refractometers to biosensors. *Biosensors, 7*(2), 23.

Chiavaioli, F., Zubiate, P., Del Villar, I., Zamarreño, C. R., Giannetti, A., Tombelli, S., ... Baldini, F. (2018). Femtomolar detection by nanocoated fiber label-free biosensors. *ACS Sensors, 3*(5), 936–943.

Del Villar, I. (2015). Ultrahigh-sensitivity sensors based on thin-film coated long period gratings with reduced diameter, in transition mode and near the dispersion turning point. *Optics Express, 23*(7), 8389–8398.

Fan, S. Y., Chiu, H. S., Lin, D. Y., Liao, A., & Liao, K. C. (2016). Percutaneous fiber-optic biosensor for immediate evaluation of chemotherapy efficacy in vivo (Part II): In vitro and in vivo characterization. *Sensors and Actuators B: Chemical, 222*, 579–587.

Froggatt, M., & Moore, J. (1998). High-spatial-resolution distributed strain measurement in optical fiber with Rayleigh scatter. *Applied Optics, 37*(10), 1735–1740.

Gong, Z., Xiang, Z., OuYang, X., Zhang, J., Lau, N., Zhou, J., & Chan, C. C. (2019). Wearable fiber optic technology based on smart textile: A review. *Materials, 12*(20), 3311.

Gono, K. (2008). Multifunctional endoscopic imaging system for support of early cancer diagnosis. *IEEE Journal of Selected Topics in Quantum Electronics, 14*(1), 62–69.

Guo, T., González-Vila, Á., Loyez, M., & Caucheteur, C. (2017). Plasmonic optical fiber-grating immunosensing: A review. *Sensors, 17*(12), 2732.

Guo, T., Liu, F., Liang, X., Qiu, X., Huang, Y., Xie, C., ... Albert, J. (2016). Highly sensitive detection of urinary protein variations using tilted fiber grating sensors with plasmonic nanocoatings. *Biosensors and Bioelectronics, 78*, 221–228, Apr 15.

Gupta, S., & Madoff, D. C. (2007). Image-guided percutaneous needle biopsy in cancer diagnosis and staging. *Techniques in Vascular and Interventional Radiology, 10*(2), 88–101.

Han, L., Guo, T., Xie, C., Xu, P., Lao, J., Zhang, X., ... Mao, W. (2017). Specific detection of aquaporin-2 using plasmonic tilted fiber grating sensors. *Journal of Lightwave Technology, 35*(16), 3360–3365.

Khan, F., Denasi, A., Barrera, D., Madrigal, J., Sales, S., & Misra, S. (2019). Multi-core optical fibers with Bragg gratings as shape sensor for flexible medical instruments. *IEEE Sensors Journal, 19*(14), 5878–5884.

Kim, J. S., & Kim, B. W. (2017). Training in endoscopy: Esophagogastroduodenoscopy. *Clinical Endoscopy, 50*(4), 318.

Kosma, K., Zito, G., Schuster, K., & Pissadakis, S. (2013). Whispering gallery mode microsphere resonator integrated inside a microstructured optical fiber. *Optics Letters, 38*(8), 1301–1303.

Kuipers, E. J., & Haringsma, J. (2005). Diagnostic and therapeutic endoscopy. *Journal of Surgical Oncology, 92*(3), 203–209.

Kumar, S., Kaushik, B. K., Singh, R., Chen, N. K., Yang, Q. S., Zhang, X., ... Zhang, B. (2019). LSPR-based cholesterol biosensor using a tapered optical fiber structure. *Biomedical Optics Express, 10*(5), 2150–2160.

Liao, K. C., Chiu, H. S., Fan, S. Y., Tseng, Y. D., & Lu, P. H. (2016). Percutaneous fiber-optic biosensor for immediate evaluation of chemotherapy efficacy in vivo (part I): Strategy of assay design for monitoring non-homogeneously distributed biomarkers. *Sensors and Actuators B: Chemical, 222*, 544–550.

Liao, K. C., Hogen-Esch, T., Richmond, F. J., Marcu, L., Clifton, W., & Loeb, G. E. (2008). Percutaneous fiber-optic sensor for chronic glucose monitoring in vivo. *Biosensors and Bioelectronics, 23*(10), 1458–1465, May 15.

Liu, Z. L., Liu, Y. X., Tang, Y., Zhang, N., Wu, F. P., & Zhang, B. (2017). Fabrication and application of a non-contact double-tapered optical fiber tweezers. *Optics Express, 25*(19), 22480–22489.

Loyez, M., Hassan, E. M., Lobry, M., Liu, F., Caucheteur, C., Wattiez, R., ... Albert, J. (2020). Rapid detection of circulating breast cancer cells using a multiresonant optical fiber aptasensor with plasmonic amplification. *ACS Sensors, 5*(2), 454–463.

Loyez, M., Larrieu, J. C., Chevineau, S., Remmelink, M., Leduc, D., Bondue, B., ... Caucheteur, C. (2019). In situ cancer diagnosis through online plasmonics. *Biosensors and Bioelectronics, 131*, 104–112, Apr 15.

Poeggel, S., Duraibabu, D., Tosi, D., Leen, G., Lewis, E., McGrath, D., ... Mirone, V. (2015). Differential in vivo urodynamic measurement in a single thin catheter based on two optical fiber pressure sensors. *Journal of Biomedical Optics, 20*(3), 037005.

Poeggel, S., Tosi, D., Fusco, F., Ippolito, J., Lupoli, L., Mirone, V., ... Lewis, E. (2014). Fiber-optic EFPI pressure sensors for in vivo urodynamic analysis. *IEEE Sensors Journal, 14*(7), 2335–2340, Mar 11.

Ribaut, C., Loyez, M., Larrieu, J. C., Chevineau, S., Lambert, P., Remmelink, M., ... Caucheteur, C. (2017). Cancer biomarker sensing using packaged plasmonic optical fiber gratings: Towards in vivo diagnosis. *Biosensors and Bioelectronics, 92*, 449–456.

Sansone, L., Macchia, E., Taddei, C., Torsi, L., & Giordano, M. (2018). Label-free optical biosensing at femtomolar detection limit. *Sensors and Actuators B: Chemical, 255*, 1097–1104.

Shaimerdenova, M., Ayupova, T., Sypabekova, M., & Tosi, D. (2020). Fiber optic refractive index sensors based on a ball resonator and optical backscatter interrogation. *Sensors, 20* (21), 6199.

Shen, S. C., & Huang, J. C. (2009). Rapid fabrication of a micro-ball lens array by extrusion for optical fiber applications. *Optics Express, 17*(15), 13122–13127.

Śmietana, M., Koba, M., Mikulic, P., & Bock, W. J. (2016). Towards refractive index sensitivity of long-period gratings at level of tens of µm per refractive index unit: Fiber cladding etching and nano-coating deposition. *Optics Express, 24*(11), 11897–11904.

Śmietana, M., Koba, M., Sezemsky, P., Szot-Karpińska, K., Burnat, D., Stranak, V., ... Bogdanowicz, R. (2020). Simultaneous optical and electrochemical label-free biosensing with ITO-coated lossy-mode resonance sensor. *Biosensors and Bioelectronics, 154*, 112050.

Sun, D., Sun, L. P., Guo, T., & Guan, B. O. (2018). Label-free thrombin detection using a tapered fiber-optic interferometric aptasensor. *Journal of Lightwave Technology, 37*(11), 2756–2761.

Sypabekova, M., Aitkulov, A., Blanc, W., & Tosi, D. (2020). Reflector-less nanoparticles doped optical fiber biosensor for the detection of proteins: Case thrombin. *Biosensors and Bioelectronics, 165*, 112365.

Sypabekova, M., Korganbayev, S., Blanc, W., Ayupova, T., Bekmurzayeva, A., Shaimerdenova, M., ... Tosi, D. (2018). Fiber optic refractive index sensors through spectral detection of Rayleigh backscattering in a chemically etched MgO-based nanoparticle-doped fiber. *Optics Letters, 43*(24), 5945–5948.

Sypabekova, M., Korganbayev, S., González-Vila, Á., Caucheteur, C., Shaimerdenova, M., Ayupova, T., ... Tosi, D. (2019). Functionalized etched tilted fiber Bragg grating aptasensor for label-free protein detection. *Biosensors and Bioelectronics, 146*, 111765.

Zhao, Y., Tong, R. J., Xia, F., & Peng, Y. (2019). Current status of optical fiber biosensor based on surface plasmon resonance. *Biosensors and Bioelectronics, 142*, 111505.

Index

Note: Page numbers followed by "*f*" and "*t*" refer to figures and tables, respectively.

Index

P

FSC
www.fsc.org
MIX
Papier | Fördert
gute Waldnutzung
FSC® C083411

Kolibri 360 GmbH
Ferdinand-Jühlke-Straße 7
99095 Erfurt, Deutschland
produktsicherheit@kolibri360.de